Praise for Robert Paarlberg's

RESETTING THE TABLE

"A cogent, revealing look at the future of food." —*Kirkus Reviews*

"A terrific book. *Resetting the Table* shows how the whole world can be fed without environmental harm, and that's worth listening to. . . . Urgent yet reasonable at the same time."

—Gregg Easterbrook, author of
It's Better Than It Looks

"A clear-eyed look at the present and future of food production. . . . Paarlberg places the blame for our current epidemic of obesity and diet-related health problems firmly on the shoulders of food manufacturing, grocery stores, and restaurants for their promotion of unhealthy food." —*Library Journal*

"A fresh, deeply researched, and courageous study of the unprecedented challenge of ensuring a healthful diet. . . . [Paarlberg] provides much-needed context for all those concerned with bringing the food system in line with human needs." —Rachel Laudan, author of
Cuisine and Empire

"[An] astute look at food production in the U.S. Noting that food sources and producers—Big Ag, trans fats, GMOs, beef production, the sugar lobby, and farm subsidies—have been charged as contributors to the shortcomings of America's food system, [Paarlberg] redirects the blame, instead, to Big Food—a term for the powerful and persuasive industry that manufactures and markets what people consume." —*Publishers Weekly*

"Gutsy, objective, and beautifully written. Paarlberg advocates 'ecomodern'—sensible—farming practices that benefit farmers, the environment, animals, and consumers. . . . Must-reading for anyone seeking to understand controversies over food and farming."

—Michael F. Jacobson, PhD, cofounder of the Center for Science in the Public Interest

"Jam-packed . . . with scientific data and recent improvements to the agricultural complex." —*San Francisco Book Review*

"On a topic all too often subject to wild claims, emotional argument, and rejection of evidence in favor of prejudice, Robert Paarlberg brings welcome good sense, a wealth of facts, and an eloquent use of language." —Matt Ridley, author of *How Innovation Works*

"[A] broadly and deeply informed discussion of the life-and-death issues over how we grow, process, and consume our food. . . . An almost indispensable guide to our food system—and how to make that system work better." —*Booklist* (starred review)

"In *Resetting the Table*, Robert Paarlberg fact-checks the most central myths of the modern food movement. Paarlberg's firm grasp on the realities of modern agriculture lend credence to his insights on how we might take meaningful steps toward solving our dietary and environmental ills. He argues that food policy, rather than farm policy, should serve as the focal point of action. In doing so, he offers valuable straight talk to commercial farmers and highlights the critical importance of continued innovation and entrepreneurship in agricultural production. This is a must-read book for anyone interested in understanding where their food comes from and the policies that affect how we eat."

—Jayson Lusk, distinguished professor and head, Department of Agricultural Economics, Purdue University

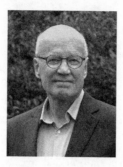

Robert Paarlberg

RESETTING THE TABLE

Robert Paarlberg is an associate at Harvard's Weatherhead Center for International Affairs, and has been a professor of political science at Wellesley College, and an adjunct professor of public policy at the Harvard Kennedy School. A consultant to the International Food Policy Research Institute, the U.S. Agency for International Development, and the Bill & Melinda Gates Foundation, he has chaired the Independent Steering Committee for a global research program, Agriculture for Nutrition and Health (A4NH). He is the author of *Starved for Science, Food Politics*, and *The United States of Excess*. He lives in Massachusetts.

RESETTING
THE TABLE

RESETTING THE TABLE

Straight Talk About the Food
We Grow and Eat

Robert Paarlberg

VINTAGE BOOKS
A Division of Penguin Random House LLC
New York

FIRST VINTAGE BOOKS EDITION, FEBRUARY 2022

Copyright © 2021 by Robert Paarlberg

All rights reserved. Published in the United States by Vintage Books,
a division of Penguin Random House LLC, New York, and distributed
in Canada by Penguin Random House Canada Limited, Toronto. Originally
published in hardcover in the United States by Alfred A. Knopf, a division
of Penguin Random House LLC, New York, in 2021.

Vintage and colophon are registered
trademarks of Penguin Random House LLC.

Pages 353–54 constitute an extension of this copyright page.

The Library of Congress has cataloged the Knopf edition as follows:
Names: Paarlberg, Robert L., author.
Title: Resetting the table : straight talk about the food we grow and eat /
Robert Paarlberg.
Description: First edition. | New York : Alfred A. Knopf, 2020. |
Includes index.
Identifiers: LCCN 2019050600
Subjects: LCSH: Food industry and trade—United States. | Farms—
United States. | Agriculture—Economic aspects—United States.
Classification: LCC HD9005 .P25 2020 | DDC 338.1/973—dc23
LC record available at https://lccn.loc.gov/2019050600

Vintage Books Trade Paperback ISBN: 978-0-525-56681-6
eBook ISBN: 978-0-525-65645-6

Author photograph © Marianne Perlak
Book design by Betty Lew

www.vintagebooks.com

Printed in the United States of America
1st Printing

To Marianne,

for absolutely everything

Surely, I said, knowledge is
the food of the soul.

—*Socrates*

Contents

Introduction   *3*

CHAPTER 1: Testing the Case Against Industrial Farming   *17*

CHAPTER 2: Food Swamp Nation   *45*

CHAPTER 3: The Limits of Local Food   *77*

CHAPTER 4: The Panic for Organic   *112*

CHAPTER 5: Should Peasants Stay Poor?   *139*

CHAPTER 6: Rejecting Biotech Food   *168*

CHAPTER 7: The Fate of Farm Animals   *195*

CHAPTER 8: The Brave New Future of Food   *228*

EPILOGUE: Straight Talk to Commercial Farmers   *267*

Acknowledgments   *277*

Notes   *281*

Index   *333*

RESETTING
THE TABLE

Introduction

❧

I n 2008, I was attending a panel discussion on "sustainable food" at Harvard University, in the storied Faculty Room of University Hall. The purpose of the panel was to promote and celebrate good food, so we were served tasty hors d'oeuvres carefully sourced from local farmers and fishermen, beginning with demitasse cups of a delicious scallop chowder from Cape Cod Bay. The featured speakers were a celebrity restaurateur from the San Francisco Bay Area, a playwright from New York, and the young leader of Slow Food USA. It didn't take long for all three to reach a lockstep conclusion: In the future, they said, sustainable food would have to be organic, local, and "slow," definitely not fast or industrial.

Those at the event nodded their heads in assent, but I had a different take, having just returned from a research trip to rural Africa. I had been interviewing farmers in Uganda who were trapped inside a food system that was entirely organic, local, and slow. The women I had spoken with (most African farmers are women) did not know it, but they were living an extreme version of the Harvard dream. They were organic because they could not afford any nitrogen fertilizer; their food was all local because the rutted dirt roads made transport almost impossible during the rainy season; and their daily food preparation tasks were laboriously slow. Before cooking a porridge meal for their family these women had to strip, soak, dry, and then pound the maize kernels into flour, then carry in wood to build a fire plus

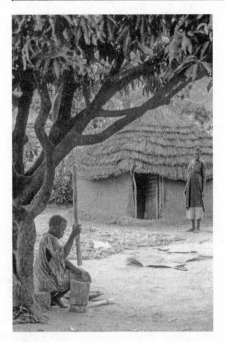

Pounding maize in Uganda, where slow food preparation is an everyday experience, and a daily burden for women and girls.

water for the pot. Despite these efforts, many of their children were stunted from poor nutrition.

Farmers are important to me for personal as well as professional reasons. Both of my parents were from a farming background, and as a young teenager in the summer months I worked on my uncle's Indiana farm, alongside my older brother and two cousins. We got up early to feed the cattle and hogs in the dark, before sitting down to our own breakfast. My cousins were still too young to drive a car, but they were handling powered machinery, working with animals four times their size, and they already knew things about farming well beyond the ken of most playwrights or big-city restaurateurs.

Discussions of food today can quickly turn into discussions about farming. Consumers not only want food to be tasty, safe, nutritious, and affordable; they also want it to come from farms that protect the natural environment, respect the welfare of animals, help sustain rural communities, and give hired workers a living wage. I share all of these goals, but my prescriptions differ from the Harvard panel's dream. My research experience tells me not to yearn for an organic, local, or slow food system, since that would mean abandoning a century's worth of modern science. It would force farmers to accept more toil and less income, consumers would be given fewer nutritious food choices, and greater destruction would be done to the natural environment. All this will be explained.

The use of modern science is broadly welcomed in medicine, transport, and communications, yet it has become strangely controversial in food production. Many of my friends in Massachusetts, where I live and work, hold a view that modern farming has become far too "industrial." They agree with Mark Bittman, a former *New York Times* columnist, who blames industrial farming for having "spawned an obesity crisis, poisoned countless volumes of land and water, wasted energy, tortured billions of animals." They would also agree with Philip Lymbery, the author of *Farmageddon,* who concludes that "every day there is a new confirmation of how destructive, inefficient, wasteful, cruel and unhealthy the industrial agriculture machine is. We need a total rethink of our food and farming systems before it's too late."

As their preferred alternative, many of my friends imagine a return to small, local, and chemical-free (organic) farms. These farms should produce a traditional mix of both crops and animals, as opposed to the specialized, industrial-scale farms that today produce just one or two crops and probably have no animals at all. When it comes to buying food, my friends would rather not be seen shopping in supermarkets, since too many items on the shelf are heavily processed or have traveled too many "food miles." Their ideal, when they have plenty of time, is to buy unprocessed foods directly from local growers at a farmers market, or from a community supported agriculture (CSA) farm. They admire Alice Waters, proprietor of the acclaimed Chez Panisse restaurant in Berkeley (she was one of the speakers on the 2008 Harvard panel), who states with pride that she has not set foot in a supermarket for the past twenty-five years.

I hear all this, but I'm not persuaded. I want a food solution that works for all, including people who live on a budget and those without a lot of spare time. Dinners at Chez Panisse must be a wonderful experience, but they start at more than a hundred dollars, not including the wine. Buying fresh produce at a farmers market is rewarding in season, but even then it means a separate trip to get needed products local farms don't grow. Assembling healthy meals from fresh, unprocessed ingredients is a joy for many, but the time required for shopping, preparation, and cleanup may be too much for a single parent with school-age kids.

Food solutions should also make sense for farmers. Here is where the organic approach creates problems, since it tells farmers they cannot use manufactured nitrogen fertilizers. True, *all* farming worked that way before synthetic fertilizers were first developed early in the twentieth century—but it made food production less abundant and needlessly laborious. Most farmers in the United States don't want to turn the clock back, which is why only 1 percent of their land has been converted to organic production methods.

Problems would also arise if we "relocalized" our food system. Dietary health would decline because fresh fruits and vegetables would become scarce for many consumers in the cold winter months. Because transport costs have continued to fall, the dominant food system trend continues to be globalization, not localization. Traditional methods might at least seem a better way to protect the welfare of farm animals, given the abuses they suffer inside today's "factory farm" confinement systems, but these traditional methods could not begin to meet today's greatly expanded market demand for animal products. Total meat consumption in the United States is now five times as high as it was in 1940, and trying to meet this demand with traditional pasture and barnyard methods would be impossible. It will be better to follow Europe's example and tighten welfare regulations for the farm animals we raise indoors, all the while developing better imitation meat products to reverse the growth of the livestock industry.

My realistic approach to such matters is one I learned from my father, who grew up on a small family farm in Indiana. After starting college late, he went on to earn a Ph.D. in agricultural economics, in order to learn why making a living on farms had suddenly become more difficult in the 1930s. My dad could be sentimental, but he always warned me not to romanticize the hard physical labor required by traditional farming.

My own career choice was also shaped by an early life experience, a trip to India and Nepal to visit my brother, who was serving in the Peace Corps. I had seen poverty in America, mostly in cities, but the extreme rural poverty I encountered on this trip to Asia left me angered and upset, yet also motivated. I have studied international food and agriculture in part to learn how poor farmers might better their lives. I have worked over the years in seven Asian countries, five countries in Latin America, and sixteen countries in Africa. My research has been financed entirely by international institutes, government agencies, my own academic institutions, and philanthropic foundations, not by any private corporations. I learned early on that big international agribusiness companies usually pay scant attention to poor farmers, since they are such bad customers for what the companies have to sell.

My colleagues and I who work in global food and farming can celebrate a considerable reduction in rural hunger and poverty in recent decades, especially in Asia. This progress has been sustained, in most cases, by making modern science-based farming methods available to the rural poor. This good news is surprisingly difficult to communicate back home, where science-based farming is routinely criticized for being too "industrial," and where a long list of nationally known food writers, journalists, and academics now promote distinctly preindustrial alternatives. Many in this group, including writers such as Alice Waters, Michael Pollan, Mark Bittman, Barbara Kingsolver, and others, see themselves as the leaders of a new social movement to reverse the direction of modern farming. Pollan, in a 2010 essay titled "The Food Movement, Rising," explained it was time to reform industrial food and food production because "its social/ environmental/public health/animal welfare/gastronomic costs are too high."

Many elite institutions have embraced this thinking. Beginning in 2001, Waters worked through Yale University to help build a new sustainable food program that included a college farm, university composting, and a shift by the dining services toward sourcing local organic food. Not wanting to be left behind, Harvard began fertilizing the grass in Harvard Yard using only organic methods, then it put up signs to let people know.

Influential national media outlets have offered mostly uncritical support. Pollan, with remarkable candor, described it this way to an audience in Santa Cruz, California, in 2013:

> In the elite media, the critique of industrial food has gotten plenty of play. The media has really been on our side for the most part. I know this from writing for the *New York Times,* where I've written about a lot of other topics, but when I wrote about food I never had to give equal time to the other side. I could say whatever I thought and offer my own conclusions. Say you should buy grass fed beef, and organic is better, and these editors in New York didn't realize there is anyone who disagrees with that point of view. So I felt like I got a free ride for a long time.

Pollan's 2006 best-selling book *The Omnivore's Dilemma* became something of a sacred text for this new food movement. It was adopted as mandatory summer reading for incoming students at numerous colleges and universities, where the author himself led at least a dozen different freshman readings. A streamlined version of the book pitched to "young readers" came out in 2009, along with a documentary film based on the book titled *Food, Inc.* Hollywood gave the film an Academy Award nomination.

In 2007, Barbara Kingsolver wrote her own bestselling book, one that recorded a personal decision to move to Virginia and eat only locally grown food for an entire year (except for grains and olive oil). Also in 2007, the *New Oxford American Dictionary* selected *locavore* as its Word of the Year. By 2009, the new food movement even gained official endorsement from the White House. First Lady Michelle Obama arranged to be photographed shopping at a farmers market, and at the urging of Waters she planted an organic garden on the White House lawn. Barack Obama's Department of Agriculture also began promoting local food by initiating a "Know Your Farmer, Know Your Food" program.

This new food movement deserves credit for the valuable alert it sent on America's bad eating habits, which had led to heavier burdens of chronic disease. By 2018, 42 percent of American adults were clinically obese. Food movement leaders correctly blamed some of this on the corporate actors between farm and table—food manufacturing companies, supermarkets, restaurant chains—but they also began promoting a view that our farms, or at least our farm subsidy policies, shared much of the blame as well.

Farm subsidies were said to be ruining the nation's diet by encouraging too much corn and soy production, as opposed to fruits and vegetables. I am generally opposed to farm subsidies, because they are wasteful and poorly targeted, but there is no good evidence that they have made us fat. Agricultural economists know that farm subsidies do not make obesity-inducing foods artificially cheap. Corn, soy, sugar, and dairy products are all artificially expensive because of federal policy, not artificially cheap. The reasons will be explained.

Industrial farming hurts the environment, but mostly because of how much food is produced, not how it is produced. If we tried to produce as much as we do today using preindustrial methods, the damage would be far more extreme. Modern industrial farming did become too chemical intensive after the Second World War, but more recently, thanks to the emergence of "precision agriculture," chemical use on farms has decreased significantly, not just relative to output but often in absolute terms as well. Fertilizer use on America's farms has remained flat for the past four decades while total production was increasing more than 40 percent, and total insecticide use on farms is now more than 80 percent lower than in 1972.

With satellite positioning, drone-based sensors, big data, robotics, and now machine learning as well, a modern revolution in precision farming has made possible the production of more food while using less land, less water, less energy, and fewer chemicals, implying large benefits to the natural environment. This promising new path to environmental protection has been dubbed *ecomodernism,* since it works not by producing less, or returning to the past, but by using new technologies that can produce more with fewer resources.

One exciting ecomodernist project now under way is the use of molecular science to develop imitation products that substitute for meat, milk, and eggs, making it unnecessary to raise and feed so many farm animals. If we can produce comparably delicious simulated meats from plant materials, or perhaps from cell cultures in a lab, fewer greenhouse gasses will enter the atmosphere, more farming and grazing lands can be returned to nature, and fewer animals will have to experience mistreatment at our hands.

A return to preindustrial food and farming methods can work on a small scale for those with plenty of money to spend, *but it will never be a society-wide solution.* Scaling up to supply most of the market may not really be a food movement goal. Alice Waters puts a higher value on her culinary integrity, and derides "scaling" as a term from fast-food culture. Other celebrity chefs also seem comfortable with exclusivity; they advise us to eat seasonally, but then they fly off to Sicily in April to give cooking workshops where they won't have to suffer with late-winter vegetables. The Blue Hill restaurant, at the picturesque Stone Barns Center for Food and Agriculture, thirty miles north of Manhattan, promotes delicious farm-to-table meals sourced from the Hudson Valley, but the fixed-price menu is $258 per guest, and that's exclusive of beverage, tax, and a 20 percent "administrative fee" in lieu of tips.

The food movement vision is culturally fashionable, but it hasn't managed a significant scale-up in the marketplace so far. Consider organic food. The latest official data from the Department of Agriculture show that fewer than 2 percent of farm commodities produced in the United States are produced organically, and less than 1 percent of harvested cropland in America is organically certified. Big food companies continue adding organic choices to their product lines, yet fewer than 6 percent of total retail food sales in the United States were organic as of 2018.

Likewise for local food. If we consider all sales at farmers markets, as well as CSA, pick-your-own, roadside stands, farm-to-school and farm-to-restaurant sales, and then add in local food hubs, the total sales in 2017 came to less than 1 percent of all farm sales. The dominant trend has not been toward local food, but toward more global food. In the 1990s, 11 percent of food in America was imported; today that share is up to 20 percent.

A return to small, artisanal farms is comforting to contemplate, since it conforms to what we still learn about farms from happy children's songs and nursery rhymes. Nobody will ever try to make a happy children's song about modern industrial farming, where big machines do the work and most of the animals are raised indoors. When city people take a drive through the countryside, they would naturally prefer to see traditional farms, with wooden barns and cows in the pasture, not modern farms.

Such urban affections for a dimly remembered rural past are well intended, but good intentions alone can bring serious trouble when it comes to producing food. In June 1843, Bronson Alcott, a progressive educational reformer, the father of Louisa May Alcott, and an early opponent of slavery, moved his wife and three young daughters from Concord, Massachusetts, to a nearby ninety-acre farm, hoping to create a modern Garden of Eden. He called his little utopian community Fruitlands, but it hardly lived up to the name.

Alcott's strict ethical standards did not allow the "enslaving" of any animals, so he and his followers used hand tools only, and some ate only the "aspiring vegetables" that grew upward toward heaven, ruling out root crops like potatoes and carrots. Alcott was often away giving lectures, so he did little of the physical farm work himself. Louisa May, who would grow up to write *Little Women*, was only ten at the time, but she later recalled that her father's recruits "began by spading garden and field; but a few days of it lessened their ardor amazingly."

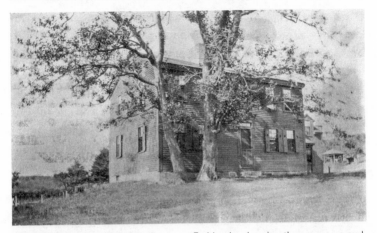

A 1915 image of the old Alcott house at Fruitlands, showing the grown-up mulberry trees Bronson had planted too close to the front door. Fruitlands ran short of food long before the trees produced any silkworms.

In the end, they did not produce enough food, Louisa May became ill, and the misguided experiment folded after seven months.

Most Americans today know even less about food production than Bronson Alcott. Back in 1950, 16 percent of Americans lived on farms, but now it's fewer than 2 percent. Many nonfarmers have experience growing vegetables in a backyard garden, but this is a labor of love that can skew thinking about what commercial agriculture should look like. A clear understanding of what commercial farming requires is hard to gain without some direct exposure to America's agricultural regions, located at a distance from most of us, in sparsely populated "flyover" country.

Growing numbers of my East Coast students are now interested in farming, and many have even worked on the local farms near where they live in New England, but this is usually just one step up from gardening and can't count as exposure to modern commercial agriculture. New England farms frequently fit the food movement ideal: most are very small, quite a few are organically certified, and they often sell what they grow through local roadside farm stands, farmers markets, or community supported agriculture. In our national marketplace, though, they are close to insignificant. The total commercial sales made by all of the farms in Massachusetts, Connecticut, Maine, New Hampshire, Vermont, and Rhode Island put together make up less than 1 percent of total national farm sales.

I will agree here that most of our processed industrial foods are making an unfortunate contribution to the eating environment, but industrial farms, for the most part, are not. This distinction goes against food movement fashion, but it follows from the evidence. Industrial farming's biggest problem is its mistreatment of food animals, but even here a return to preindustrial systems—the food movement's favorite solution—would not be an affordable option. Tighter regulation and continued innovation are the better way forward.

In the pages that follow we will first visit an "industrial" corn and soybean farm in eastern Indiana to meet a fifth-generation family farmer who has gone digital. He uses computer-programmed and satellite-guided machines that operate with extreme precision, cutting wasteful fertilizer use without any loss of yield. We will explore whether large farms such as his, producing mostly corn and soy, can be blamed for America's bad diet. We will also contemplate the social consequences of allowing large, specialized farms to replace small, traditional farms.

Then we confront the eating environment in America, one now swamped with unhealthy choices designed, manufactured, and marketed by large food companies, retailers, and restaurant chains. We will meet a food-marketing expert who has worked for a major retail chain but now promotes a nutrition-guidance system for use on supermarket shelves. We will also share a lunch at Applebee's with a consultant to the food service industry, gaining an insider's view on the future of restaurants, including their impact on dietary health. We then review some policy options to moderate the damage being done by these corporate actors, such as mandatory calorie counts on restaurant menus, taxes on sugary beverages, and restrictions on food ads to children.

Next we will explore the recent popularity of local food, starting with a visit to a successful CSA farm. Farmers markets, CSA farms, local food hubs, and farm-to-school arrangements enjoy wide popularity, yet, as I have said, the commercial space they occupy in America's food system remains tiny. I will show why trying to grow more food locally—including in urban settings—encounters so many economic, environmental, and dietary limitations.

Similar questions will be asked about organic food. Despite several decades of popularity with consumers, organic food still makes up less than 6 percent of all food sold through U.S. retail channels, and just 2 percent of all commodities produced on American farms. We will see that most farmers do not convert to organic methods because following the rules requires too much land and labor for every bushel produced. These rules also fail to deliver the promised benefits to health, nutrition, and the environment. The organic dream, hatched a century ago as a rejection of manufactured fertilizers, remains unfulfilled because of its weak scientific foundation.

We will also examine the advice now being given to poor farmers in the developing world to practice "agroecology," by avoiding purchased inputs like fertilizers and staying away from crop monocultures or specialized production systems. This alternative approach has been heavily promoted by international civil society organizations and also by the special agencies of the UN system, but farmers in poor countries show little interest because it requires too much human labor. A parallel concept also promoted by outsiders, known as "food sovereignty," has likewise failed to catch on in poor countries, despite its fashionability with advocacy organizations and some academics in rich countries.

The highly controversial subject of genetically engineered crops, known as GMOs, will be explored as well. We will see that advocacy groups opposed to GMOs have been surprisingly successful in curtailing the spread of this technology. Genetically engineered varieties of wheat, rice, and potato have been available to plant for more than two decades, but they are not grown anywhere today, primarily due to stifling regulations. We will meet a rice scientist who explains this outcome, then ask if a more recent breakthrough in crop science known as "gene editing" will be blocked in a similar fashion.

To explore animal welfare we will scrutinize modern "factory farms," the concentrated animal feeding operations (CAFOs) that keep most farm animals in excessive confinement. Insights will be gained by talking to a chicken scientist in Georgia, an animal welfare lobbyist in Sacramento, a veterinarian in Africa who works with cattle herdsmen, an innovative farmer in the Netherlands dedicated to caring for her pigs, and a progressive commercial pig farmer in the United States who puts his sows in pens instead of crates, but mistrusts the organizations trying to make this a legal requirement.

We also will look into the future, starting with the growing threat both to the climate and human health from diets too rich in animal products, especially red meat. The dietary enrichments we can expect in densely populated Asia in the years ahead will make this a global crisis. Perhaps imitation meats, made from plant materials or grown from cultured cells, will eventually provide part of the escape. Crop farming, meanwhile, is likely to become even more precise and information-driven in the years ahead, by moving further into the digital age. Robotic machines will appear in the fields able to pick even the most delicate fruits like strawberries. I will ask an engineer who designs these machines how far this robotics revolution will spread in agriculture, and then consider the social implications with a scientist who grew up as a farmworker, picking crops in California's Central Valley.

Finally, I will offer some straight talk to America's commercial farmers, advising them to spend less time supporting food companies and more time advocating for dietary health. This switch would open space to improve nutrition in America, and it might soften some of the criticism now directed at industrial farming. To make this beneficial change, farmers will have to adjust the way they present themselves, but not the way they farm.

. . .

The cultural distance in America today between commercial farmers and quality-conscious food consumers has become dangerously wide. In my own work I try to straddle this divide, but it gets more difficult all the time. My family roots are definitely on the farming side, but quality-conscious eating is also a big part of my life. The students I teach at Harvard, many from urban or suburban backgrounds, are heavily committed to healthy and ethical eating, but most arrive in my classes deeply suspicious of modern farming. My intention here is to offer one way to navigate between these different worlds, by drawing careful distinctions, painting with a finer brush, and most of all by following the evidence. The vision I offer is a mix of science, economic realism, ethical humanism, and practical politics, flavored by bits of my own personal experience. This will not be a tale of villains and victims, or a catalog of sins compiled to spark outrage. My goal is not to provoke strong emotions but to promote good results. The heroes and heroines in my story are those making practical efforts to improve our collective food future, both on the farm and at the table.

CHAPTER 1

Testing the Case Against Industrial Farming

❧

Modern industrial farming did not bring unhealthy eating to the United States. Poor nutrition has been a problem from the start, originally linked to preindustrial poverty. A century and a half ago, most American citizens had so little income they could afford only cheap stomach-filling foods like bread and potatoes. Because this was a diet lacking in protein and micronutrients, Americans remained short in stature and vulnerable to a wide variety of diet-linked ailments well into the twentieth century.

Diets finally began to diversify in the late nineteenth and early twentieth centuries, but not because farming had changed. Instead, industrial development had brought increased urbanization and higher personal income, along with improved food access thanks to innovations such as refrigerated rail cars, packaged and processed foods, and supermarkets. This gave consumers a wider range of choice, so milk and fruit consumption increased as bread and potato consumption declined. Potato consumption in the United States fell by nearly half on a per capita basis between 1909 and 1959, while flour and cereal product consumption dropped by more than half. Even so, serious nutrient deficits persisted. Pellagra, a disease caused by a niacin deficit, led to the death of 100,000 Americans during the first three decades of the twentieth century. Rickets, a deforming ailment caused by vitamin D deficiency, afflicted three-quarters of infants in New York City in 1921.

As late as the Second World War, inadequate nutrition made it hard for the army to find enough young men fit for military service. General Lewis B. Hershey, head of the Draft Board, testified that "probably one-third" of the men rejected for service in that war failed to qualify because of disabilities linked to nutrition deficits. Industrial farming was not the source of these problems, since it hadn't yet arrived. The nation's food production system was still heavily dependent on small, local, diverse farms that used few if any chemicals.

In the second half of the last century, added gains in personal income contributed to still more dietary enrichment. This, plus targeted feeding programs like Food Stamps after the 1960s, eventually corrected most of America's nutrition deficiency problems. But then, with barely a pause, America went from being underfed to being overfed. Between the early 1960s and 2018, the prevalence of obesity in the United States tripled to reach an astonishing 42 percent. Chronic ailments such as diabetes and cardiovascular disease, linked to excessive consumption of energy-dense foods and processed meats, emerged as the nation's number one public health problem. Estimates based on known diet-disease relationships suggest that twice as many Americans now die from eating processed meats as in car accidents. Nearly half of all U.S. deaths due to heart disease, stroke, and diabetes are now diet linked.

Poor diets have even returned as a national security concern, since one in three young Americans nationwide is now too fat to enlist in the military. Other wealthy countries also face dietary problems, but on the European continent, obesity rates tend to be only half as high as in the United States. In November 2018, the *Economist* Intelligence Unit published rankings of thirty-five high-income countries according to their success at meeting "nutritional challenges," and the United States came in next to last, barely ahead of Saudi Arabia.

When these problems with modern eating first emerged in America, nobody blamed industrial farming. Rather than pointing the finger at Big Ag, most critics focused correctly on Big Food. Eric Schlosser's 2001 classic, *Fast Food Nation: The Dark Side of the All-American Meal*, singled out fast-food restaurant chains. Schlosser devoted only three

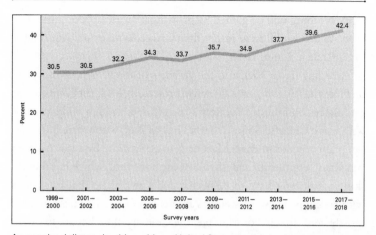

An unsolved dietary health problem. United States trends in obesity prevalence among adults ages twenty and over, 1999–2000 through 2017–2018.

of his 288 pages to farming, and the index to his book has no entry at all for "agriculture." In that same year, nutritionist Marion Nestle also produced an important book, *Food Politics: How the Food Industry Influences Nutrition and Health,* with no indexed references to either farms or farming. A subsequent book by Anthony Winson on our "industrial diet" traced poor eating not to farms or farm subsidies but to food processors and manufacturers, retailers, and restaurant chains.

On America's farms, the nutrient quality of some foods grown today has been diminished. Mark Schatzker, author of *The Dorito Effect: The Surprising New Truth About Food and Flavor,* observed that for most of the twentieth century, farm crops and farm animals were developed to deliver things like rapid growth, cosmetic appearance, shelf life, processing traits, and resistance to pests and disease. There was little or no emphasis on nutrition, or even on flavor, which is a trait associated with nutrition. One 2004 study examining the nutrient content of forty-three garden crops between 1950 and 1999 found a decline in six out of the thirteen nutrients contained in these crops, including a 38 percent drop for riboflavin. Yet Schatzker's solution is to change the way we breed crops and animals, not the way we farm. Nothing will be gained by growing a nutrient-poor variety of broccoli on a small farm rather than a large farm, or on a local farm rather than a distant farm.

Breeding flavor back into the varieties of crops and animals used on farms has now become an active project. In 2018, chef and author Dan Barber co-founded the Row 7 Seed Company to provide growers with more flavorful options. Barber has worked with Cornell University plant breeder Michael Mazourek to bring more flavor into a mini version of a butternut squash, called the honeynut, which has thinner skin so it doesn't have to be peeled and a sweetness that intensifies with cooking. These new efforts are heavily focused on taste and are mostly chef driven. For example, the Culinary Breeding Network in Oregon now connects chefs to breeders and hosts public tastings to demonstrate the delicious result. At one showcase event in New York City attended by four hundred people, the new varieties available to taste included a blue fenugreek that smelled like maple syrup, a new Primero Red chili for hot taco sauce, and leaves from a new variety of amaranth.

The diminished nutrient content of food needs correcting, but the excess calories we consume are far more damaging to our health. Average per capita food calorie consumption in the United States (based on calories available adjusted for spoilage and other waste) increased 25 percent between 1970 and 2002. Physical activity levels declined at the same time, but this was not the heart of the problem according to Marion Nestle. "Large portions are a sufficient explanation for why people are gaining weight. It's not because of lack of exercise; it's because we're eating more." Portion sizes in restaurants are one contributor. Compared to 1986, average entrée portions in fast-food chains by 2016 were delivering ninety more calories. Nutritionist Lisa Young (known as the "portion teller") famously dramatized this historical increase in serving sizes for bagels, hamburgers, and soda in the film *Super-Size Me*.

It takes surprisingly little time for a simple reduction in food intake to begin bringing health improvements. In one study with 143 healthy men and women between twenty-one and fifty years of age, all were

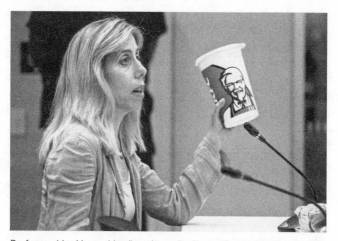

Professor Lisa Young (the "portion teller") testifies in 2012 to support a proposed New York City ban on sales of sugary drinks in sizes larger than 16 ounces.

allowed to choose their own variety of foods but half were asked to reduce total calorie intake. Over a two-year period the restricted group reduced total calorie intake by only 12 percent yet still lost an average of sixteen pounds. Those on calorie restriction also saw many of their cardiovascular and metabolic health markers improve, even though all had started within the normal range.

Increased calorie consumption in America was also caused in part by unsound medical advice. In the 1970s, physicians and nutrition experts told us to minimize consumption of saturated fats to protect against heart disease. Research would later reveal that saturated fats had a relatively weak link to heart disease, falling somewhere between good fats (monounsaturated and polyunsaturated) and the bad industrial-made trans fats. But the damage had already been done; the fat avoidance recommendations had driven eaters to consume far too many carbohydrates instead. These carbs tended to leave the body less satiated, so hunger returned sooner and still more calories were then consumed.

In addition to being excessive, American eating is badly unbalanced across different food groups and nutrient categories. Every five years the USDA and the Department of Health and Human Services promulgate their "Dietary Guidelines for Americans," intended as a common standard for what a balanced diet should look like. It is revealing to compare these guidelines to America's actual eating patterns, as measured in the National Health and Nutrition Examination Survey. More than four-fifths of Americans fail to consume the recommended quantity of vegetables, and three-quarters are low in fruits, dairy, and oils. Meanwhile, more than half *exceed* the recommended intake limits for grain and protein foods, nearly two-thirds consume too much added sugar and saturated fat, and almost nine out of ten consume too much salt.

C ritics of industrial agriculture have tried to trace this imbalance in what we eat to an imbalance in what America's farms produce. Corn and soybean production currently takes up more than half of all farmland area in the United States, and both of these crops are used to feed the cattle and pigs that give us too much meat, as well as the cows that give us ice cream and cheese. These crops are also key ingredients in energy-dense snack and junk foods, and the syrup made from corn sweetens our drinks. The critics say our diet would improve if our farmers grew less corn and soy, and more fruits and vegetables.

Michael Pollan traces this imbalance to farm subsidies encouraging too much commodity crop production: "We create incentives for our farmers to grow huge quantities of corn and soy, mostly in the Midwest," he told one university audience in 2017. "Corn and soy is really where the calories in most of the junk food come from . . . we have inadvertently created a system where the cheapest calories in the supermarket are the least healthy." Food consumers, according to Pollan, have been suffering from a "plague of cheap corn." This theme was picked up and amplified in popular films like *King Corn*, and *Food, Inc.*, the latter being nominated in 2009 for an Academy Award.

The American diet is not, however, determined by what America's farms grow. Our farms do produce a lot of corn, but more than one-third of it never enters the human food supply because it is used to make ethanol, an alcohol we mix with gasoline for auto fuel. Another 14 percent of our corn crop is exported to foreign livestock producers, along with 52 percent of America's soybeans, so none of this enters America's food supply either. Corn and soy are principally animal feeds, and we grow more of these crops today because rising incomes, particularly in East Asia, have driven up consumer demand for meat, milk, and eggs in the global marketplace.

Meanwhile, America's lower production of fruits and vegetables is corrected through imports. More than half of America's fresh fruit consumption is now imported, along with almost a third of its fresh vegetables. Four-fifths of America's fish consumption is also imported. Is this a bad thing? In 2018 Pollan told the *New York Times*, "I had no idea that more than half our fruit is imported, and it shocks me that this has happened so quickly." Without these imports America's diet would be much further out of balance, so shock may not be the proper reaction.

In addition to missing the role of imports, exports, and the use of so much corn for fuel, most critics misunderstand the operation of farm subsidies. They assume farm subsidies are making food artificially cheap when they actually do the opposite. The purpose of these subsidies has always been to increase the income of farmers, and one simple way to do this is to push *up* the price that farmers get for their crops, and this is what typically happens. One study by three independent agricultural economists published in the journal *Food Policy* in 2008 showed that market prices for soybeans, rice, sugar, fruits, vegetables, beef, pork, and milk were all being propped up— not pushed down—by federal farm subsidy policies.

Food prices are sometimes pushed up by restricting imports from abroad, sometimes by paying farmers to take land out of production, and sometimes by mandating the purchase of farm commodities for things like ethanol production or foreign food aid. The result in each case will be fewer commodities left in the American market, not more, and hence a higher price paid by domestic consumers.

One interesting case is sugar, a commodity two-thirds of Americans currently consume to excess. We would be consuming even more sugar if the federal government weren't propping up the price through a tariff rate quota on imports of sugar from abroad. These import restrictions, which have existed in one form or another since the 1930s, increase not only the domestic price of sugar, but also the price of other sweeteners such as high-fructose corn syrup. Between 1982 and 2012, thanks to this restrictive import policy, the average price of sugar inside the U.S. market was 64 percent higher than on the international market.

This policy is enacted by Congress in response to a well-organized sugar lobby that represents not just sugarcane producers in Florida (politically important as a swing state) but also sugarbeet producers in Minnesota, Idaho, North Dakota, and Michigan. Florida sugar barons like the Fanjul brothers have routinely used political access at the highest levels of government to keep the import restrictions in place. Their access and influence are legendary. During the 1998 impeachment effort against President Bill Clinton, Monica Lewinsky testified under oath that the president had been willing to interrupt one of his private Oval Office sessions with her to take a phone call from Alfonso Fanjul.

The federal government also pushes up wheat prices, by paying farmers in Kansas and other states to take land out of production under the so-called Conservation Reserve Program (CRP). This makes bread more expensive. In 2006, when Michael Pollan was claiming that farm subsidies made food cheap, the CRP was idling thirty-seven million acres of cropland, an area larger than the entire state of Iowa, thus keeping food prices high.

Pollan's 2006 account also misconstrued a policy change in 1973 that ended some Depression-era "supply control" measures and some programs for the purchase and storage of surplus production. According to Pollan, President Nixon's secretary of agriculture, Earl Butz, devised these changes to make farm commodities cheaper, to benefit food processing and manufacturing companies, livestock industries, and also grain-exporting firms like Cargill that could use the lower prices to undersell foreign competitors. It certainly sounded like something the Nixon administration would do. But the 1973 changes were instead triggered by a sudden upward spike in the price of farm commodities, so they were undertaken not to ensure low food prices but to avoid disastrously high prices.

In a single month in the summer of 1973, the price of a bushel of wheat jumped from $2.47 to $4.45. The principal cause was an inflationary cheap-money policy by the Federal Reserve, which brought on higher commodity prices across the board, not just for food but also for oil, copper, tin, and bauxite. To help contain a further food price increase, the government did, temporarily, encourage more farm production, but only for a brief interlude. When monetary policy was eventually tightened in the 1980s, crop prices tumbled back down and the USDA reintroduced both its land-idling and government purchase programs.

New price-propping measures were undertaken in the 1980s as well. A conservation reserve was devised to restrict wheat acreage, along with the so-called Payment in Kind program to idle still more land. As a result, wheat producers reduced their plantings by more than a fifth, corn production fell by almost half, and the United States was soon idling more cropland than all of Western Europe was still planting. All this was being done, once again, to prop commodity prices up, not push them down.

The idea that government policies give us cheap corn is particularly far-fetched. Government policy drives *up* corn prices by mandating that a large part of the harvest be used to produce auto fuel. A panic over foreign fuel dependence early in the 2000s inspired a government-mandated doubling of corn ethanol production, causing corn prices to double as well, up from two dollars to four dollars per bushel by 2007. This was hardly a plague of cheap corn. By 2018, 38 percent of the entire U.S. corn crop was used to make ethanol.

One common suggestion from critics of industrial farming is to switch the subsidy programs from corn and soy to fruits and vegetables. Ironically, assuming the same policy instruments were used, namely import restrictions, land idling, and mandated purchases for non-food uses, fruit and vegetable prices would go up as a result and consumption would go down, not the desired outcome. Direct payments to fruit and vegetable farmers might be an alternative option, but the USDA already does this through the Specialty Crop Research Initiative and a Specialty Crop Block Grant Program. The 2014 farm bill increased funding levels for these specialty crop programs by more than half, to about $4 billion over ten years.

While farm subsidies haven't made food cheap, some other programs contained in the farm bill do cheapen food for low-income consumers. The Supplemental Nutrition Assistance Program (SNAP), previously known as Food Stamps, provides roughly $70 billion in food purchase credits every year to low-income Americans, increasing the amount of food they can afford to purchase. In addition, the Women, Infants, and Children (WIC) nutrition program provides roughly $6 billion every year, both in food and cash-value food vouchers, to low-income women, infants, and children, and the National School Lunch Program makes free or inexpensive school meals available to low-income schoolchildren at an annual cost of $13 billion. In all, the farm bill is now allocating four times as much money to cheapen food for poor consumers as it is spending to boost the income of farmers.

This allocation of public spending makes good sense, since America's poor consumers are in far greater need of income support than commercial farmers. Yet the SNAP program isn't perfect, since it can be used to purchase things like sugary beverages, junk foods, and candy. Advocates for improved nutrition attempted in 2018 to change the rules of SNAP, restricting purchases of sugary beverages, but this effort failed when anti-hunger groups, in denial about the health problems linked to excess calorie consumption, joined in a tacit alliance with the beverage industry to defeat the idea.

The poet and agrarian advocate Wendell Berry has famously said "eating is an agricultural act." This was once the case, but little of our food today comes to us directly from farmers. More than 90 percent of all commercial value added in America's food supply now comes not from farms but from food processing, packaging, trans-

Where America's Food Dollar Went, 2017

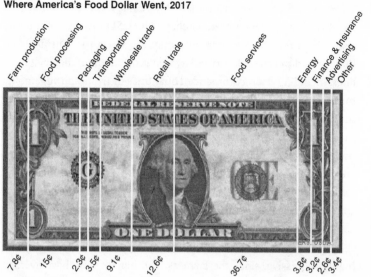

Farm production Food processing Packaging Transportation Wholesale trade Retail trade Food services Energy Finance & Insurance Advertising Other

7.8¢   15¢   2.3¢ 3.5¢ 9.1¢   12.6¢   36.7¢   3.8¢ 3.2¢ 2.6¢ 3.4¢

Note: "Other" includes two industry groups: Agribusiness plus Legal & Accounting.
Source: USDA, Economic Research Service, Food Dollar Series.

Less than 8 percent of the consumer's "food dollar" goes for farm production, making "Big Ag" look not so big after all.

port, wholesale trade, retail, advertising, finance and insurance, energy, and the restaurant sector. Big Food, in fact, is almost seven times as large now as Big Ag.

Because Big Food is good at cutting costs to compete, the retail price paid by consumers for food has been in a long-term decline. It isn't just the junk foods that are getting cheaper. Between 1980 and 2006, the average inflation-adjusted price for calorie-dense foods like chocolate chip cookies, cola, ice cream, and potato chips, and for healthy foods like apples, bananas, lettuce, and dry beans, fell at essentially the same rate when adjusted for quality and seasonality. As a result, healthy food in America today tends to be just as cheap as unhealthy food. For example, when the USDA compared dollar costs among different snack foods, it found the cost per portion for twenty healthy fruit and vegetable snacks averaged 2 cents *less* than for twenty food snacks that were less nutritious.

Healthy food is now particularly affordable for those with time to shop, cook, and clean up the kitchen. The USDA calculated in 2013 that a hypothetical four-person family following its "Thrifty Food Plan" could purchase foods that would satisfy federal dietary guidelines, including the recommended quantities of fruits and vegetables, for only $145.86 per week, or less than two dollars per person per meal. Dollar costs are not what stop most of us from consuming these healthy meals; instead it is a combination of time costs and taste preferences. Too many Americans simply prefer pizza, beef jerky, ice cream, and potato chips to green vegetables. These industrial food temptations do not come from farms, however; all are concocted and sold by food manufacturers, retailers, or restaurant chains.

The fact that farm subsidies are not making us fat does not make these policies a good idea. They have become both unnecessary and highly regressive, since the farmers who benefit now have average income levels substantially higher than the consumers and taxpayers footing the bill. The average income for all family farms in America in 2016 was 42 percent above the national household average. In 2017, the American Enterprise Institute published a study advising Congress to terminate many farm subsidy programs, since they sent taxpayer-funded checks to wealthy individuals, wasted scarce economic resources, and raised food prices for consumers. This advice was ignored in 2018, when Congress passed yet another farm bill renewing these programs.

M odern industrial farming is also depicted by critics as damaging to the natural environment. The Union of Concerned Scientists has observed that all forms of agriculture impact the natural environment, but it calls industrial agriculture a special case, since "it damages the soil, water, and even the climate on an unprecedented scale."

The scale of the damage is indeed quite large, but this is due to the expanded quantity of food now being produced, *not* the way it is produced. This is an essential distinction seldom drawn by the critics, who should pause to consider the much larger environmental cost if today's output were produced using yesterday's preindustrial methods. When total production quantities are taken into account, we discover that modern methods are doing a significantly better job of protecting nature.

Farms in America in 1870 produced less than one-tenth the output of today. Average corn yields at that time were only twenty to thirty bushels an acre, roughly one-tenth the yield today on well-run farms. If we tried to use these earlier methods to produce what the market asks for today, the cultivated area planted with corn would have to expand roughly tenfold. Likewise for most other crops. If we went down this path, fragile and sloping lands would have to be plowed up and ruined, and much of our remaining forestland would disappear.

Low-yield preindustrial farming methods were becoming environmentally unsustainable even back in 1870. In geographer Stanley Trimble's words, farming at that time was based on "a widespread attitude that land could be used, exhausted, or destroyed as the case may be, and then abandoned for new land." Trimble points out that such a system existed well into the twentieth century in much of the southeastern United States, "and the depredations on the landscape are still visible today." Recall that it was a heedless expansion of low-yield farming onto the southern plains early in the twentieth century that led to the disastrous Dust Bowl of the 1930s, creating a *Grapes of Wrath* generation of environmental refugees.

This kind of environmental damage was not contained until a mid-twentieth-century transition toward farming methods based on the latest science. Rather than expanding onto more fragile lands, farmers made existing fields more productive by using things like manufactured fertilizers and hybrid seeds. As these innovations spread, total farmland area in the United States finally stabilized and stopped increasing by 1950, even as total agricultural output continued to more than double over the next five decades.

Economists call this *productivity*, which is different from just producing more. It means producing more without using more resources, or it can mean using fewer resources to produce the same amount,

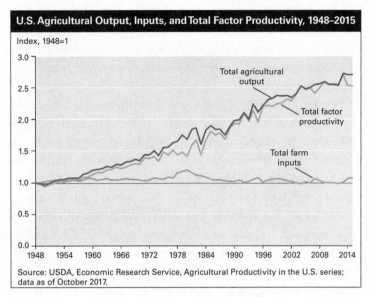

U.S. Agricultural Output, Inputs, and Total Factor Productivity, 1948–2015

Index, 1948=1

Total agricultural output

Total factor productivity

Total farm inputs

Source: USDA, Economic Research Service, Agricultural Productivity in the U.S. series; data as of October 2017.

Total U.S. farm output (top line) has more than doubled since 1948, while total farm inputs have scarcely increased at all. Modern science progressively "decouples" farm production from heavy resource use.

delivering enormous benefits to the natural environment. Farm productivity gains have continued into the twenty-first century, thanks to the introduction of GPS satellites, remote sensors, and also modern biotechnology, all of which allow farmers to increase their production while consuming many fewer material resources. To illustrate, pay a visit to John Nidlinger's farm in eastern Indiana.

The Nidlinger farm, with its large equipment barn and tall shiny grain bins, can be seen from a considerable distance across a flat landscape. In early October, when I visited, the corn harvest was underway. John Nidlinger, the farm's owner and operator, was honored as an Indiana Master Farmer in 2016—jointly with his wife, Nan—so I would see modern commercial farming at its best. John had agreed to share with me his experience in using what is called pre-

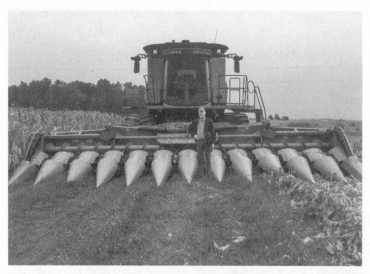

The author is dwarfed by John Nidlinger's satellite-steered twelve-row combine harvester. Only a century ago, corn was still picked by hand.

cision agriculture (PA) to optimize crop yields while reducing chemical use.

We talked while John worked, seated in the cab of his wide Case combine harvester. John would take manual control only long enough to engage the auto-steer system guided by GPS satellites, one that uses navigation software similar to that of a modern airliner. With his left hand on a button-studded joystick, John steered the pointed dividers on his combine into the field between the next twelve rows of brown corn stalks, which held plump ears of ripened corn. A sound like a metallic "ching" meant the satellite guidance system had taken control, and we made our first pass through the field at a brisk walking pace. Rather than clipping the stalks like a mower, the harvesting head pulls the stalks down through a narrow channel, stripping off the ears of corn and tumbling them onto an unseen threshing drum beneath our seats where the kernels will be separated from the husks and cobs. The separated grain is captured in a tank in the machine's belly, while the cobs and chaff are pushed out the back.

The yield monitor at John's right elbow gave him a continuous read on how much corn was coming in. This would be his payoff for a season of work, so he watched it closely. The monitor was bouncing back and forth between 220 and 240 bushels an acre, well above the recent national average of 177 bushels per acre. John's yield was also more than double the national average of the 1980s, and four times what my uncle's Indiana farm could do back in 1960. When we reached the end of the row, John reclaimed manual control, turned the machine around, reengaged with his GPS satellites, and resumed the harvest going in the opposite direction.

A century ago corn was picked and husked by hand. Harvesting today has indeed become an industrial process, but John does not see his farm as "industrial." This is because growing the corn (farmers like to call themselves growers) is still essentially a biological process, one that cannot be made uniform since even within the same field conditions will constantly vary. Growers confront surprising differences in soil moisture and soil chemistry location by location, along with variations as a crop responds to flooding and drought, heat and frost, and also insect damage, crop disease, and weed competition.

Today's most successful commercial farmers have learned to master these challenges by collecting and using more and better data and real-time information. With digitized soil maps, GPS signals, remote sensors, drones, and big data, farmers can bring more location-specific, real-time information to bear on their operations. Machines still do the work, but they are smart machines, guided by onboard computers programmed to do different things at different locations as they move through the field. This allows farmers to cut down on the wasteful use of water and chemicals, delivering corollary benefits to the natural environment downstream.

Farm crops are still grown from seeds, but now even the seeds are smart. Since the 1990s, new applications of molecular biology have given farmers like John Nidlinger corn plants able to protect themselves from insects with fewer chemical sprays. The plant tissues have been engineered to carry proteins that butterfly and moth caterpillars cannot digest. This saves the farmer money by reducing chemical and diesel fuel costs, but it also protects innocent life in the field since only the caterpillars trying to eat the crop will be harmed. Duane Kiess is vice president of Nidlinger Farms. He coordinates precision farming activities, including the GPS data systems and the variable rate application systems that continuously alter chemical applications to match variations in soil and plant needs. John's son, J.D., is responsible for purchasing seeds and chemicals, for fertilizer and lime applications, for the ditching of fields to insert underground drainage tiles, and also for soybean planting.

I asked Duane if the farm was using big data to optimize chemical fertilizer applications, reducing waste and runoff. He said they used a service named Encirca, but added that the farm also relies on its own data collection and conducts its own analysis. "With the technology we've got now, every field is a test plot," said Duane. "We're recording everything. We can look at every acre in every field." Records are kept of which strips in a field were given a fungicide treatment and which were not, with the differential impacts on yield analyzed at harvest time. The Nidlinger farm does not use drones yet, but some neighbors do, and Duane expressed an interest.

John planted the previous spring using a GPS-steered twenty-four-row planter, a smart machine preprogrammed by J.D. to put down seeds with variable spacing *within* rows, matched precisely to the variable water-holding capacities of the soil, and matched also to the small variations in elevation that make some parts of the field drier than others. Critics of industrial farming claim that it tries to impose uniformity on nature, but this planter delivers a continuously variable seeding pattern tailored precisely to location-specific needs. A base station on the farm is capable of logging small errors in the incoming GPS satellite data, then sending correction signals to roving equipment in the field via radio or cellular modem. This allows the position of the field equipment to be known, in real time, with sub-inch accuracy. Sub-inch accuracy, in a cornfield.

John also uses precision when fertilizing his corn. Rather than spreading uniform quantities of nitrogen, phosphorus, and potash, John's equipment applies these chemicals at variable rates, based on

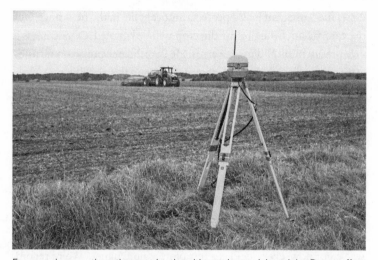

For cropping practices that require the ultimate in precision, John Deere offers the StarFire 3000 RTK receiver, which can correct GPS satellite signals to plus or minus one inch accuracy.

previously mapped variations in the chemistry of the soil. During the growing season, John also uses tissue samples from his plants to calibrate when and where to add a bit more nitrogen, or when and where to treat against fungus.

By adopting these modern PA methods, John Nidlinger has been able to reduce his nitrogen use for each bushel of corn harvested by more than one-third since the 1980s. This saves him money on chemical costs, but it also reduces chemical runoff into the local water supply. This is a collateral benefit to all who are downstream, including people in Toledo at the western tip of Lake Erie. John monitors his nitrogen use closely. "I'm concerned with the water in Toledo, and I don't want to be spending money on nutrients if I don't need to," he says. Duane is also hungry for better information and is thinking about installing in-field sensors to gather real-time nitrogen, moisture, and even chlorophyll readings.

Critics of modern farming in the United States like to imagine that as corn production has increased the land area planted with corn has increased as well. Not so. Since 1940, corn production in the United

States increased fivefold yet the total acreage planted to corn *declined* by one-fifth. Producing five times as much while using fewer acres is a good way to spare land for wildlife habitat.

Modern farming protects the environment not only by using less land compared to several decades ago; it also uses less water, less fossil energy, and fewer chemicals for every bushel produced. One major contributor here is no-till farming, which is a method for planting seeds in unplowed fields. This method requires specialized equipment, but it reduces soil erosion, protects soil moisture, sequesters carbon, and requires much less burning of diesel fuel, which is why farmers began doing it in the 1970s, a decade of high fuel prices. According to the latest USDA Census of Agriculture, more than twice as much cropland is now under no-till or reduced-till compared to intensive tillage. In parallel fashion, new irrigation systems such as center-pivot and drip have replaced simple flooding, thus conserving water. Lasers are employed to help level farm fields, which eliminates surface runoff. GPS auto-steering eliminates wasteful overlaps in the field. Genetically engineered seeds help farmers protect against insects and weeds with fewer and less toxic chemical sprays.

One of the first studies to measure the emerging environmental gains from innovations such as these was published in 2008 by the Organisation for Economic Co-operation and Development in Paris. This report, titled "The Environmental Performance of Agriculture," looked at the world's thirty most advanced industrial countries and found a surprising result. In 2004, compared to 1990, these countries were producing 5 percent more food but with diminished environmental impacts across the board. The land area used by agriculture had fallen 4 percent, soil erosion from both wind and water had diminished, water use on irrigated lands had declined 9 percent, and greenhouse gas emissions from farming were down 3 percent. Herbicide and insecticide spraying had declined 5 percent, and the excessive use of nitrogen fertilizer had declined 17 percent. Meanwhile, biodiversity on farms had increased, as a wider variety of both livestock breeds and crops had come into use.

Similar results have been documented specifically for the United

States. In 2015, Professor Jesse Ausubel at Rockefeller University reported that America's NPK fertilizer use (nitrogen, phosphorus, and potassium) had increased sharply from almost zero in 1940, but then it plateaued in the 1980s while production continued to increase. Data from the Environmental Protection Agency confirm that total fertilizer use on American farms peaked in 1981 and has remained essentially flat in the decades since, even as total crop production grew 44 percent. Total insecticide use in American farming peaked in 1972, and now it has fallen by more than 80 percent.

One more confirmation that science-intensive farming can help save nature is found in a 2016 study provided by the Field to Market organization, an alliance of private companies and civil society organizations promoting science-based pathways to sustainable agriculture. This study used crop data from the USDA to monitor a number of environmental indicators in American farming between 1980 and 2015. For wheat production, land use per bushel of production was down 22 percent over this period, soil loss per acre down 28 percent, irrigation water use per bushel down 26 percent, energy use per bushel down 22 percent, and greenhouse gas emissions per bushel down 9 percent. For corn, the reduction percentages per bushel were 41 percent for land, 46 percent for irrigation water, 41 percent for energy use, and 31 percent for greenhouse gas emissions. Similar environmental savings per unit of production were seen in cotton, potatoes, rice, soybeans, and sugar beets. These environmental gains were achieved not by a return to preindustrial farming systems but instead by incorporating more modern science, by going postindustrial and digital.

Casual observers fail to notice these environmental gains from modern farming because continued increases in total production have offset some of the benefit, and also because some of the damage done previously has yet to be repaired. Water use efficiency in irrigation has dramatically improved, but some prominent groundwater aquifers—like the massive Ogalalla, which irrigates portions of eight states in the central and southern plains—remain diminished and are far from being stabilized. Fertilizer use per bushel of production in the

Midwest has come down over the past four decades, but because of increased total production the annual runoff remains high enough to continue polluting downstream. In 2017 the dead zone at the mouth of the Mississippi River grew to cover an area of 8,776 square miles, the largest recorded in thirty-two years of monitoring. "The bottom line," said an aquatic ecologist at the University of Michigan, "is that we will never reach the dead zone reduction target of 1,900 square miles until more serious actions are taken to reduce the loss of Midwest fertilizers into the Mississippi River system."

John Nidlinger's farm has cut nitrogen use per bushel of production by about one-third since the 1980s, but he and his neighbors still haven't done enough to reduce phosphorus runoff into the Maumee River watershed flowing into Lake Erie, leading to blue-green algae blooms that contaminate drinking water and diminish lake tourism. The amount of phosphorus in this watershed dipped briefly in 2016, but only because there were fewer storms that year to wash excess fertilizer off of fields or through underground drains.

The citizens of Toledo tried to fight back in a special election in 2019, by adding a Lake Erie Bill of Rights to the city charter, allowing citizens to file lawsuits against polluters of the lake, including farmers. In December 2019, a federal judge struck down the measure, but if it ever went into operation livestock farms in Ohio would become the first target. The number of animals being raised in the Maumee watershed has more than doubled in recent years, and more than two-thirds of the phosphorus added to the watershed each year is suspected to come from livestock farms.

We have focused so far on modern crop farming, yet environmental impacts from livestock production can be a bigger challenge. The Chesapeake Bay, for example, has long been contaminated by wastewater drainage plus chicken waste from poultry farming. Thanks to an upgrading of wastewater treatment plants, progress was made, and by 2016 almost 40 percent of the bay and its tidal tributaries met standards for water clarity and algae growth, as well as for oxygen. Less progress was made for farm runoff, and in 2018 the bay's cleanup scorecard dropped from a C– to a D+. To reach their goals by 2025,

Maryland and Virginia will have to increase current rates of nitrogen reduction from farmland sixfold and fourteenfold, respectively. Modern industrial farming, including livestock farming (a topic addressed in a later chapter), needs to move much faster down the ecomodernist path.

Another charge against modern industrial farming is the harm it does to traditional rural communities. This is personal for me, and for others whose parents or grandparents grew up on the land but then left when traditional small farms were squeezed out by highly specialized, industrial-scale operations. Over time, the demographic shock became seismic. America's farm population fell in the twentieth century from twenty-nine million down to just five million, and this happened despite a tripling of the nation's population overall during that period. Between 1910 and 2002, the total number of farms in America fell by nearly two-thirds, while average farm size more than doubled. At the beginning of the twentieth century, farms employed close to half of the entire U.S. workforce, but now it's just 2 percent.

The change was actually more dramatic than these numbers suggest, since the official definition of what constitutes a farm was getting more lenient all the time. The USDA defines a food-growing operation as a "farm" if it produces and sells (or if it "normally would have sold") at least $1,000 worth of agricultural output over a twelve-month period. Congress set this threshold at a low level back in 1975 so as to exaggerate the nation's farm population, in hopes this would help justify the continued existence of a separate cabinet-level Department of Agriculture. Thanks to currency inflation since then, the threshold today is 80 percent lower in real terms, so it now takes almost nothing to be classified as a farmer. You can qualify by grazing and shearing just a few dozen sheep, or by selling the apples from several backyard trees at a stand by the road. Because the official dividing line continues to fall in real terms, every year more hobby gardeners come to be counted as farmers for official purposes.

Many of these over-counted farms contribute very little to food production. Of America's two million official farms today, more than four out of five are either retirement farms, part-time farms, or tiny farms with few sales. It is America's larger farms—the 146,568 farms with annual sales above $500,000—that account for the most production. They make 81 percent of all national product sales, despite representing just 7 percent of all farms. These are the modern "industrial" farms that draw the most criticism.

A century ago, smaller full-time family farms dominated the landscape of rural America. They generated only modest incomes, yet they were a preserve of important social values including personal dignity, mutual respect, family solidarity, self-reliance, basic equity, and local pride. When smaller farms began selling out to their larger neighbors, some of these important values were put at risk. The farm families that once shopped in town moved away, school enrollments fell, and barbershops and grocery stores shut down. A recent book by Ted Genoways, *This Blessed Earth: A Year in the Life of an American Family Farm*, describes what the loss of small family farms did to the town of Benedict, Nebraska:

> The school stands empty and abandoned; the only restaurant has been for sale for years. There's a grain elevator, two well drillers, a feedlot outside of town, but otherwise there's no work, nothing to do, no reason to be there instead of anywhere else.

Hollowed-out rural towns like Benedict are a challenge to my personal optimism about modern farming. When I return to Indiana now to visit relatives, my back-country detours take me through some small towns that have virtually disappeared, depopulated rural hamlets with names like Barnard, Raccoon, Parkersburg, and Lapland. There is still a road sign pointing toward Raccoon, but the post office closed in 1934 during the Depression and the town itself has long been abandoned. In the towns still struggling to hang on, fragments of the past can be seen at church on Sunday morning, or in the main-street café where locals still stop for coffee and a sandwich, but it seems only a matter of time before these too will be gone.

This represents a social loss, but measuring the magnitude of that loss is a challenge, because the rural communities that grew up around small traditional farms had drawbacks as well as virtues. For the farmers themselves, unrelenting physical labor could deaden both mind and spirit. Albert Sanford's 1916 book *The Story of Agriculture in the United States* records this truth through the eyes of a young boy. He saw his mother, "sober faced and weary, dragging herself, day by day, about the house with her entire life centered upon the drudgery of her kitchen, and all the rest of the world a closed book to her." The boy saw his father "broken down with long hours and hard work, finally relieved of the task of paying for the old place—just a few months before he died."

Traditional family farming trapped large numbers of Americans in deep poverty. In 1910, the average household income on farms was less than two-thirds of the nonfarm level. In the 1930s, it briefly dropped to just one-third the nonfarm level. In the 1920s, only one in ten farms in America had indoor plumbing. On my grandfather's farm in 1932, despite the uncompensated help provided all year by my dad and his three brothers, the net return to labor and management was a *loss* of $1,203.

Some of the cultural values intrinsic to small, traditional family farms also had a downside. Education was sacrificed because children were frequently valued more for their labor than their learning. As late as 1950, farm children still received, on average, three fewer years of schooling than urban children. The social isolation brought on by geographic dispersion was only partly relieved with the arrival of paved roads and personal automobiles. Electricity came late to rural America; by the 1920s most cities and towns had electricity, but as late as 1932, 90 percent of rural America still had none. Traditional farming was also physically unsafe, with roughly three thousand deaths every year from farm accidents as late as the 1950s.

Farming communities in rural America also lacked racial and cultural diversity. The biggest cultural divide was sometimes between the Germans and the Scandinavians, or between the Methodists and Presbyterians. It was also a world with an unhealthy degree of racial prejudice, with descendents of white Europeans looking down on everybody else. At one point in 1920, 15 percent of all farm operators in America were nonwhites, but three-quarters of these were impoverished tenant farmers or sharecroppers in the South, working land they did not own. Currently, 95 percent of farm producers in the United States are white.

Women always did their share of the work on farms, but a century ago the role of farm operator was almost always reserved for the man. A popular newspaper described life on one early Illinois farm as "a perfect paradise for men and horses, but death on women and oxen." Farm women were expected to produce children in large numbers, and in 1900, they were raising twice as many children as their urban counterparts. Women were consistently more likely than men to leave farming, and less likely to come back.

The modernization of American farming in the twentieth century—call it industrialization, if you wish—helped alleviate many of these social ills. When powered machinery came into use in the 1920s, the physical burdens of farm life began to diminish. Tractors and combines were expensive, but they paid for themselves quickly on farms large enough to keep them in regular use, which is why bigger farms mechanized first and then bought out their neighbors and grew bigger still. Larger tractors, multi-row planters, and powered combine harvesters made it possible for fewer individual farmers to operate much bigger farms, causing average farm size to double after the 1950s.

This consolidation process was accompanied by increased specialization. The number of different commodities produced on farms fell from an average of five in 1900, to four by 1950, and to about one by 2000. My grandfather in the 1930s took the traditional view that specialization in farming was risky, so his farm grew corn, oats, hay for the cows and horses, soybeans, onion sets, asparagus, cabbage, sweet corn, tomatoes, and potatoes. He also raised cattle, hogs, chickens, sheep on one occasion, and kept a small dairy herd. The animals kept his spouse and four sons working all the time.

Traditional farms at that time all had livestock as well as crops, and the daily feeding, watering, and cleaning up after these animals was a time-consuming chore, frequently assigned to the children. One popular Depression-era rhyme tried to make light of this burden:

> Down on the farm about half past four,
> I slip on my pants and sneak out the door;
> Out through the yard I run like the dickens,
> to milk ten cows and feed all the chickens;
> Clean out the barn, curry Nancy and Jigs,
> separate the cream and slop all the pigs.
> Work two hours, then eat like a Turk,
> and now I'm ready for a full day's work.

Modern livestock systems are built around specialization and tighter confinement, plus new genetics, better feeds, and automation. This reduced labor requirements dramatically, which is why it happened. In 1910, it took more than three hours of human labor to produce 100 pounds of milk, but by 1986 that had fallen to just twelve minutes. In the late 1930s it required eight and a half hours of human labor to produce 100 pounds of broiler chickens, but by the early 1980s that had fallen to just six minutes.

With this shrinkage in farm labor requirements, children were able to spend more time in school, leave the farm, and find better-paying work in town, including new factory jobs with better hours, union contracts, and even summer vacations. The larger, consolidated farms that remained did better as well, so everyone's income usually went up. The process sometimes turned cruel, like in the 1980s when high interest rates, low crop prices, and dropping land values all hit at the same time. Debts couldn't be paid, and hardworking families were forced to give up farming under a stigma of failure. Foreclosure auctions conducted on the front lawn of the family homestead became the final humiliation. The farm consolidations that took place in better times caused far less distress, because the younger generation usually had already left for town, and the older generation was more than ready to retire. One 1959 study found that "the social and psychic costs of the move to the city are not of great consequence."

The social loss brought on by the consolidation of commercial farms was also contained because some families were able to remain on the land with income from something other than farming. Many rented or sold their fields but continued living in the farmhouse where they grew up. Some farmed only part-time, while a spouse commuted to a job in town. In 1929, only 6 percent of American farms reported 200 days of work off the farm every year, but by 1997 this had increased to 35 percent. By 2016, three out of five farms in America were either pure retirement farms with little or no farming income, or they were farms where agricultural production was not the primary occupation. Many are commercial farms in name only, but they remain home for a valued share of America's rural population.

This has brought us to an interesting outcome. Most of our food production today may be "industrial," but most of our farms and farmers are not. As noted earlier, 81 percent of agricultural sales today are made by just 7 percent of farms. The other 93 percent of our farms are not a part of Big Ag, but they make big contributions to the social health of rural America.

Rural America has multiple problems today, including job loss in manufacturing and services, social breakdown, and substance abuse, problems often traceable to the automation or outsourcing of jobs—but these were almost all nonfarm jobs. These are all serious problems, but they do not reflect an impoverishment of farming. There is a great deal of deep poverty in rural America, but farms—even small farms—usually avoid this fate thanks to retirement assets, rental income from the land, or income from a working spouse. Only 2 percent of America's farm households fall below the poverty line today, compared to 14 percent of all U.S. households. The average income for farm families in America in 2016 was 42 percent above the average for nonfarm households, and the median net worth of households operating farms in America was an impressive $912,000. Some of the small farms you see in rural Indiana today may look poor from the road, but every acre of average-quality farmland in the state is worth about $7,000, so even a small patch of land debt-free can represent a comfortable cushion of wealth. Farmers like to joke about living poor but dying rich.

Consider one more benefit from this growing split in rural America between large commercial farms and smaller lifestyle farms. It means most of our crops are being grown on the bigger farms, those capable of using advanced precision farming techniques, which brings both reduced production cost and a smaller environmental impact. Meanwhile, others can continue living on much smaller farms, financed by off-farm work, retirement savings, and sometimes even agritourism (barn weddings have become a significant money-maker). These smaller farms grow very little food, but they support the preferred lifestyle of their owners while helping to boost the social health of rural communities. We could label such an outcome "multi-agriculturalism."

While bringing an abundance of social change to rural America, modern industrial farming has done little to alter one of the most distinctive features of our nation's farm system. The USDA considers a "family farm" to be one where the majority of the business is owned by the operator or individuals related to the operator, even if some may not live in the operator's household. By this definition, 96 percent of American farms and ranches today are still family owned, including not just the small lifestyle farms and the more traditional midsize farms, but also the larger operations, including the Nidlinger farm. We all should be pleased to see that this valued tradition has survived.

CHAPTER 2

Food Swamp Nation

❦

America's children in the 1970s enjoyed, on average, just a single snack every day. By 2012 three snacks daily was the norm, adding almost two hundred calories to the daily diet. Snacking has now become nearly a $90 billion industry in the United States, and it continues growing at a 3 percent annual rate.

As we've seen, this risk to dietary health did not come from America's farms. What changed was the eating environment, which became a swamp of affordable food products surrounding us all day long. The products were designed by corporate scientists to be irresistible, and they have been relentlessly promoted by food manufacturing companies, food retail stores, and large restaurant chains. It is probably in our nature to overeat when surrounded by such an abundance of tasty and affordable food, but corporate strategies ruthlessly exploit this human weakness. Food products laden with sugar, salt, and fat are now deliberately formulated to ensure eaters will crave them; then they are promoted as innocent fun and placed within easy reach, pushing personal consumption into the danger zone.

Private companies have always known how to make people buy things they don't really need, such as too many shoes, too many appliances, and too many children's toys. This is wasteful, but it does not lead to a public health crisis. When companies use the same tricks to sell us too much food, they take us down a road to chronic disease. The principal promoters of excessive eating today are the large com-

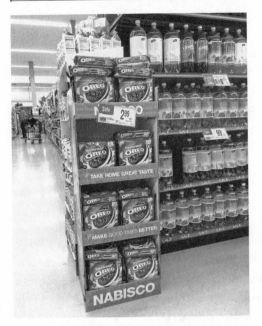

A prestocked endcap display provided by Nabisco promoting impulse buys of Oreo cookies. Subliminal background messaging says "joy," "laugh," and "entertaining."

panies that occupy most of the commercial space between our farms and tables. Containing the behavior of these companies has become an important public health challenge.

Julie Greene was a senior marketing executive and director of health and nutrition at Ahold Delhaize, a Dutch retail firm operating more than six thousand food stores in eleven countries around the world, including supermarket chains in the United States such as Giant Food, Stop & Shop, Hannaford, Food Lion, Giant Martins, and Peapod. One afternoon she gave me a personal tour through a handsome new Hannaford supermarket in Scarborough, Maine. Greene had earlier worked directly for Hannaford, where she helped launch a nutrition guidance program for retail stores called "Guiding Stars." She knows that retail practices have been a significant source of America's unhealthy eating.

Walking past Hannaford's checkout area, a prime marketing space, Julie spotted a colorful display stacked with small packets of snack products: Cheetos, Doritos, and Tostitos tortilla chips. Companies like Frito-Lay pay stores to place such products in "endcap" displays, facing outward to tempt shoppers into whim purchases. "I've got a fifteen-year-old boy," said Julie, "and his friends are going to come over tonight and hang out; I'd love to grab some snacks I could live with, but I'm not buying any of this. This is garbage, they don't need this; they've got a soccer game tomorrow. I'd buy popcorn, or some fun sparkling water, whatever. To me there's an opportunity here that's not being captured."

We passed an attractive seasonal display of Courtland apples, good for baking. An adjacent companion display was pushing a highly sugared apple crisp dessert mix. Julie wished the store had taken a different autumn-themed approach. "Instead of this, let's put some oatmeal next to the apples, then say 'Bring your favorite season into breakfast.' If you chop up an apple and throw it into your oatmeal for the last minute as you cook, then add some cinnamon, it will be just like the topping on your crisp. Trying to get five servings of fruit a day? Well, you're missing out on something if you don't have any for breakfast."

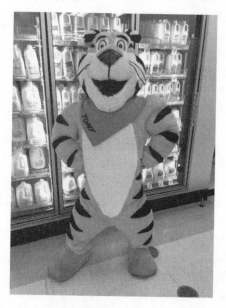

Kellogg's sends Tony the Tiger into supermarkets to promote Frosted Flakes.

It doesn't take a marketing professional like Julie Greene to notice how food manufacturing companies and retailers have teamed up to surround shoppers with unhealthy temptations. Candy bar companies pay the store to put their products in the checkout aisle, directly opposite the cash register, because the companies know a significant segment of our population will not be able to resist. As one former marketing executive at Coca-Cola described it, "We wanted to have Coke next to the deli sandwiches. We wanted Coke in a cooler at checkout, we wanted an endcap, we wanted a vending machine. We wanted to have ten or twenty places at a single grocery store." The company referred to this concept as always having Coke "within an arm's reach of desire," and paying the retailers to make it happen.

Pepsi has gone one step further to keep its products within arm's reach. In 2019 it introduced snack delivery robots—Snackbots—on college campuses, starting in California at the University of the Pacific. If no vending machine is handy, students can use their new Snackbot app to summon Pepsi products to any one of fifty designated drop points on campus.

One week after my visit with Julie Greene I was back at my own local Stop & Shop in Massachusetts, looking for paper towels, laundry detergent, and some milk. I was still thinking about in-store food promotions when I spotted a six-foot-tall Tony the Tiger swaggering toward me wearing a bright orange-and-white mascot suit. He had big yellow cartoon eyes, a blue nose, a red bandanna, a happy smile, and was waving his two front paws to the shoppers and their kids. A public address system then came on to tell us Tony was in the store to promote a special on Kellogg's Frosted Flakes, and he was eager to shake hands and have his picture taken. I checked the Fooducate app on my phone and found that Frosted Flakes earned only a C– because each serving had 3 teaspoons of added sugar and contained a controversial additive known as butylated hydroxytoluene.

How can we protect ourselves, and our children, from this kind of aggressive marketing? The Alice Waters strategy of never setting foot inside a supermarket is no longer enough, since unhealthy foods are now displayed and marketed nearly everywhere, including in convenience stores, gas stations, department stores, and pharmacies. The Target store in my local mall has a "grocery" section selling thirteen different categories of chips, snacks, and cookies. When I go to my local CVS for a prescription, I walk through an aisle stocked with cookies, crackers, chips, bread, ice cream, cereal, salted nuts, snacks, juice, and soda before I finally get to the pharmacy counter. In a single visit, CVS patrons can now guard their health and ruin their health at the same time.

It was not always this way. Just outside of Washington, D.C., where I lived when I was in junior high school, my friends and I had easy access to candy at the Rexall drugstore on the way home from school, but actual food marketing was mostly restricted to just two grocery chains—Giant and Safeway. Giant and Safeway are still there today, but so is Walmart, Costco, Aldi, Lidl, Whole Foods, Wegmans, Trader Joe's, and Target. If you want Asian food, you can find an H Mart or a Lotte. And even with all this, the third-largest grocery retailer in the region isn't a supermarket at all; it's CVS Pharmacy, which has 133 stores in the District of Columbia alone.

People shopping for groceries now routinely stop to eat some food as part of the experience. Ninety-six percent of supermarkets today are "grocerants," offering prepared meals with in-store seating, and most have their own chefs to oversee food preparation. In Fairfax, Virginia, one local Whole Foods has a wine bar, a sports bar, a ramen bar, a seafood eatery, and a barbecue smokehouse. Food courts were originally introduced into shopping malls to help make the retail stores a destination, but now supermarkets have copied this eating strategy to lure in customers. The Wegmans in Lanham, Maryland, just outside the D.C. Beltway, is designed as a food-themed social center. One member of a high-spirited social group called Women of Wegmans raves about the experience. "You have everything. . . . You can find prepared food items. If you want to sit and have a meeting or play chess or backgammon, you can. My husband and I use [the store] for date night on Saturday because they have jazz. And they have some of the best ice-cream custard I've ever had."

Some think Americans are being forced into unhealthy eating

because they do not have enough access to supermarkets and are thus living in "food deserts." First Lady Michelle Obama bought into this argument, and as one part of her campaign against childhood obesity in 2009 she worked to persuade Walmart, Walgreens, SuperValu, and other grocers to locate more stores in low-income neighborhoods. One grocery industry group, supported by banks and health-care organizations, responded by committing $200 million to eliminating food deserts in California. These were well-intentioned efforts, but the food desert hypothesis was suspect from the start.

The real problem has not been a lack of access to healthy foods, but a dramatically increased exposure to unhealthy foods from fast-food restaurants, corner mini-marts, take-out pizza joints—and also, alas, from supermarkets. Low-income Americans are in trouble not because they are stranded in food deserts but because they are drowning in food swamps.

One 2017 study defined a food swamp as a neighborhood with a high ratio of fast-food restaurants and convenience stores to supermarkets and grocery stores. If a neighborhood had four unhealthy places to buy food for every one that was deemed healthy it was classified as a swamp. By contrast, food deserts were mapped out based on the share of the population with both low income and low access to supermarkets or grocery stores in terms of physical distance (one mile in urban areas and ten miles in rural areas). This study found that food swamps were a stronger predictor of obesity than food deserts. In fact, the contribution of food deserts to obesity became statistically insignificant once you controlled for food swamps.

Even without this study, strong evidence had earlier cropped up against the food desert argument. Researchers in 2011 examined fifteen years of data on five thousand people in five cities and found no connection between grocery store access and healthful diets. A 2014 study at Tufts University found that low-income, obesity-prone Americans actually enjoyed a closer proximity to supermarkets than Americans who were not so poor. A 2019 study in the *Quarterly Journal of Economics* found that access to supermarkets explains, *at most,*

1.5 percent of the difference in healthy eating patterns between high-versus low-income households.

The unhealthy products flooding into our food swamps come from private food manufacturing companies that design them for taste, aroma, texture, color, shelf life, convenience, low manufacturing cost, and basic safety, but seldom for nutrient value. The goal is to make these products as difficult as possible for consumers to resist, and this often means adding fat, salt, and sugar. The Frito-Lay snack products on the Hannaford endcap display—called "garbage" by Julie Greene—were designed by food scientists working at a corporate research complex near Dallas that employs nearly five hundred chemists, technicians, and psychologists.

Every aspect of a chip is carefully considered, including mouthfeel and crunch. As reported by Michael Moss in 2013, Frito-Lay uses a $40,000 device that simulates a chewing mouth, so as to determine a perfect break point, which turns out to be about four pounds of pressure per square inch. Food companies then pay ordinary consumers to smell, touch, sip, and taste different versions of their products, using computerized algorithms to map out the most promising ingredient mix. Finding the optimal recipe for a single new Cadbury cola product—the Cherry Vanilla Dr Pepper—involved testing sixty-one slightly different mixes at a total of 3,904 tastings organized in four different cities. The tasters were told to rest five minutes between each sip, in order to reset their taste buds.

Food company defenders depict all this as an innocent attempt to give consumers exactly what they want, implying the consumer is at fault for any adverse health outcome. Yet the companies are not just responding to bad eating preferences; they are conditioning and enabling our behavior by designing foods and food environments that promote some preferences over others. The companies do this first by adding sugars and refined carbohydrates to foods. Added sugars are found in nearly 70 percent of packaged foods, including breads, yogurts, sauces, and even "health foods." This makes them more palatable, but it also leads to spikes in insulin levels, causing more calories to be stored in fat cells instead of in the blood. This fools the brain into thinking the body is still hungry, triggering still more calorie consumption. The companies may not fully comprehend all the metabolic details, but they welcome the result.

Food companies have also discovered precise mixtures, textures, and ingredients in foods that will trigger a dopamine high, one that teaches the reward circuit in our brains to crave such foods. Food scientist Howard Moskowitz was the first to describe this as a "bliss point," one that sends intense reward sensations to our brain. The brain remembers the sensation, associates it with the product, and any future connection with that product will cue a brain-driven desire to consume again, whether or not the stomach needs the food.

David Kessler, a former commissioner of the Food and Drug Administration, describes how companies use bliss-point food formulations, together with marketing, to trigger excessive consumption:

> I give you a package of sugar and I say, go have a good time. You're going to say, what are you talking about? Add to that sugar fat, add texture, add temperature, add color, add the emotional gloss of advertising—put it on every corner, say you can have it 24/7. It's socially acceptable to eat and we can make it into entertainment. And what do we end up with? One of the great public health crises of our time.

The mere presence of a craveable food such as Lay's potato chips or Oreo cookies, or just an advertisement for such a food, will be enough to trigger the cycle. This is why food companies advertise heavily, and why they want their products always to be "within an arm's reach of desire." The brain science behind food cravings is still in its infancy, but brain helmets with functional magnetic resonance imaging, adapted from medicine, are producing brain scans that reveal more all the time.

Not all eaters are equally susceptible to these body and brain inducements. At one extreme there are disciplined, health-conscious, and often better-educated consumers who know to avoid the most addictive processed foods and beverages. For this segment, the advertising may go completely unnoticed. At the other extreme is an "eat, drink, and be merry" segment that would overindulge even without corporate conditioning or advertising. The segment of greatest interest to food companies is the "movable middle" of our population, those who can be nudged from a safe place to excessive food product consumption.

Judging from how they use their advertising budgets, food companies have decided to focus on minority children and teens as part of this movable middle. A 2017 study of TV advertising by thirty-two major food brands found that black children and teens saw an average of more than sixteen food-related ads a day, roughly twice the number seen by white children and teens. Black children and teens viewed about two and a half times more candy ads than their white peers. In TV programming where black consumers made up a majority of the audience, 86 percent of the food ad spending was for fast food, candy, sugary drinks, and unhealthy snack brands.

The targeted eaters in the middle sometimes work hard to resist. An estimated ninety-seven million Americans are actively dieting, and every year consumers hand over $66 billion to the weight-loss industry. It is usually a losing battle. A 2015 study of 176,000 higher-weight people found that more than 95 percent of those who lost weight dieting gained it all back within five years. More than three-quarters of consumers also profess to be nutrition conscious when buying food. In 2017 the Food Marketing Institute asked shoppers if they were either somewhat concerned or very concerned about the "nutritional content of their food," and the responses were almost half "somewhat" and 29 percent "very." Use of the "Nutrition Facts" label on packaged foods is another indicator. A survey in 2016 revealed that nearly two-thirds of shoppers did occasionally read the "Nutrition Facts" label, and almost half said they avoided some foods based on the label.

While some in the movable middle have been trying to fight back against food swamp temptations, it isn't really a fair fight. Hank Cardello, a former director for marketing at Coca-Cola USA and a former brand manager for General Mills, wrote a book in 2009 describing how food companies keep the upper hand:

> In practice, personal responsibility accounts for only a small fraction of the decision making that goes into what you eat. . . . What do you do when a company's focus-grouped, test-marketed, $20 million advertising campaign for doughnuts is designed to ensure that people in your precise demographic will struggle to select a healthier alternative over their product?

In their defense, food manufacturing companies can show it is a commercial risk to switch to more healthful offerings. Once the consuming public has been conditioned to seek out oversweetened and oversalted foods, individual companies can lose market share if they go in another direction. Geoffrey Bible, a former chairman of the board of Kraft Foods recalls these internal pressures:

> People could point to these things and say, "They've got too much sugar, they've got too much salt." Well, that's what the consumer wants, and we're not putting a gun to their head to eat it. That's what they want. If we give them less, they'll buy less, and the competitor will get our market. So you're sort of trapped.

The long-run implications of this trap first emerged as an internal food industry debate more than two decades ago. In 1999, the heads of eleven major American food companies met at Pillsbury's headquarters in Minneapolis to confront the fact of increasing obesity. They heard a presentation from a vice president at Kraft named Michael Mudd, who warned that doing nothing would eventually leave the industry vulnerable to the same kinds of taxes and regulations that eventually reined in cigarette manufacturers. Mudd's view was immediately challenged by Stephen Sanger, CEO of General Mills, a company that had recently strengthened its bottom line by adding a sugary yogurt product named Yoplait. Hiding behind a healthy yogurt image, this product was delivering annual sales above

$500 million, even though it gave consumers twice the sugar per serving as Lucky Charms, a marshmallow cereal.

Investigative reporter Michael Moss from the *New York Times* later learned what Sanger had said to the group. "Don't talk to me about nutrition," said the General Mills man. "Talk to me about taste, and if this stuff tastes better, don't run around trying to sell stuff that doesn't taste good." As a top Pillsbury executive later recalled, "Sanger was trying to say, 'Look, we're not going to screw around with the company jewels here and change the formulations because a bunch of guys in white coats are worried about obesity.'"

Two decades have now passed, the obesity crisis has dramatically worsened, and the pressure has grown on companies to make healthful product changes. Some have responded. Smuckers now has twenty-two different jam and jelly products that are reduced in sugar or sugar free. The Kraft Heinz company has introduced a no-added-sugars version of Capri Sun, Oscar Mayer hot dogs without meat by-products, and even a mac-and-cheese product with no artificial coloring. Frito-Lay is introducing healthier versions of its chips to limit sodium and saturated fat, while adding more fiber, whole grains, vegetables, and protein. In 2016, according to the Consumer Goods Forum, food companies improved the health profile of about 180,000 products, compared to 80,000 in the previous year.

There are limits, however, to the changes consumers will tolerate. When General Mills tried to replace the artificial coloring in Trix cereal with natural coloring in 2016, consumers complained that without the classic neon blues and greens it looked "depressing." After customer frustrations poured out on social media, the company brought back the synthetic original.

Food companies are good at adapting to evolving consumer preferences. A 2017 survey released by the Food Information Council Foundation found that 45 percent of consumers between the ages of eighteen and thirty-four were following specialty diets such as ketogenic, paleo, gluten-free, or the Whole30 program. Food companies had responded by offering keto-friendly Dang Bars sweetened with stevia extract, and gluten-free everything. Online food delivery services such as Factor 75, Ice Age Meals, Keto Fridge, and Kettle-bell Kitchen now provide entire meals that are keto-compliant. Far from trying to homogenize the way Americans eat, food companies eagerly proliferate new offerings, trying to satisfy everybody. Indra Nooyi, the former CEO of PepsiCo, was asked in 2019 why, if she was committed to health, her company kept selling soda and chips. She responded, "I'm not here to tell you what to eat or drink. My job is to give you a choice—between fun for you, better for you, and good for you. I'll give you low calorie products. I'll give you indulgent products."

The indulgent products tend to win out. A comprehensive study in 2018 funded by the Robert Wood Johnson Foundation rated the product offerings of America's ten largest food and beverage manufacturers: Conagra, Kraft Heinz, General Mills, Kellogg, Nestlé, PepsiCo, Unilever, Coca-Cola, Dr Pepper Snapple, and Mars. Only 30 percent of the assessed products from these companies were judged to be healthy, and these healthy products contributed less than a quarter to the sales of the companies. In addition, only 14 percent of the companies' products were deemed nutritious enough to merit marketing to children. A majority of the companies had pledged to market responsibly, but their voluntary commitments did not cover mobile and digital media, and they made only limited commitments regarding marketing in schools. Shiriki Kumanyika, chair of the Nutrition Index Expert Group, which produced this study, said the leading companies were making efforts to improve but were "not harnessing the significant opportunities they have to help families across our country make the kind of healthy food and beverage choices that will enable them to live healthier lives."

Since food companies shy away from making healthier products for fear of losing market share, government actions will be needed to move them together to a higher standard. We know this can work for sugary beverages. Taxes designed to reduce the consumption of sugar-sweetened beverages are now in place in France, Hungary, Catalonia, Malaysia, Mexico, Norway, Portugal, South Africa, Panama,

Peru, the Philippines, and the United Kingdom, and they are working as intended. In 2013, Mexico passed an excise tax of one peso per liter, or roughly 10 percent, on sugar-sweetened beverages. After one year, a proportionate decline in purchases of these taxed beverages was seen overall, offset by increased purchases of plain water. Norway, which recently raised its levy on sugary drinks by 42 percent, has seen sales of soft drinks fall from 93 liters per person in the late 1990s to just 47 liters by 2018.

In the United States, economic modeling suggests that a dedicated tax on sugary beverages at a penny an ounce (enough to raise the price to consumers by slightly less than one-fifth) would reduce consumption among adults by about 15 percent, and this, in turn, could prevent 2.4 million person-years of diabetes, 95,000 coronary heart events, 8,000 strokes, and 26,000 premature deaths, while reducing direct medical costs by $17 billion. The tax would deliver an added benefit if it were focused more narrowly on the sugar content of drinks; this would induce the beverage industry to reformulate away from sugar.

Britain began taxing the sugar content of soda in 2018, causing a number of large beverage manufacturers to reformulate even before the tax took effect. Coca-Cola in Britain changed the recipe for Fanta, and the sugar content of San Pellegrino soda was cut by 40 percent. Purchases of Coke Zero Sugar also increased by half. In July 2018, when France refocused its beverage tax on sugar content, manufacturers there also reformulated popular beverages. Americans concerned with public health should be asking themselves why we aren't doing the same thing here.

Congress has shunned taxes on sugary beverages thanks to beverage industry lobbying plus a political fear that such taxes would be seen as regressive on the poor. In 2009, a number of public health advocates suggested that Congress impose a soda tax to help pay for Obamacare, but this proposal was rejected by President Obama himself, since he had pledged in his 2008 campaign not to raise "any form" of taxes on families making less than $250,000 a year. Twenty-one different beverage companies, not wanting to take any chances, spent $24 million early in 2009 to oppose soda taxes, and by November nobody in Congress was talking about this option anymore.

The companies that manufacture nonalcoholic beverages in the United States make roughly $200 billion in domestic sales every year, enough to fund a continuous lobby presence both in Congress and in most state legislatures. Nonetheless, some political space for change has recently been found at the municipal level. In 2014 the city of Berkeley, California, enacted a sugary beverage tax, and similar local soda tax enactments followed in 2016 in Philadelphia, San Francisco, Oakland, Albany (California), Boulder, and Cook County, Illinois (which includes Chicago). The Cook County decision was later reversed, and a local tax effort failed in Santa Fe in May 2017, but Seattle joined those opting for a soda tax the following month. These successful municipal tax efforts all had three things in common: strong Democratic Party control over city government, an announced plan to dedicate the tax revenues to a specific purpose other than deficit reduction, and external financial support for the campaign from private foundations, especially Bloomberg Philanthropies.

Municipal soda taxes produce results. Soda consumption was cut by one-fifth in Berkeley, and in Philadelphia soda sales fell by 38 percent in 2017, even when increased purchases in neighboring towns are taken into account. Purchases in Seattle dropped 30 percent in the months after the tax took effect. Results like these are why the beverage industry is fighting back hard. It has used its political influence with state legislatures to enact state laws preempting city taxes on soda. In the summer of 2018, the beverage industry pressured the California legislature to enact a twelve-year statewide moratorium on new soda taxes. The industry then sponsored similar preemption measures in Oregon and Washington, disguising them as campaigns to prevent city taxes on "groceries," even though no such grocery tax had been proposed anywhere. The preemption measure was defeated in Oregon, but a $20 million beverage industry campaign in the state of Washington produced a victory there.

America should support taxes and regulations designed to nudge consumers toward healthy purchases, and also to nudge food companies toward healthier product offerings, but this will be a difficult political struggle. At the state level the most critical variable will be political party control. So long as anti-tax and pro-industry Republicans continue to dominate America's state legislatures, only limited progress will be possible. Democrats did well in the 2018 elections, but Republicans were still left in control of sixty-two legislative chambers nationwide, compared to just thirty-seven for Democrats.

M ost of the products created by food manufacturing companies reach consumers through supermarkets, so the behavior of food retail chains is another part of America's dietary health challenge. Retailers have been timid about initiating changes on their own, much like the food manufacturers. If a store decides to fill the checkout area with healthy items that are less crave-worthy or from companies that won't pay a fee, revenues will be lost. Competition in food retail has recently intensified with the arrival of new supercenters, warehouses, limited assortment stores, online shopping, home deliveries, and meal kits. The supermarket share of all retail food sales fell from more than two-thirds in 2005 to just under half by 2017.

Online purchases are disrupting retail everywhere. In food, they recently represented only 6 percent of total household grocery spending, but were growing at a 15 percent annual rate even before the COVID-19 crisis. Among shoppers with children under eighteen years of age, and those with annual household incomes above $100,000, almost one in five were ordering groceries online at least once a month. When the COVID-19 crisis broke in March 2020, the online grocer Peapod saw its orders increase by 33 percent, and daily downloads from Instacart and Walmart Grocery doubled. In one week in March 2020, e-commerce sales of consumer packaged goods rose 91 percent from a year earlier. Walmart embraced e-commerce aggressively, offering grocery pickup services at three thousand of its stores and grocery delivery at sixteen hundred.

Online shopping will reduce in-store marketing opportunities for food companies. Candy companies cannot count on impulse purchases if a customer no longer has to walk past their products on the way to checkout, so the Hershey candy company now has a chief digital commerce officer exploring ways to sustain impulse purchases online for candies and snacks. Even in-store impulse purchases will be harder to influence once checkout lines themselves disappear, as is likely in the coming decade. Choice Market, which opened its doors in Denver in 2017, is already moving toward card-swipe or app-based checkout-free vending options. In 2019, Ahold Delhaize began piloting a checkout-free technology in Quincy, Massachusetts, and in early 2020 a checkout-free Amazon Go Grocery opened in Seattle.

Supermarkets have recently gained some leverage over food manufacturers, thanks to retail chain consolidations plus rapidly increasing sales of private-label store brands, optimized now through better in-store data collection. They have used this leverage to extract larger fees from the companies for placing products in the eye-level "strike zone" locations. By one calculation, supermarkets have been collecting more than $50 billion a year in fees or discounts from food and beverage companies. Such fees can add up to as much as one-fifth of a food manufacturer's total costs, but they are worth paying if they can lock up valuable real estate in stores and prevent smaller up-start competitors from breaking in.

With so many of America's consumers currently addicted to unhealthy products, moving our nexus of codependent retailers and food manufacturers toward more healthful offerings will require efforts on several fronts, but getting better information to shoppers in the movable middle is one place to start. Since 1990 the FDA has required food companies to disclose the nutrition content of their products on the standardized "Nutrition Facts" label on the side of the package, but the label is all fine print and numbers and not easy to use. The format will be updated in 2020 to show calorie counts in larger type, provide more realistic serving sizes, and supply new information such as amounts of added sugars, but it still won't be on the *front* of the package and it won't make summary judgments.

Summary ratings of the healthfulness of individual food products are resisted by the FDA and USDA, since both insist that only an entire diet can be given an overall health rating. They have a point, and for this reason federal nutrition advice takes the form of *dietary* guidelines based on quantities and balances among food groups. The food companies are comfortable with this approach, since it protects them from harsh individual product judgments. Since the food companies are comfortable, so are most politicians. But without summary ratings for individual products, many shoppers will remain poorly informed.

Other countries can show us a better way. Since 2013, Britain's Food Standards Agency has issued guidance to food companies for nutrition labels on the front of food packages, not the side, including color-coded messages easier for shoppers to take in. Separate numerical totals are still there for calories, grams of fat, saturated fat, sugars, and salt, just as in the United States, but these are rated as either high, medium, or low, and then shaded red, amber, or green in traffic-light fashion to allow faster comprehension for shoppers. The labeling standards remain voluntary, in part because Britain was a member of the European Union in 2013 and nutrition labeling regulations fell under the jurisdiction of Brussels, but most companies have nonetheless complied, including nineteen out of Britain's twenty-five cereal manufacturers. The system implicitly rewards companies that are willing to reformulate their products away from the red label category, toward amber or green. In 2020, Mexico mandated its own front-of-pack warning sign on products with high amounts of sugar, sodium, and saturated fats.

The United States government has not been able to create even a voluntary rating system for the front of packages. In October 2009, President Obama's FDA commissioner, Margaret Hamburg, signaled her intent to develop the criteria for such a system, but progress then stalled. America's grocery manufacturers and retailers, partly to hold off any new federal standard, launched a voluntary system of their own in 2011, called Facts Up Front. This system was parallel in many ways to the UK system, but it lacked the color code, a critical omission. More than one hundred companies agreed to use the Facts Up Front labels on their products, but they had slight impact absent the at-a-glance color-code. The FDA said it would monitor and assess the performance of this voluntary industry system "over time," but has signaled nothing more.

To get around bureaucratic caution at FDA, and also to finesse resistance from food manufacturing companies, private retail chains are now stepping in to provide their own summarized nutrition guidance to shoppers, placing nutrition messages not on the front of the packages but on the front of their own retail shelves, just below each product on display. One of these shelf tag systems, designed in 2006, came from a team of nutrition experts led by David Katz at the Yale-Griffin Prevention Research Center. It was based on an algorithm that rated products for nutrition by dividing the good attributes (like vitamins, minerals, and fiber) by the bad attributes (like sugar, sodium, and saturated fats), generating a numerical score from 1 to 100 for each product. The research team offered its algorithm to the FDA, hoping for an official endorsement, but according to Katz, "the system went beyond what the agency was willing to do at the time." One FDA scientist told Katz that neither of them would live long enough to see the federal government "put such brutal honesty about the food supply on routine display."

Unable to get government support, Katz and his team decided to form a private company named NuVal, and begin licensing the rating system directly to supermarkets. The uptake was encouraging, with at least sixteen hundred supermarkets using the NuVal shelf tags at one point, but then problems were encountered. The USDA told NuVal it could not put its ratings on packaged meats, and an organization named the National Consumers League filed a complaint with the FDA in 2012, calling the NuVal algorithm "fatally flawed." Katz dismissed the National Consumers League as "a shell organization" mostly supportive of the consumer packaged goods industry, but a wider distrust emerged when NuVal gave some snack chips higher ratings than canned fruits and vegetables. The fact that the algorithm was never made public heightened suspicions, and the system was quietly discontinued in 2017.

A rival front-of-shelf nutrition rating system named Guiding Stars hopes to have more staying power. This system, originally launched in 2006 by the Hannaford supermarket chain, calculates the nutrient density of foods per 100 calories, then awards stars—one, two or three—to those above a certain threshold. Guiding Stars avoided some of NuVal's mistakes by publishing its algorithm, and also by giving no rating at all to foods below the minimum threshold. Saying nothing at all about such foods made the honesty slightly less brutal. The shelf tags for products above the threshold have no numerical scores, displaying instead a blue cartoon figure running after one, two, or three yellow stars. This is an easy-to-spot signifier of nutrition value and an easy-to-comprehend gradient of praise for the products awarded stars.

The founding director of Guiding Stars was Jim McBride, who held corporate positions at Hannaford for more than three decades and designed the Guiding Stars nutrition database (which now has ratings for fifty thousand food products). He also helped the program's scientific advisers develop the original nutrition algorithm. The Hannaford chain decided to launch Guiding Stars after the board of its parent company, the Delhaize Group in Brussels, challenged group members to do a better job addressing customer health concerns. Hannaford responded by designing and then extending the Guiding Stars shelf tags to the 150 supermarkets within its own chain.

Building on this modest start, the system spread to thirteen hundred Food Lion markets in 2007, also part of Delhaize America, and in 2012 it was licensed to a Canadian grocer, Loblaw. When Delhaize was purchased in 2016 by Ahold, a Dutch retail company, a larger Ahold Delhaize Group of supermarket chains was created that also included Stop & Shop, Giant, Giant/Martin's, and Peapod. In April 2018, Ahold Delhaize announced a plan to implement Guiding Stars within this entire group, and by the end of 2019 the system was available in 2,500 retail locations. This scale up will require added mana-

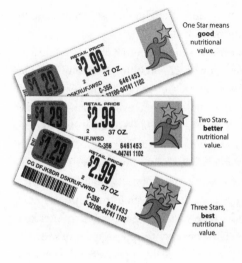

One Star means **good** nutritional value.

Two Stars, **better** nutritional value.

Three Stars, **best** nutritional value.

The Guiding Stars shelf tag system provides at-a-glance nutrition guidance. A majority of packaged products in stores earn no stars at all, a sign that the grading system is honest.

gerial effort at the store level, plus staff time to put the shelf tags in the right place, keep them there, and then explain what they mean to shoppers.

How easy is it for food products to get at least one Guiding Star? McBride told me that when the program was first launched, three-quarters of Hannaford's products got no stars at all. All of the fresh fruits and vegetables got at least one star, but only half of milks and juices did, only about a third of baked and canned goods, and only about a quarter of meats. Hannaford had no commercial motive to be this honest. Jim said the ratings were based on independent scientific judgments, which the company decided to honor.

Do the Guiding Stars shelf tags influence shopper choices? Several academic studies have shown small but significant reductions in the share of zero-star products purchased after the system is implemented. A 2017 study observed that even such small changes, if spread across enough shoppers, "could have sizeable population effects on diet-related health conditions."

To ensure wider and more effective use, Guiding Stars could use a government push. McBride did coordinate closely with the Institute of Medicine, a component of the National Academies of Science, when designing the system, and the U.S. Surgeon General gave it a public endorsement at a national conference on the "Weight of the Nation" in July 2009, but the FDA and USDA have not joined in. The FDA is holding back because it does not want to be seen favoring one legally marketed product over another. Meanwhile, the Grocery Manufacturers Association and the Food Marketing Institute remained wedded to their weaker Facts Up Front approach. In 2018 these two industry associations began promoting a SmartLabel system, with smartphone-scannable matrix barcodes on packages, providing more raw information to deeply curious shoppers, but still no summary ratings at a glance. Meanwhile, Guiding Stars continues to update its algorithm to remain current with federal dietary guidelines, and also to reflect the latest in nutrition science on things like omega-3 fatty acids.

Food service companies, especially chain restaurants, also make a contribution to unhealthy eating in America, a problem that will continue, assuming restaurant use bounces back following the COVID-19 crisis. Before that crisis, even households at or below the poverty line had turned to restaurants more than four times a week on average. Spending for food prepared away from the home—either eaten at restaurants or taken away—grew to roughly equal the total spending for meals prepared in the home. The National Restaurant Association calculated total restaurant industry sales in 2017 at $799 billion, nearly identical at the time to annual grocery sales.

Regrettably, a majority of these restaurant meals have worsened the nation's overall diet. Compared to meals prepared from purchased groceries, restaurant meals tend to have less calcium, iron, and fiber, and more saturated fats and sodium. They are also higher in calories. In the late 1970s, only 17 percent of total average daily calorie intake came from foods prepared away from the home; by 2012 that had doubled. Quick-service chains (fast food) and full-service chains (order from the table) are both implicated in this excess. Fine dining is not the issue here; what the industry calls "white table cloth" dining makes up only 2 percent of total restaurant use.

Many fast-food establishments assemble and heat meals that were actually cooked somewhere else. The meal components are prepared off-site by a manufacturer, shipped to a distributor, and then sent to individual restaurants for little more than a final heat and serve. McDonald's restaurants once made their own fries, but now these items are manufactured at a large plant in Idaho, because that's the best place to source potatoes. The standard recipe for these fries includes dimethylpolysiloxane, the same silicone used in Silly Putty. Full-service restaurants do more real cooking, but sometimes only a bit more, and the meals themselves are seldom more healthful. If restaurants began making meals that were less caloric and more nutritious, it might compensate for some of the unhealthy eating and snacking that takes place inside so many American homes. Is it foolish to hope this might happen someday?

Applebee's—with roughly eighteen hundred sites in the United States—has been a leader for more than three decades in the "casual dining" segment of the full-service restaurant industry, alongside other chains like Ruby Tuesday, TGI Fridays, Chili's, and Red Lobster. "Eatin' Good in the Neighborhood" is Applebee's slogan. The menu features appetizers galore, combo meals, salads, chicken and burger dishes, and a signature treat known as "riblets." The food-blogging YouTube star Nikocado Avocado (not his real name) raves about Applebee's fried mozzarella cheese sticks, but makes a telling side comment about the calories: "There's gonna come a time when I stop apologizing for the double chin."

Applebee's isn't alone in serving fat-laden, high-calorie fare. When the sociologist Anthony Winson examined typical meals (a dinner entrée, a side dish, and a dessert, excluding beverage) from Red Lobster, Olive Garden, and Chili's, he found that in all these restaurants a typical single meal delivered more saturated fat than is recommended for an entire day, and at Olive Garden and Chili's it was twice the recommended daily level. A brief published in the *Journal of Nutrition*

Education and Behavior in 2014 found from a study of twenty-one full-service chain menus in Philadelphia that the average meal—consisting of an adult entrée, side dish, and shared appetizer—delivered 1,495 calories, 28 grams of saturated fat, and 3,312 milligrams of sodium. If a nonalcoholic beverage and shared dessert are added, the calorie total for a single meal goes above two thousand. A 2012 study in the journal *Public Health and Nutrition* found that entrées at full-service family restaurants consistently had more calories, fat, and sodium than at fast-food restaurants. Other studies confirm that compared to fast-food restaurants, the full-service chains also deliver larger portion sizes, offer a lower proportion of healthier items, and make children's entrées that are less healthy.

Just like food companies and retailers, restaurants can feel trapped by customer preferences for sugar, salt, and fat over green vegetables. When Applebee's recently attempted a menu change to emphasize more healthy offerings, business sagged and they reverted to form. In the view of one professional restaurant analyst, "They tried to pursue a customer who wasn't going to Applebee's anyway." After sales flopped, John Cywinski took over as Applebee's new president in March 2018 and returned the chain to its traditional emphasis on eating for pleasure. "Americans are stressed," Cywinski explained to CNN Business. "When stressed, they tend to go to comfort food . . . and we're pretty darn good at comfort food. That's the role we play."

To promote its revival of feel-good food, Applebee's ramped up drink promotions ("Dollaritas") and broadcast close-up TV ads that panned slowly over creamy pasta dishes with the silky voice of Etta James in the background singing "At Last." The chain also brought back its popular all-you-can-eat offering of riblets and chicken tenders, plus shrimp, priced at just $14.99. It worked. In the third quarter of that year Applebee's U.S. sales set a fourteen-year record. Many full-service chains do offer "lighter fare" items for those who are trying to cut calories, yet even these may pack a day's worth of sodium. Only half of the chains highlight such items on the menu, and they make up just 15 percent of total sales.

I ate at an Applebee's Bar & Grill in a shopping mall outside of

Boston with Bill Hale, founding president of the Hale Group, a firm that publishes well-researched white papers peering into the future of the food service industry. Bill is a senior consultant to the NRA (the National Restaurant Association, not the gun group), and also to individual food manufacturers, retailers, and restaurant chains. Seated in our comfortable booth, we were handed menus that featured large-format glossy photos of colorful plated meals. Bill ordered the double-crunch fried shrimp, served with fries, cole slaw, and separate cups of cocktail and tartar sauce—1,320 calories in all, for just $14.29. I went with the cedar-grilled lemon chicken dish, on cranberry-pecan rice, with quinoa and a Granny Smith apple relish. A small green heart on the menu had helped guide me to this option, and with water to drink, and no appetizer or dessert, my meal would total just 600 calories, and cost only $12.49.

Bill explained that the "combo" meals on the menu were there

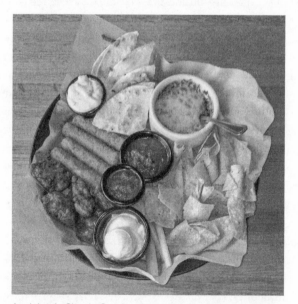

Applebee's Classic Combo platter. This "appetizer" dish has boneless buffalo wings, spinach and artichoke dip, chicken quesadilla, mozzarella sticks, corn chips, and salsa—2,180 calories for $14.39.

to nudge customers toward the fries and drinks, since that's where the biggest profit margins reside. Potatoes are a moneymaker since you buy them by the pound then sell them by the portion. Bill also pointed to the electronic touch tablet on our table that allowed us to pay at any time without having to flag down our server. Bill explained it was there primarily to save labor costs for the company. "More people can be served by fewer staff. The server saves three trips to your table: she doesn't have to give you the paper check, or return to take your credit card, or bring the card and check back for you to sign. Each staff member now can cover eight tables."

The biggest labor savings were being captured in the kitchen, which Bill referred to as the "back room." When my chicken breast arrived it was nice and hot, with authentic-looking blackened grill marks, but Bill said, "These are reconstituted products, preprepared and preseasoned. Tyson can supply them with or without the grill marks." Bill's shrimp had also been prebreaded off-site, then delivered to the restaurant for a quick par-fry. "Not a lot of creative cooking going on in the back room," said Bill. Restaurant chains try to avoid a large on-site kitchen staff because of payroll costs, rapid turnover, and low dependability.

Restaurants have long used prepared foods in the back room to save on labor, but these days, according to Bill, "they can't afford to *look* like prepared foods." Millennials want authenticity, so some "micro-chain" restaurants have even moved back toward on-site cooking, preparing in the morning the products they estimate they will need later in the day. If a customer must later be told a dish has sold out, that simply adds to the authenticity.

Customers are also demanding more nonmeat choices. Bill had just come from a meeting in Arkansas sponsored by Tyson Foods where he moderated a roundtable discussion among fifteen presidents of smaller micro-chain or metro-chain restaurant companies. "One of the guys who has a successful business said, 'I used to have only one vegetarian plant-based offering on my menu. Now I need to have at least three.'" Tyson has recently placed some bets of its own on plant protein, initially by investing in plant-based Beyond Burgers and then moving to develop its own independent line of animal-free imitation meat options.

Will the more progressive tastes of today's younger eaters eventually inspire a competition among big restaurant chains to prepare and promote lighter and more nutritious menu items? Will our restaurants take the lead in improving America's diet? Bill's answer was "Probably not." Beverage offerings are part of the problem. One 2019 study in the *American Journal of Preventive Medicine* compared the 2017 offerings from 63 restaurant chains to 2012, and found the number of different sugary beverages available—sodas, fruit drinks, sports drinks—had increased by more than 80 percent.

Some restaurant patrons do seek better nutrition, but for most this has not been the priority. Bill mentioned industry research from Datassential suggesting restaurant goers can be sorted into four broad categories. First are the Basic Eaters, who use restaurants regularly out of necessity and are looking for affordability. They tend to favor fast food. Second are the Experientialists, who also use restaurants frequently, but for social ambience or novelty, so once again nutrition and health are not the first priority. A third group are the Quality Essentialists, who do look for food quality, but mostly in terms of ingredients, careful preparation, seasoning, and taste, largely apart from nutrition or health. Only then do we come to the Progressives, who do make choices based on nutrition and health, but they are influenced by food fads and fashions as well.

These Progressives are pushing restaurant chains toward more plant-based items today, but when Applebee's made changes to attract more Progressives it drove away the Experientialists and Essentialists. Full-service restaurant chains in the upscale urban settings attractive to today's millennials are wise to offer more healthy fare, but less so elsewhere.

Progressive change might actually come more quickly from some innovative fast-food chains. Taco Bell has developed an entire menu of vegetarian options, and Pizza Hut is reducing sodium in its products while removing artificial flavors, colors, and monosodium glutamate. The Food Network now endorses twenty-three different fast-food chains as healthy. One of these, Little Beet, chases fashion with a gluten-free and largely paleo menu, but with plenty of vegan options as well. Globally influenced creations can also be found, like grilled avocado garnished with "super seeds," but until recently only those living in New York or Washington, D.C., could find a Little Beet. More widely available is Veggie Grill, with its quick-service menu revolving around plant-based items such as tempeh, pea proteins, and supergrains. Veggie Grill got started in Irvine, California, and now has multiple locations on both coasts.

Another new chain focused on health is Sweetgreen, which features assembly-line ordering, scratch cooking, and local sourcing, all similar to Chipotle, but with no soft drinks, no red meats, and mostly salad greens and veggie ingredients. The chain currently operates just one hundred stores in nine cities but hopes to double its size by 2023. The emphasis at Sweetgreen is on health, delicious taste, and high-tech convenience, with a website option to order ahead for either delivery or pickup (more than half of total order volume was online even before COVID-19). A Sweetgreen salad costs roughly twice as much as a Big Mac, but this isn't the only thing limiting scale-up potential. No matter how convenient they become, salads will never be as filling as sandwiches, or as popular as beef and pork—or as addictive and stimulating as Starbucks coffee.

On balance and over the longer run, fast food meals have not been improving. Healthier items have come onto the menus, but the benefit is usually offset by larger portion sizes, more fat, and more salt. A 2019 study from the *Journal of the Academy of Nutrition and Dietetics* compared items served in 2016 versus thirty years earlier, at ten top fast-food chains. Across the ten chains, the average entrée in 2016 weighed thirty-nine grams more and had ninety more calories. It delivered more than 40 percent of the recommended daily allowance for salt, an increase from less than 30 percent. Desserts had 186 more calories than the average dessert three decades earlier.

Many restaurant menus are in constant flux, driven by fads and fashions, and sometimes this does move the industry in a healthy direction. When Chipotle and Panera started providing chicken meat that was antibiotic free (ABF), others quickly followed. Soon, four-teen of the top twenty-five fast-food and casual dining companies had made ABF promises of their own, including KFC, Burger King, Starbucks, Dunkin' Donuts, and Jack in the Box. McDonald's met its target for ABF chickens nine months ahead of its own original deadline, then said late in 2018 it would also reduce the use of medi-cally important antibiotics in the beef it served. New food service practices of this kind will oblige livestock producers to adjust as well, an added bonus.

One recent fad in food service that preceded COVID-19 had noth-ing to do with nutritious eating. To satisfy customers who want to stay at home, restaurants are now delivering meals prepared in "ghost kitchens" that serve no walk-in customers at all. Orders are taken online then delivered using mobile apps like Uber Eats, Grubhub, or DoorDash. Money is saved because a single kitchen location can cook for multiple restaurant brands, with no need for waiters, tables, chairs, a parking lot, or an attractive décor. A ghost kitchen can be built in an unused warehouse for as little as $30,000, while outfitting a traditional restaurant usually costs thirty times that much.

Nutrition, in any case, is seldom the focus. The celebrity chefs who influence restaurant menus could be playing a positive role, but too often they just go for novelty and taste. One study in the *Food and Public Health Journal* tested nine hundred recipes from twenty-six famous chefs and found that nearly nine out of ten fell short of healthy eating guidelines.

On the positive side, consumers with an interest in dietary health have recently been given a better way to inform themselves about chain restaurant meals. Since May 2018, restaurants with twenty or more locations and standardized menus have been required under federal law to post calorie counts for all food items on menus and menu boards. This rule also applies to foods on display in supermar-kets, convenience stores, and movie theaters, plus nearly all of the nation's five to six million vending machines.

It took fifteen years of political struggle against industry resistance to enact this new rule. A national "menu labeling" law originally introduced in 2003 was finally passed by Congress in 2010 as part of the Affordable Care Act. The NRA had initially blocked the measure, but relented after more than twenty separate states including California—plus major cities including New York City—began enacting their own separate menu labeling requirements. At this point the NRA decided that a single nationwide rule would be better than a patchwork of different state and local menu labeling requirements. The FDA took three years to finalize the regulations, then almost four more years of delay ensued before the measure finally came into effect. Federal rules governing food service tend to change, when they change at all, at a snail's pace.

We do not yet know what difference calorie counts on menus will make. Some customers may adjust their eating habits once they learn a single pumpkin muffin at Dunkin' delivers 550 calories. At the Cheesecake Factory, some diners may begin to select the Four Cheese Pasta with 1,190 calories over the Louisiana Chicken Pasta with 2,330 calories. On the other hand, those most in need of changing their habits may ignore the new information. One local study by researchers at New York University in 2016 found nearly two-thirds of customers surveyed had not noticed menu calorie counts. A review

Required calorie counts on menus now tell eaters the Cheesy Double Beef Burrito has almost three times the calories as a Crunchy Taco.

published in *Nutrients* in 2017 found that outside of laboratory settings, menu labeling resulted in "no significant change" in reported calories ordered or consumed. Yet a Cochrane Collaboration review of calorie counts in restaurants, coffee shops, and cafeterias found that people did reduce calorie consumption, on average by forty-eight calories per meal, or about 8 percent, suggesting the new rule will bring some benefit nationwide.

Many dietitians promote "intuitive eating" over counting calories, and some fear unintended consequences from the menu calorie counts. A 2017 study in the *International Journal of Eating Disorders* suggested that women with anorexia might order fewer calories in response to menu labels, while those with binge-eating disorders might order more. If menu labeling does deliver a healthy eating payoff, it will partly come through decisions by restaurants to reduce the calories in their meals. One Seattle study found that chain restaurants did reduce calories in their offerings after a local menu labeling law went into effect there.

The news from America's food swamp was recently both good and bad. In 2018, FDA commissioner Scott Gottlieb admitted that obesity rates had continued to rise, and that more than one out of five deaths in America was attributable to poor dietary factors. But then he pointed to some promising trends:

> From 1999 to 2010, researchers have observed a steady improvement in the average quality of the American diet, as more people reduced intake of trans fat and reduced consumption of sugar sweetened beverages and fruit juices, while increasing consumption of whole fruit, whole grains, polyunsaturated fatty acids and nuts and legumes.

The research study Gottlieb referred to was a Harvard School of Public Health report in 2014 that rated dietary quality on an index scale from zero to 110. The index score for 2010 was 46.8, significantly higher than the 1999 score of 39.9. More than half the improvement had come from reduced consumption of trans fats. In the case of trans fats, America's food companies, supermarkets, and restaurant chains went along with positive change. When scientists concluded in 1990 that partially hydrogenated oils (PHOs) were causing millions of premature deaths, food companies like Unilever invested in ways to deliver products like margarine that had no trans fat. City governments eventually played a constructive role as well. In 2006, New York mayor Michael Bloomberg banned trans fats in city restaurants, and by 2015 even the cautious regulators at the FDA were on board, moving toward an effective trans fat ban by declaring that PHOs would no longer be considered "Generally Recognized as Safe." In 2018, despite backsliding seen elsewhere under the Trump administration, the FDA announced a plan to revoke all remaining sanctioned uses of PHOs.

America's declining sugary beverage consumption has been another healthy turn. Sales of nondiet carbonated soft drinks fell 27 percent by volume on a per-person basis between 1998 and 2017. This drop, together with reduced trans fat consumption, helped to reverse national trends in the incidence of diabetes, after a long period of dangerous increase. The beverage industry will continue to fight against government soda taxes, but they also respond to evolving consumer tastes. Bottled water sales in America now exceed sales of carbonated soft drinks.

Another recent trend is less promising. Americans with higher income and higher educational attainment are improving their diets far more rapidly than lower-income citizens with less education, so the diet quality gap between rich and poor Americans has continued to widen. Food companies, retailers, and restaurant chains have shown little interest in closing this gap. They are content to promote healthy foods for better-educated eaters along with plenty of unhealthy food for the less privileged majority. Food companies and supermarkets put more healthy foods on the shelf, but the unhealthy products are not taken away. Restaurants add plant-based items to the menu but continue to offer the riblets in all-you-can-eat portions.

America's growing dietary divide is not like the farming divide described earlier. In farming, both the large commercial farms at one end of the spectrum and the smaller lifestyle farms at the other end have found a good enough place to land. Not so with America's eaters, where the widening gap leaves some with improved nutrition and health, while so many others struggle with high rates of chronic disease. In terms of dietary health there are now two Americas, a majority who are stuck in the constantly spreading swamp and only a minority safely on dry land.

Some have imagined a bold solution to this problem. If food companies, retailers, and restaurants are not doing enough to correct these eating problems, maybe we should bypass the corporate middlemen altogether, get off the supermarket grid, and start purchasing unprocessed foods directly from local farmers. Let's take a closer look at that possibility.

CHAPTER 3

The Limits of Local Food

When summering in Maine, I enjoy getting off the supermarket grid. Our traditional Fourth of July clambake, hosted by close friends just down the shore, includes enough freshly caught lobsters from our own bay to feed a dozen or more hungry celebrants just before the local fireworks.

To cook the meal properly you find a sheet of steel nearly as big as a door and balance it on top of an open-faced oven, hand built at low tide from the rounded rocks on the beach. The oven fire burns hot, fueled with cedar shakes and scrap wood. We layer the lobsters, corn, and potatoes between freshly gathered bunches of dark-green rockweed, then cover it all with a canvas sailcloth doused occasionally with salt water, generating a hiss of steam. When we are done eating, the lobster shells can be tossed right back into the bay, making cleanup easy, and the rising tide eventually smothers any smoldering coals remaining from the fire. The meal is always finished off with home-baked blueberry pie.

Eating this way isn't for every day. You need someone experienced to take charge, plus access to a rocky coastline, a lobster co-op nearby, a trunk-load of firewood, plenty of muscle to handle the heavy steel, and time to gather the rockweed and build the oven. Also, because the meal lacks green vegetables and requires a great deal of melted butter, it's far from healthy. Nor is it entirely local, since local corn is not ripe in Maine on the Fourth of July. The corn usually comes in from Georgia, and the fresh blueberries from somewhere in South America.

The blueberries tell an important story. The imported share of total food consumption in the United States has increased since the 1990s, almost doubling to one-fifth. Just since 2008, the imported share of plant-based foods has increased from 19 to 24 percent. So instead of becoming more local, America's food system continued to become more global.

Local food has been culturally popular and heavily promoted for more than a decade, yet it makes up only a minuscule portion of our national diet. When the USDA adds up all direct farm-to-consumer sales made through farmers markets, CSA farms, roadside stands, pick your own, and on-farm stores, the total retail value in 2017 came to less than 1 percent of all farm sales, as previously noted. The local share is a bit larger if we add in local farm sales that are semidirect, made from farms to consumers through local retail outlets, local institutions, or food hubs for "local or regionally branded products," but even then the total retail value is just $11.8 billion, still less than 1 percent of all sales.

Measuring the local food sector is a challenge because there is no settled definition of *local*. Should it be based on how far the food has traveled, or how it is sold, or both? Jessica Prentice, the Berkeley-based chef and writer who coined the term *locavore* in 2005, said local should mean grown within a one-hundred-mile radius of the eater, whether it was sold directly from a farm or not. Others have embraced distance-based definitions that are far more lenient. The USDA decided *local* should mean within a four-hundred-mile radius, or simply in-state, but that could mean nearly eight hundred miles in a big north-to-south state like California. The retail chain Whole Foods defines local in terms of time in transit: seven or fewer hours of travel by car or truck. At sixty-five miles an hour, that might be as far away as 455 miles.

If all the supermarket food sales that retail chains advertise as local are added in, the local share of total retail sales does get larger. Packaged Facts, a market research firm, expected that by 2020 this larger category of local food sales would reach $20 billion, four times the 2008 total but still only a bit more than 1 percent of total U.S. food and beverage spending.

Committed advocates want local food to become far more than just a tiny add-on. Jessica Prentice imagines a food system that is almost entirely local, with exceptions only for tropical products that can't be grown in the United States. Importing coffee, coconuts, and chocolate would be fine, but in the spirit of her locavore vision she advises that even these items be enjoyed sparingly:

> If you spend a few weeks each year without the pleasures of imported delicacies, you really do learn a whole lot about your foodshed, about your place, about what you're swallowing on a daily basis. . . . Once upon a time, all human beings were locavores, and everything we ate was a gift of the Earth.

Most farmers would object to calling the food they work long hours to produce a "gift of the Earth," but America's food was indeed primarily local right up to the middle of the nineteenth century. All this changed once the Industrial Revolution began moving people off of farms and into cities, and once rail transport made long-distance food sales more affordable. At this point food companies began to process farm commodities into shelf-stable packaged goods, suitable for long-distance shipment on ships and rail cars just like other industrial products.

Advocates for local food view this move toward nonlocal, industrial food as a fall from grace. Michael Pollan in his book *In Defense of Food* gives this advice: "Don't eat anything your great-grandmother wouldn't recognize as food." When an interviewer told Pollan this statement made him sound like a reactionary, he did not deny it:

> Yeah, I'm a little freaked out about how reactionary this book is in some ways. I am, you know, but the more I study food, the more I see that most of the innovations have not been very positive, beginning in about 1880.

Pollan's statement prompts me to consider my own great-grandmother on my father's side, Pietertje In't Hout, an immigrant from Holland who raised eleven children. She knew quite a bit about the food of her day, not only from preparing meals for her family but also from running a grocery store together with her husband, Corstiaan, in Oak Glen, Illinois. The children were put to work in the store as soon as they could handle a broom. We know the complete inventory of foods available for purchase in her store on May 3, 1888, thanks to a list penned and signed by Corstiaan.

The store had exactly fourteen different items for sale: coffee, sugar, rice, soap, tea, raisins, butter, cheese, eggs, flour, barley, starch, prunes, and apples. Early in May in northern Illinois there were still no green vegetables. It was the job of women and girls to turn these mostly unprocessed foods into plated meals, which meant plenty of time spent peeling, chopping, soaking, mixing, cooking, and baking. Groceries back then also cost much more relative to the meager incomes of the day. The In't Hout apples were selling at twice today's retail price, corrected for inflation.

The store was located in a farming community, so it was better stocked than most. For city-dwelling laborers in the nineteenth century, food choices were sometimes restricted just to bread and potatoes, with a bit of molasses as a sweetener. Another common working-class meal was "blood pudding," which consisted of pig or cow blood mixed with ground pork, paired with butter crackers. Those living on farms had more variety, but the farm food was completely unprocessed, so the daughters and wives had to churn their own butter after milking the cow, then they had to knead the dough for half an hour before baking bread.

Today's enthusiasts for local food sometimes enjoy reenacting such preindustrial agrarian chores. In the Sustainable Food Program at Yale University, students started a farm of their own fifteen minutes from campus, where they knead their own pizza dough, then bake it in a wood-fired oven. This is a good learning experience, as long as it includes learning that today's commercial pizza restaurants could never afford to hire all that manual labor.

Part of the attraction of local food may be pure nostalgia. The pick-your-own apple orchards in Massachusetts are fun because you get to ride in a hay wagon then pick from an old-style pointed wooden tree ladder. In less than an hour you and your family can leave with several peck bags of ripe apples, imagining that traditional farm work must have been great fun. To trigger more imagined agrarian memories, New England tourists head upcountry to stay in rustic B&B's, purchasing artisanal foods at local farmers markets. The food is local even if those buying it are not. One study of farmers market patrons in Vermont in the summer found that more than half were not year-round residents. When I visit my local farmers market in Maine in August, most of the cars parked by the roadside have license plates from Massachusetts, New York, Pennsylvania, or beyond.

Buying food from local farms feels like a reconnection with agrarian tradition, but many of the local farmers are far from traditional agrarians. One study of CSA farmers revealed that almost three-quarters of them had a college degree and nearly one-third had a graduate or professional degree. Both the growers and the shoppers at farmers markets will also, most likely, be white. This is not a surprise, since for most African Americans the agrarian past meant either slavery or impoverished sharecropping in the Jim Crow South, neither a source of fond memories. For too many Hispanic Americans, harvesting crops by hand under the hot sun is not a memory at all, but a current reality they would prefer to escape.

America's most prominent champion of agrarian localism is the poet and novelist Wendell Berry, a native of rural Kentucky. Berry is hardly a lifelong agrarian, since he left home early to earn a master's degree in English, study creative writing at Stanford, accept a Guggenheim in Italy and France, then work briefly in New York. When he returned home to teach at the University of Kentucky, he moved onto a small farm. He wrote twenty-five books of poems, sixteen volumes of essays, and eleven novels or short story collections, so he wasn't farming all the time.

Berry is a fierce critic of modernity, and to make his point he decided to farm like his grandfather, using a team of horses rather than a tractor to do field work. In one early essay he even objected to weather forecasts, since they preempted the farmer's traditional reliance on experience and intuition. At a deeper level, Berry saw the traditions of agrarian localism as the best way to fight back against the ravages of industrial capitalism:

> The only conceivable defense against so great an economic force, which has always been "global," is a local economy founded upon local land, local nature, and the cooperation and mutual trust of local producers and consumers. The establishment of a local economy, then, involves the establishment or re-establishment of the local community.

Most champions of local food today do not want to abandon all of industrial capitalism since that would mean abandoning far more than just modern commercial farms and supermarkets, but they admire Berry for putting the idea in play.

Local food is promoted for reasons that go far beyond yearnings for a dimly remembered agrarian past. Some see it as a way to ensure food will be tasty and fresh, safer to eat, or grown with less harm to the natural environment. Yet if local food can deliver all these tangible benefits, why does it fail to grow in the marketplace above low single digits? To investigate this question, I visited Andrew Rodgers, a farmer who pursues the local food vision with energy, skill, and significant commercial success. Andrew is the manager of Clark Farm, located in the semirural town of Carlisle, Massachusetts, about twenty-five miles west of Boston. He produces certified organic vegetables, eggs, and meat on forty-five acres, for roughly three hundred local CSA subscribers, plus farmstand customers and some local farm-to-table restaurants and retailers. Carlisle is right next to Concord, home to Bronson Alcott, and the town where America's revolution began in 1775. Some could see Andrew's farm as the leading edge of a new revolution, aimed at rebuilding ties between eaters and small local farms.

Andrew grew up in suburban Newton, Massachusetts, became an English major in college, married, then took a job on the West Coast with a market research company, conducting focus groups for high-tech firms. His spouse, Diana, earned her undergraduate degree in art education, then got a job doing brand strategy with an advertising agency. She always had a personal interest in nutrition, and she and Andrew both enjoyed the outdoors and were concerned about the environment, so they gravitated away from the corporate world. They began looking for a small farm where they could grow nutritious food while at the same time protecting the land from unsustainable development.

Andrew came back east first to do graduate work in soil science, and then took an apprenticeship on an organic farm. He moved up to managing the Green Meadows Farm in Hamilton, Massachusetts, then, in 2012, took over Clark Farm in Carlisle, where he and Diana raised their two children. They also have two border collies, named Chase and Fly, who help with the sheep and keep hawks away from the chickens.

Clark Farm is on land continuously used for food production since early in the eighteenth century. It supported dairy cows until 1985 but was then purchased by a couple who put it into an agricultural easement, to block any future sale for commercial or residential development. Clark Farm today has an antique feel, with a picturesque 150-year-old wooden barn and a white silo capped by a conical red roof. Behind the barn is a low flat field containing row crops and some mobile chicken coops, spreading away for a considerable distance, sealed off from neighboring properties by mature pine and hardwood trees. Everything feels neatly contained, like a diorama display in an agricultural history museum.

For the past several years I have been taking students to visit Clark Farm in early autumn to learn about the CSA farming model. On one recent visit in October the farm worked its magic on my students, even though the peak growing season had passed. Dazzling red-orange leaves on sugar maples, back-lit in the morning sun, fluttered beneath a powder-blue sky. After Andrew explained the business side of the operation, he walked us into the old barn. We were hit by the perfumed smell of hay, like I remembered from the haymow of my uncle's barn in Indiana.

Most of the vegetables in the fields were gone by October, but the pastured hens were still picking bugs from the thick green grass, attended by a rooster. Several dozen good-sized pigs roamed under the trees behind a low fence. Andrew and Diana are quick to defend selling and eating the meat from these animals, since they are humanely raised and slaughtered, and the Rodgers family itself consumes about two pigs' worth of meat a year. Diana's interest in nutrition led her to a career as a registered dietitian, and she recently authored *The Homegrown Paleo Cookbook,* which emphasized the role animal products can play in a nutritious diet.

Andrew raises sheep, which spend the winter in the barn, where lambing usually starts the first week in February. "I keep them inside, in the barn, close to Mom. They fatten up, there's no parasite load to deal with, there's no coyote to get them. You take them for some walks, but overall they just get to relax, and the lambs come out so much bigger and better." He also grows microgreens in a hoop house for direct sale to local restaurants, bringing in about 6 percent of the farm's total revenue, and he has started offering microgreens in a new experimental winter share to forty of his CSA members.

The microgreens bring in some money in the winter, but Clark Farm delivers its main harvest of vegetables, pork, lamb, goat meat, eggs from pastured hens, blueberries, strawberries, and raspberries during the twenty-four weeks between mid-June and November. Andrew also sells flowers, and he partners with other local growers to sell mushrooms, tree fruit, and even fish. All of Clark Farm's products are certified organic, and all of the animals are pastured rather than tightly confined, so he can charge a higher price.

The eggs sell for seven dollars a dozen, more than three times the price for conventional supermarket eggs. Andrew dislikes such comparisons, because he says his eggs are better than anything you can get in a supermarket. On animal welfare grounds, he is right. Using the animal welfare rating system employed by Whole Foods, his pastured pork and eggs would earn a top score of five, which is higher than the ratings found on most animal products sold by Whole Foods itself.

For a small operation, Clark Farm generates impressive sales. The eighty to ninety members who buy the large annual food shares for $900 provide the farm with $81,000 in revenue, while the other 220 members buying smaller shares for $630 generate $138,600. If you add in the revenue from farm-stand sales, farm-to-restaurant and local retail sales, and now the new winter shares, Clark Farm falls into a respectably high sales class for an American farm.

The farming is labor-intensive. Andrew plants and harvests some of his best crop beds four times every year. Clark Farm has twelve acres of row crops, with forty beds in each acre and with rows two hundred feet long. Each bed might have six hundred heads of organic lettuce, which sell for two dollars each, roughly twice the supermarket price for conventional lettuce. Farming this way requires continuous human labor because organic certification does not allow the use of manufactured fertilizers or pesticides. Andrew makes his own compost for fertilizer, fights insect and fungus pests with nonsynthetic pesticides, and hires high school students at minimum wage in the summer to help keep weeds under control. He also hires an assistant farm manager plus several foreign workers on J1 Exchange Visitor visas, which are available to those who want to work on organic farms. In recent years he has employed summer crew members from Brazil, Kenya, and Ecuador.

After each visit to Clark Farm, my students inevitably ask why this can't be the future of farming everywhere in America, and this is indeed the central question. I later asked Andrew how much potential for expansion he sees in CSA farming, either through more numerous small farms like his, or perhaps bigger and more specialized farms. As for bigger, he was not sure. He has considered increasing his own revenue by selling more shares every year, but then he would need to hire a larger crew and would not have the satisfaction of knowing all his subscribers personally. He could also scale up by becoming less diverse, selling a higher volume of just one or two specialty products like microgreens, using intermediate distribution hubs rather than selling directly to subscribers. This would still be off the supermarket grid and the sales would mostly remain local, but Andrew says he does not want to specialize:

> I could easily follow the numbers and scale up the microgreens business, but if I did that and had five greenhouses, and delivery trucks, and all the logistics going on, I'm not going to enjoy it very much. It's no longer being a small-scale farmer, where I come in and do all the seeding myself with a small crew that's dynamic and interesting for me to hang out with. I know a lot of growers who have scaled up to a point where they don't farm anymore— they sit in an office. I get to farm, and be in the fields, and that's what I want to do.

A better option, says Andrew, would be an increased number of small and fully diversified farms such as his, enough so everyone in the community could belong to a CSA. He admits this vision is still quite a ways off. When I asked how many CSA farms there were altogether in Carlisle, a town of roughly five thousand inhabitants, he answered, "Uh . . . one."

Economists would have no trouble explaining the limited growth of CSA farming so far, since it restricts consumer choice and asks more in terms of consumer time. The only items available are those grown locally, and only when seasonally ripe. Separate supermarket trips will still be necessary for CSA members to get things like milk, rice, pasta, canned goods, paper products, and cleansers. CSA farms located close to a metropolitan area must also charge more, since wages and land costs will be much higher in such areas. If the owners of Clark Farm had not restricted the land to agricultural use in order to get a tax easement, the property would probably have been sold by now for residential development. Carlisle is an affluent town with

a median home value of $795,000. Clark Farm's affluent local cus-
tomer base clearly makes it easier for the farm to sell its high-priced
organic and pastured products, but Andrew points out that some of
his most loyal members are actually recent immigrants who grew up
without supermarket food, and who therefore appreciate the fresh,
hand-grown quality of what he sells.

Before COVID-19, restaurant sales were a significant growth
opportunity for local food, since chefs with high standards are ready
to pay more for quality and freshness. In the Metro Atlanta area,
the number of farm-to-table restaurants more than doubled to reach
seventy-eight after 2006. One local chef explained why: "You have to
source the best ingredients if you want to make the best food possible," not what he called "some garbage from Nicaragua or something that has been in transport for weeks and picked un-ripened."

Even so growers face financial challenges, and CSA farmers must
sometimes shortchange themselves to help make ends meet. One ten-
year study of twenty-four CSA farmers in Minnesota and Wisconsin
found that most lacked health-care coverage, or funds for retirement,
and only fourteen were still involved with CSA at the end of the study
period. One 2005 study found that most CSA farms in the Northeast
can only cover their costs when compensation to the farm operator
is not included. With these costs included, net income becomes negative. One coalition of CSA farms outside of Chicago recently saw six
of its members go out of business, and a semifamous pioneer of the
CSA movement in Illinois, John Peterson, was selling a quarter fewer
weekly boxes compared to previous years. Cheryl Brown and Stacy
Miller at West Virginia University concluded from such findings that
"CSA farms will probably never be more than a small part of the
food system."

Andrew Rodgers is not so pessimistic. He believes the strong
appeal of local food, especially when organic, can ensure continued
growth for the CSA model. Small-scale specialization might be one
key. "There's going to be a niche for really small CSAs. I wouldn't
be surprised if fresh produce in the future comes more from micro

farms, with people growing stuff in their backyards, then selling it to a co-op or a restaurant. Maybe you just grow really great hot peppers, and for just one small part of your income."

Andrew takes quickly to challenges and thinks all the time about boosting his own efficiency. Like all vegetable growers, he worries about spoilage before his produce can be sold. He knows this risk will increase under the CSA model if he gets a bumper crop, since he sells to a relatively fixed number of customers every season. In these situations he feeds the surplus to his pigs or spades it into the ground to enrich the soil, but these are suboptimal commercial strategies. Andrew fantasizes about refrigerated trucks pulling up to his farm on a weekly basis to take his surplus production for delivery to paying customers, but he hasn't gone in this direction so far.

For larger produce farms that sell into a national market it's easier to avoid spoilage. A picked vegetable will rot only half as fast if it can be kept at 40 degrees Fahrenheit versus 60 degrees, and on large farms the vegetables will be refrigerated in the field, packed at a low temperature, transported in a refrigerated truck, stored in a refrigerated warehouse, then put out for final sale in a chilled display case. Andrew's packing shed has good refrigeration, but small local growers that sell through farmers markets often experience serious losses at the marketing stage. If the temperature reaches 80 degrees, vegetables on open display without refrigeration rot four times as fast as at 40 degrees, and the produce not sold by the end of the day may be impossible to market later.

I asked Andrew if raising pigs so close to a residential community had ever caused trouble with his neighbors. He reminded me that his small numbers of pastured pigs make almost no smell at all, something I had noticed myself. What he worries about are his hens polluting the local water system by putting too much phosphorus into the soil. Phosphorus runoff from livestock operations was also a problem for the Chesapeake Bay and for the Maumee watershed where John Nidlinger farms. Andrew does his own soil testing and knows it would be irresponsible to increase the number of hens on his farm. "I sell out of eggs all the time, so the market is telling me to

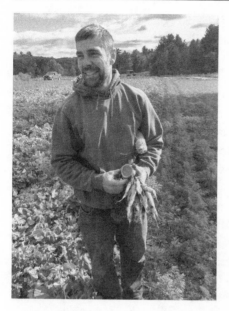

Andrew Rodgers, manager of a successful CSA farm, showing off the organic carrots and radishes he has just pulled from the ground.

grow more chickens, but I can't. Three hundred birds, that's all I can do on my thirty acres of pasture. That's it." If the hens were confined indoors, their waste could be contained, but that's not a compromise Andrew is willing to make.

Andrew's breadth of technical knowledge is impressive, along with the respect he shows for his animals, his community, and the natural environment. There is so much to like about Clark Farm, I wish more of our food could be produced this way. Preventing this are prohibitive land and labor costs plus too little consumer choice and convenience. Farms like this will continue to produce high-quality local food in season for a small segment of the market. Consumers who want year-round variety and time-saving convenience will continue finding most of their food elsewhere.

Nearly all of America's food was grown locally on small family farms two centuries ago. As with Clark Farm, fresh fruits and vegetables were available only in season, and tropical fruits could not be had at all. America's diet did not significantly diversify until the food system began to delocalize, following the advent of canals, railroads, and refrigeration. When the Erie Canal opened in 1825, connecting the Hudson River to the Great Lakes, transport costs between the East Coast and the agricultural Midwest were dramatically reduced, allowing more city dwellers to be supplied from farms on the rich soils of the Ohio Valley.

A second canal that was completed in 1848 connected Lake Michigan to the Illinois and Mississippi Rivers, enabling barge transport all the way to the Gulf of Mexico. Steam railroads became the primary means for moving agricultural products overland after 1860, and this gave northern cities wintertime access to fresh produce such as New Orleans peas or peaches from the Carolinas and Georgia. Food-processing industries sprang up along these rail lines and began producing boxed breakfast cereals, canned fruits, sliced breads, frozen beans, and many other items suited to long-distance rail travel. Once iceboxes were introduced into rail cars, and then into private homes as well, even highly perishable foods could travel a greater distance moving from farm to table.

Anthropologists Gretel and Pertti Pelto have described the process of food system delocalization as a "fundamental, apparently unidirectional tendency in human history." This delocalization process accelerated in the twentieth century when many more farm dwellers moved to the city. Between 1920 and today, the share of Americans living on farms fell from 30 percent to just 2 percent. Once this new nonfarming population owned personal automobiles and electric refrigerators, supermarket shopping took off, and the supermarkets naturally wanted to source from the most reliable bulk suppliers. This meant big wholesalers linked to distant farms and large food companies, not small local farms. By sourcing from a distance, wholesalers could get a wider variety of fresh fruits and vegetables during more months of the year, and they could take advantage of regional growing specialties: peanuts in the South, wheat in the Plains states, and apples in the Pacific Northwest.

Food from far away became even more affordable once the Interstate Highway System, started in 1956 and completed in 1992, sharply reduced long-distance trucking costs, transforming California's Central Valley into America's salad bowl. The Central Valley was well designed to supply fruits and vegetables to the rest of the country. It offered level land, a nearly year-round growing season, dry air to keep down crop pests, water for irrigation, and clear skies with bright sunshine hitting the ground during four-fifths of all daylight hours. International shipping costs also dropped steadily. Between 1930 and 2000, average ocean freight shipping costs per ton fell by 75 percent, and average air transport costs fell 90 percent. With refrigerated shipping containers and commercial jet aviation, fresh produce could be sourced not just from California and Florida, but also from Guatemala, Chile, and China.

Increasing farm wages also pushed the sourcing of food to more distant places. The Pioneer Valley along the Connecticut River was once called the "asparagus capital of the world" because it had well-drained sandy soils ideally suited to this crop. The sandy soils are still there, but the asparagus disappeared when farm labor costs in Massachusetts became too high. Asparagus is a fast-growing perennial crop sending out multiple spears that must be separately snipped every day by hand, which calls for backbreaking stoop labor. More than nine out of ten asparagus servings in America now come from other countries, including Peru and Mexico, where people can still be hired to do this kind of work.

For all these reasons, America's imports of fruits and vegetables have continued to increase. In 1990, imports provided only about a third of total domestic fresh fruit consumption, but by 2013 the imported share had increased to half. In 2000, imports of fresh and processed vegetables made up 12 percent of domestic consumption, but by 2016 it was almost double that for processed vegetables and close to triple that for fresh vegetables. Roughly 80 percent of America's seafood is now imported as well, so relocalizing our food system would mean doing without seafood in large parts of the country.

The twentieth-century shift away from local food brought Americans steady benefits in terms of healthy food choices. Over a single decade in the 1990s, the average number of produce items sold in America's supermarkets doubled. Fresh fruit availability per capita in the United States increased by 40 percent between 1970 and 2014, even after adjusting for spoilage, plate waste, and other losses along the supply chain. The total availability of fresh vegetables per person increased 21 percent. The availability of fresh tomatoes nearly doubled, fresh cucumbers nearly tripled, fresh bell pepper availability increased nearly fivefold, and fresh broccoli availability increased more than thirteenfold. Relocalizing America's food system would reverse all these advantageous trends.

Local foods are less likely to be processed, but even in Greatgrandmother's day most foods would be processed eventually, through laborious work done inside the home. Meats were dried, smoked, and salted; spices and seasonings were ground by hand; cream was separated from milk and then churned by hand into butter; fruits and vegetables from the garden were "put up" for the winter in thick glass mason jars. All this work came in addition to meal preparation and cleanup, consuming forty person-hours a week on average, a full-time job by itself.

This is why the arrival of already processed nonlocal foods was welcomed as something close to a miracle in the mid-twentieth century. As Dylan Gordon has written,

> Owning, consuming, preparing, and eating these technological marvels was downright aspirational. Food in its natural state, meanwhile, meant uncertain availability, inconsistent quality, backbreaking labor, and the threat of disease and decay.

In many notable instances, the new processed foods did compromise on nutrition. Wonder Bread, first sold in Indianapolis in 1921, surged to nationwide popularity in the 1930s because it was already sliced. In addition it was so soft you barely had to chew, so children

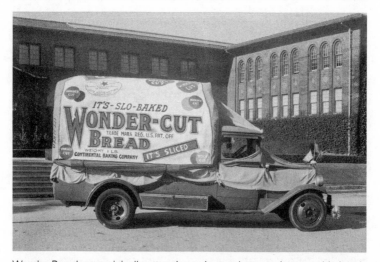

Wonder Bread was originally attractive to buyers because it was sold already sliced. It was "Wonder Cut," but not so wonderful for nutrition.

would eat it. But it was ultraprocessed, low in fiber and nutrients, and lacking in whole grains. Fooducate today rates classic Wonder Bread as a C–, its lowest score for any kind of baked bread, and just as bad as Frosted Flakes. The makers of Wonder Bread tried to offset these nutrient deficits by fortifying the white flour with added vitamins and minerals, brazenly bragging the bread would therefore "build strong bodies eight ways." Buffalo Bob, host of the *Howdy Doody* children's TV show in the 1950s, drummed this message into the heads of young baby boomers five days a week. When boomer tastes eventually matured, the brand went into steep decline. Wonder Bread tried to recover by coming out with a whole-grain white bread, baked from an albino variety of wheat, but to no avail.

Some processed foods introduced in the twentieth century were actually more nutritious, thanks to added vitamins and minerals. Beginning in the 1940s, the fortification of milk with vitamin D was an important step toward ending the threat of rickets. Enriching bread flour with niacin almost completely eliminated the pellagra problem. Following a presidential wartime directive in 1941, flour was enriched with vitamins and iron, and folic acid is now routinely added to grain and cereal products to prevent neural tube defects. Iron-fortified infant cereals, margarine fortified with vitamin A, and processed foods prepared with iodized salt have also been good for dietary health. If this kind of processing to enrich and fortify foods were discontinued, significant percentages of the population would lack an adequate intake of vitamins A, C, D, and E, plus thiamin, folate, calcium, magnesium, and iron.

Processing can reduce the nutrient content of fresh vegetables, but this will also happen to unprocessed vegetables if they are kept too long without refrigeration. In some cases, blanching and freezing (of peas, for example) makes prolonged storage possible without any reduction in iron, zinc, magnesium, calcium, or dietary fiber. Because processed fruits and vegetables are easier to store and transport, they can remain within easy reach of consumers all winter long. This means more nutrient consumption overall, even when the nutrients in each serving have been slightly diminished. Processed foods that are actually a superior choice on nutrition grounds include probiotic yogurts, canned beans with plant-based protein and fiber, jarred spaghetti sauce where cooking has improved the quality of the antioxidant carotenoids, and peanut butters containing heart-healthy fats along with protein.

Food processing also deserves credit for reducing spoilage and waste. Volunteer "gleaners" visit farm fields these days to gather unpicked or unmarketable produce for donation to poor communities, and they also work with supermarkets to "rescue" products that have gone past their sell-by date. These are excellent things to do, but without modern processing far more food would need to be rescued. Vegetables grown for processing seldom need rescue; they are typically shipped within hours of picking and sent straight to an industrial facility to be promptly frozen or canned, which stabilizes them for months or even years. The growers coordinate planting schedules in advance with processors to ensure adequate space on the line when the peas or beans arrive. Unprocessed vegetables move more slowly from the field to the packing shed, then to the warehouse, then to a truck, next to the distribution center, and finally to a supermarket, with losses at every step along the way, due to routine temperature or handling stress as well as time delays. Further loss occurs when cosmetic imperfections cause some of these fresh vegetables to be thrown out. Cosmetic appearance is not a barrier for vegetables destined to be chopped up or blanched anyway.

While some processing can be good, too much becomes a serious dietary problem. Ultraprocessed foods are a risk to personal health, in part because they cause us to eat too fast, and hence too much. A fascinating study published in the journal *Cell Metabolism* in 2019 mapped the food intake of inpatient volunteers given a sequence of diets. For two weeks one group was offered unlimited quantities of ultraprocessed foods, while a second group was offered the same foods but minimally processed. After two weeks the diets offered were reversed. Even though the two different diets had similar densities of sugar, sodium, fat, fiber, macronutrients, and calories, the individuals on the ultraprocessed diet consumed an average of 508 more calories per day and as a result gained an average of two pounds; on the minimally processed diet, they lost an average of two pounds. The higher intake of calories was correlated with a faster rate of eating. According to participant surveys, the ultraprocessed foods did not "taste" any better, but they went down faster due to less chewing, giving the stomach too little time to warn the brain it had been satisfied.

Ultraprocessed foods are surprisingly pervasive today. The NOVA Food Classification System, developed in Brazil, defines ultraprocessed foods as "industrial formulations made entirely or mostly from substances extracted from foods (oils, fats, sugar, starch, and proteins)." Using this definition, one study at Northwestern University in 2019 examined the top twenty-five food manufacturing companies by sales volume and found that almost nine out of ten of their products could be classified as ultraprocessed.

For formulated foods with added ingredients, artificial colors, or "stabilizers," consumers at least can learn what they are getting. All such additives to packaged foods must be listed on the "Nutrition Facts" label. Many more shoppers are now scanning this label for suspicious-sounding ingredients, so packaged food manufacturers have been modifying products to make the labels "cleaner." Scientifically, of course, we should not worry that there are "chemicals" in our food. As food scientist Robert Shewfelt points out, the most abundant chemical in our food is usually H_2O. If all the chemicals were taken out of food, there would be nothing there to eat.

Locally grown foods are sometimes touted as safer to eat than supermarket foods, because they travel a shorter distance and pass through fewer hands. Upon closer inspection, what matters most in avoiding toxins or microbial contamination in food is not the distance traveled or the number of handlers but instead the sanitary capabilities of those handlers.

Compared to small farms and local marketing systems, bigger operations are better able to detect and avoid contamination. They also have a stronger commercial incentive to do so, since they are more closely regulated and risk paying a larger penalty in the event of a contamination outbreak. The nonlocal foods sold in the United States are not always healthy or nutritious, but at the point of purchase they are nearly always "safe" to eat, and in some ways safer than local foods.

Refrigeration, milk pasteurization, and modern packaging improved food safety dramatically early in the twentieth century, and CDC surveys show that this progress has continued up to the present day, even as the food was becoming far less local. Over one fifteen-year period from 1996 to 2010, infections from E. coli O157:H7 declined by well over a third, listeria by more than one-third, and campylobacter by more than one-quarter. The contamination outbreaks that now occur are less local than in the past, so they generate greater national media attention, but a return to more localized food handling would increase the overall frequency of outbreaks and raise individual exposures to contamination.

The secret to improving food safety has been a widespread adoption of Hazard Analysis and Critical Control Point (HACCP) systems, first developed in the 1960s by the Pillsbury Company. These systems are costly because they require all operators in the food chain first to conduct a hazard analysis to identify every place where a physical, chemical, or biological contamination might be introduced. Critical control points to reduce these hazards are then located, and appropriate preventive control measures (for example, high or low temperatures) are specified for each. Monitoring procedures are then established, along with protocols for corrective action, all supported by rigorous record keeping and verification.

HACCP systems of this kind are far more affordable for large food companies than for small farms and local farmers markets. One 2013 study of farmers market managers in Georgia, Virginia, and South Carolina found more than 40 percent had no food safety standards in place at all. Fewer than one out of four had sanitized the surfaces used for marketing, and three-quarters offered no sanitation training to workers or vendors.

Careful studies are few, but one 1992 examination of over fifteen hundred samples of ten different types of vegetables at supermarkets, as opposed to farmers markets, found that the farmers market vegetables were more likely to contain campylobacter, a bacterium that can cause diarrhea, cramping, abdominal pain, and fever. A 2013 study found that chicken at farmers markets was more likely to test positive for salmonella. There is also evidence that shoppers at farmers markets are more often sickened by food-borne illness. According to one 2016 study, people who shopped or ate at farmers markets were more likely to say they had food poisoning in the past two weeks than people who did not eat or shop at a farmers market.

Local food vendors have managed to escape some of the regulations now imposed on conventional food operations. The Food Safety Modernization Law of 2011 included a new "produce rule" that tightened safety requirements on all growers with sales above

$25,000 a year, but advocates for local food secured an exemption from these requirements for farms relying primarily on direct sales to individuals, restaurants, and retail establishments within 275 miles of the farm.

Restaurants that try to source locally can incur higher food safety risks. The Chipotle chain, which originally built its brand around the promise of fresh, local ingredients, suffered losses in 2015 following outbreaks of E. coli, Norovirus, and salmonella; it happened again in 2017, when over 135 customers reported Norovirus illness, then again in 2018, when 100 people fell ill after eating at a Chipotle in Ohio. John Quelch, from the Harvard Business School, describes such problems this way:

> Local sourcing adds complexity, increases risk and fragments the supply chain. Even if you have a standard quality control procedure for all of your sources, you're not going to be able to monitor them on-site at every location. You're going to have to put your trust in the suppliers to live up to the expectations laid down in the quality control guidelines.

Food service chains that source nationally—like McDonald's or KFC—may get their chicken from a distant Tyson plant, but their own inspectors will be kept on-site continuously to maintain strict quality control. Some of this control is lost when chains try to source from multiple local suppliers.

Food safety concerns are frequently raised in response to the modern adoption of concentrated animal feeding operations (CAFOs), the "factory farms" that often house thousands of animals together in close confinement. These facilities deserve to be criticized for compromising the welfare of the animals, and also for putting human medicine at risk by feeding the animals too many antibiotics, yet compared to smaller, more local meat suppliers these CAFOs have not diminished food safety.

Meat from the muscle of livestock is of course prone to dangerous bacterial contamination if it comes into contact with the animal's hide, its manure, its intestinal tract, meat cutters, or the outside environment, but all this makes meat safety more of a slaughterhouse and packing plant problem than a CAFO problem. A 2008 Pew Charitable Trusts report, one that was otherwise critical of CAFOs, said this about food safety: "The potential advantage of [CAFOs] is that concentrated production and processing in fewer, larger facilities can result in improved product safety if regulations are properly instituted and vigilantly enforced."

Animal confinement also increases food safety by reducing animal interactions with the naturally occurring parasites and pathogens found in open environments. Tapeworm parasites were not eliminated from the meat supply in Europe and North America until small-scale pig rearing was replaced by confinement production. Between the 1940s and 1980s, better control of infections in modern pig farming also reduced the incidence of trichinosis in the United States, from four hundred clinical cases annually to sixty cases. The pathogen *T. gondii* was found in one out of five marketed hogs in the 1980s, but it has now been reduced by over 90 percent. Dr. Rodney Baker, a former president of the American Association of Swine Veterinarians, asserts, "By bringing the animals indoors and creating biosecurity, we've truly eliminated about 15 diseases and parasites we had back to the 1980s."

Likewise for other animal products. According to the USDA, the presence of E. coli O157:H7 in fresh ground beef has declined 63 percent since 2000, down to only one-third of 1 percent. Salmonella on chicken meat declined by one-fifth, and on fresh pork by 63 percent. Listeria monocytogenes declined by 74 percent on ready-to-eat meat and poultry products. Relocalizing livestock production would put some of these safety gains at risk.

Some suburbanites today, wanting to know more about where their food comes from, have begun raising chickens and ducks in the backyard, both for eggs and meat. Due to inadequate training and little or no regulation, these birds can quickly become a health risk.

Backyard poultry farming is one reason annual salmonella infections have been on the rise, with 961 known illnesses in forty-eight states over one nine-month period in 2017, leaving more than two hundred people hospitalized.

A dvocates for local food also claim it is better for the environment, since moving food over a shorter distance will require less burning of transport fuel. This "food miles" argument cannot stand up to careful scrutiny. Two Canadian researchers, Pierre Desrochers and Hiroko Shimizu, show that the total consumption of transport fuel, per pound of food delivered, depends far more on load size and mode of travel than on the distance traveled. Foods shipped in bulk by ocean freight will generate only a tiny carbon footprint per pound, no matter how far they travel, while small loads of food hauled about in a car or a pickup truck will always have a large footprint per pound even over a short driving distance. One calculation found that UK consumers who drive six miles in a personal car to buy green beans flown in from Africa will actually emit more carbon dioxide per bean than the aircraft bringing them in 4,200 miles from Nairobi.

For climate protection, how food is grown matters far more than how far it travels, or even how it travels. Of all the carbon dioxide attributable to food in the United States, 83 percent reflects what is happening on the farm, compared to only a 4 percent share attributable to transport from producer to retailer. Local tomatoes produced in a heated greenhouse generate almost four times as much carbon per pound compared to imported tomatoes grown outdoors.

A relocalization of our food system would also harm the environment by increasing land and chemical use. Bringing in food from a distance allows farms to locate where the fewest resources are needed to produce a crop. The state of Idaho has warm days and cool nights, so the yields for russet potatoes there are twice as high per acre as in Alabama. Trying to meet all of Alabama's potato needs with local production would thus require a substantial net expansion of cultivated land, a bad environmental outcome. According to one estimate based on forty major field crops and vegetables, if each state had to grow the quantity of these crops required by its own population, land use for crops nationally would have to increase by sixty million acres, an area the size of the state of Oregon. Total fertilizer and chemical use would also have to increase. Another estimate done by scientists at Michigan State University found that if Michigan decided to supply all of its own beef, broiler chickens, and eggs from in-state production, it would have to increase its current cropland, pastureland, and forage land area by half.

W endell Berry was correct to observe that buying food from local farms can bring important social benefits. Surveys confirm that farmers market patrons have more frequent personal interactions when shopping, not just with the farmers selling the food but also with other shoppers. Michael Pollan has described it well:

> Money-for-food is not the only transaction going on at the farmers' markets; indeed, it may be the least of it. Neighbors are talking to neighbors. Consumers meet producers. (Confirming the obvious, one social scientist found that people have 10 times as many conversations at the farmers' market as they do at the supermarket.) City meets country. Kids discover what food is. Activists circulate petitions. The farmers' market has become the country's liveliest new public square, an outlet for our communitarian impulses and a means of escaping, or at least complicating, the narrow role that capitalism usually assigns to us as "consumers." At the farmers' market, we are consumers, yes, but at the same time also citizens, neighbors, parents and cooks.

If this kind of shopping is to scale up, America's large cohort of millennials (born between 1981 and 1996) will have to take the lead. Farmers market and CSA shopping is said to appeal to this group, as it counteracts the feelings of disconnection associated with spending so much time online. Buying food face-to-face from a local farmer offers a welcome relief from sitting in isolation, staring at a glowing screen. Amory Starr, a sociologist at the University of California, Santa Barbara, has argued that "both CSAs and farmers' markets evoke abandonment of anonymous, defensive distance and entry into a trusting, convivial, neighborly conversation." She says the "cosmology "of the local food movement is one of food as a community, not a commodity. Of course we can't really "know our farmer" from fleeting encounters at a market, but a face-to-face interaction of any kind, with eye contact and an exchange of words, will bring more social satisfaction than pushing a cart at a supermarket alone, taking products off the shelf in silence.

Millennials may want social reconnection and authenticity, but it seems they also want convenience, so even before COVID-19 a growing number were shopping online rather than in person. Click-and-collect online locations at supermarkets grew more than 200 percent in 2018, and direct delivery offerings grew 500 percent. For tech-savvy shoppers, getting groceries in the future may involve no personal interactions at all. The move will be: "Alexa, order me bananas, Honey Nut Cheerios, and a loaf of bread." Many more meals are now being ordered and delivered in this "frictionless" fashion, especially since the COVID-19 experience. Students at the University of California at Berkeley—who technically qualify as Gen Z—are now summoning burrito lunches through Kiwi Campus, a local start-up that uses robots to deliver. The robots are preferred for reasons of hygiene, and because they don't expect a tip.

In any case, sales from farmers markets appear to have peaked nationally. In one multistate survey in the Northeast reported by Cornell University in 2019, 44 percent of the farmers and market managers responding indicated sales were down from 20 percent to 70 percent compared to peak sales. In my own neighborhood, the Copley Square Farmers Market in Boston reported a 50 percent drop in attendance in 2017. Some farmers markets even fall short on the claim of being genuinely local. In 2016 a food critic from the *Tampa Bay Times* published a seven-part exposé (titled "Farm to Fable") revealing that a number of local food claims were simply bogus. The critic Laura Reiley found local farmers markets selling produce that came from Mexico, Honduras, and Canada, and "gulf shrimp" that came in frozen from India.

Despite the many reasons not to relocalize, a surprising number of funders continue to promote the local food idea. We should expect city governments and chambers of commerce to advocate for local food as simple boosterism, but larger private foundations and even some state and federal government agencies are now doing so as well.

As one example, the state of Rhode Island has been trying to promote local farms by purchasing farmland at the appraised market value and then selling parcels back to aspiring local farmers at an 80 percent discount. Rhode Island has the most expensive farmland in the country, so this will be a costly program, but supporters say they want the state to be producing half of its own food by 2060. This is magical thinking, since Rhode Island currently produces only 1 percent of its food. Philanthropic foundations also provide money to help finance local Food Policy Councils (FPCs) that seek to revitalize local farms and food markets. The Jena and Michael King Foundation supports FPCs at the city, county, and regional level, and as of 2016 there were 263 FPCs in operation across America, compared to just 167 five years earlier.

During the presidency of Barack Obama, the federal government also became a strong champion for local food. This has happened before, for different reasons. Washington strongly promoted home gardening during both world wars, to free up commercial food production for export to Allied countries fighting in Europe. During the First World War, President Woodrow Wilson even created a School Garden Army, funded by the War Department, to mobilize children as "soldiers of the soil," and during the Second World War the Department of Agriculture promoted home "victory gardens" to help hold down the domestic price of vegetables. First Lady Eleanor

104   RESETTING THE TABLE

Roosevelt set an example by planting a kitchen garden on the White House lawn. By 1944, an estimated twenty million victory gardens were supplying more than 40 percent of all the fresh fruits and vegetables consumed in the country.

When the war ended, market forces took over again and local food production resumed its long-term decline. By 1971 it had declined so much that geographer Jayne Pyle published an article saying farmers markets might soon disappear. Pyle called them "Functional Anachronisms," and predicted they would continue to exist only if special protections and subsidies were provided by public agencies.

Sure enough, such subsidies were soon provided. Congress passed a Farmer-to-Consumer Direct Marketing Act in 1976 instructing the USDA to offer funds to states supporting farmers markets and to train more market managers. The central purpose at this time was not to provide "local food" to consumers but to help small growers who were being squeezed out of wholesale markets by large modern suppliers from states like California. This congressional measure did briefly revive some farmers market sales, but the Reagan administra-

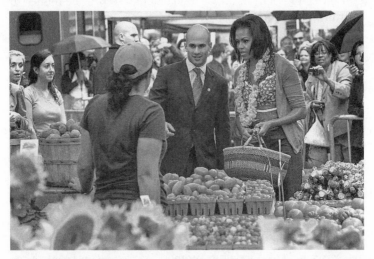

First Lady Michelle Obama, accompanied by her White House chef, promotes local food by shopping at a newly opened farmers market two blocks from the White House in 2009.

tion curtailed funding in the 1980s, and sales did not revive again until federal help was restored during the Obama administration.

President Obama's policies were also intended as help for small farmers, but the dominant theme now was getting fresh, locally grown foods to quality-conscious consumers. Prodded by Alice Waters, First Lady Michelle Obama planted an organic vegetable garden on the White House lawn and helped establish a farmers market two blocks from the White House. The Department of Agriculture then launched a "Know Your Farmer, Know Your Food" program, led by Deputy Secretary Kathleen Merrigan, who had earlier helped develop the USDA's organic certification system. Under Merrigan's leadership, the Obama administration made the promotion of local and regional food systems one of the "four pillars" of its rural development strategy, and it eventually funneled more than a billion dollars in grants to infrastructure projects for local food, and to more than forty thousand local and regional food businesses. The USDA's Agricultural Marketing Service developed the Farmers Market Promotion Program and the Local Food Promotion Program, while the Food and Nutrition Service created the Farm to School Grant Program, the Senior Farmers' Market Nutrition Program, and the WIC Farmers' Market Nutrition Program.

Democrats have always been more eager to promote local food than Republicans. The Farm to School Grant program was originally created in 2004, but money was not provided until Obama reached the White House. In 2013, when a Local Farms, Food, and Jobs Act was introduced into the House by Democrat Chellie Pingree of Maine it got zero Republican votes and failed. When Republicans gained control of both branches of government after the 2016 election, federal support for local food was dealt another blow. Alice Waters, invoking the French Resistance, vowed to fight on:

> Now is not the time. We're like the French underground. We are passing notes to each other. But soon there will be something, an event, and we will come forward together. No one knows how powerful we are. We are vigilantes.

Federal support for local food continues to depend heavily on a transactional political relationship between elected Democrats and a support base made up of small farmers, food activists, and local communities, so it waxes and wanes nationally with the fortunes of the Democratic Party. This keeps the funding modest and uncertain, which explains some of the equally modest market impact.

One surprising expression of the recent urge to relocalize food has been enthusiasm for urban agriculture. Growing food in cities goes against conventional economic logic, but at least it's not driven by nostalgia. Rather than imagining an improbable return to our agrarian past, today's urban farming pioneers are genuine innovators, and they are developing production systems never seen before. The vision is nonetheless an improbable one, since it collides with a powerful marketplace logic in favor of sourcing food where it can be produced at least cost.

One urban farming thrust is primarily social rather than commercial: community gardens created on abandoned properties and vacant lots in hollowed-out industrial cities. Another thrust has emphasized technical innovation: finding ways to produce greens on urban rooftops, devising hydroponic growing tanks in abandoned factory buildings, growing vegetables under LED lights inside shipping containers in parking lots, and stacking up greenhouse-like systems as a form of "vertical" farming. The enthusiasm has been contagious, yet economists see only limited potential. Carolyn Dimitri at New York University predicted bluntly in 2015 that agriculture in cities "isn't going to make a dent. And it's completely inefficient, economically."

The market signals are strong and clear. Production costs in urban settings are much higher than in the countryside because both land and labor are far more expensive. Within urban centers holding more than one million residents, land costs are thirty times as high as rural areas with only small towns. Urban farms can make sense as community development activities, but only if municipal authorities are willing to make land that is unused or abandoned available at virtually no cost. Even then, and even with financial support from philanthropic foundations and city budgets, urban gardens and farms produce very little food.

In hollowed-out Detroit, space has been found for thirteen hundred neighborhood gardens, and by 2014 these projects were growing four hundred thousand pounds of produce, which sounds like a lot but it was only enough to feed six hundred people, or one-half person per garden. In New Jersey, the city of Camden has forty-four community garden sites that produce enough to feed about five hundred people every day during the growing season, which is more than ten people per site, but this is still just a tiny number in a city of eighty thousand. The primary purpose of these gardens is not to grow food but to nurture community leadership, teach cooperation and discipline, and keep young people out of trouble.

These gardens survive thanks to uncompensated labor, rent-free city land, and generous foundation support. One report from a private funders' network in 2011 stated candidly, "Foundation funding is critical to the social and economic stability of urban agriculture." Among the foundations chipping in are the Claneil Foundation, the Cedar Tree Foundation, the McGregor Fund, the W. K. Kellogg Foundation, the William Penn Foundation, and the Geraldine R. Dodge Foundation.

In Pittsburgh the Hillman Foundation funds the twenty-three-acre Hilltop Farm located in a low-income housing neighborhood. In East Baltimore, the American Communities Trust has developed a $17 million "Baltimore Food Hub" with federal, state, and local funding. It will have a three-and-a-half-acre "campus" of food system facilities, including a "culinary social enterprise workforce program" and a "kitchen incubator." Charity-driven community development operations of this kind deliver valuable benefits to the participants even when they don't relocalize much food production.

In Detroit since 2010, RecoveryPark Farms has transformed a twenty-two-block area into a complex of self-heating hoop houses that grow leafy greens, herbs, and exotic vegetables for high-end restaurants. Some of the restaurants are two hundred miles away, so the eating isn't always local, but the central purpose is to provide gainful employment at eleven dollars an hour, with full health benefits, to ex-convicts and people in recovery from substance abuse. The project survives thanks to rent-free land access, a million-dollar grant from a private foundation, and bridge financing from a $400,000 state grant.

Promoting community gardens on vacant lots is far more difficult in places like New York City or San Francisco where property values are extremely high. During New York's financial crisis in the 1970s, when numerous buildings were being abandoned or torn down, the city was willing to lease empty land for as little as one dollar a year to those wishing to plant gardens. This arrangement was formalized into a GreenThumb program in 1978, funded by community development block grants from the federal government. In the 1990s, the economy recovered, land values shot up, and the city began selling the community garden sites to developers for commercial or residential use. Defenders of the gardens then mobilized and persuaded the city to preserve about four hundred sites, but a continuing real estate boom has slowed garden expansion. GreenThumb continues, but it requires several million dollars each year in public support to pay professional staff, finance training, and provide free plants, shovels, and wheelbarrows.

Urban gardening also requires public assistance in San Francisco, where wealthy landowners get some of the benefit stream. Under San Francisco's Urban Agriculture Incentive Zones Act, owners of million-dollar city lots can reduce their tax assessment to just $12,500 an acre—the same low rate that is extended to "irrigated farmland"—if they rent to gardeners. Cultural enthusiasm for local food has encouraged numerous tax breaks of this kind. The state of Maryland in 2010 authorized the mayor and the city council of Baltimore to grant tax credits to urban agricultural property. In 2011, New Jersey authorized property tax exemptions for public properties that were sold or leased to nonprofits for gardening or urban farming. In 2013 the state of Missouri authorized the establishment of Urban Agricultural Zones (UAZs), where no property taxes would be assessed for twenty-five years. Even Congress gives support to urban

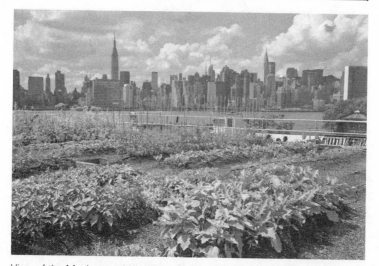

View of the Manhattan skyline from the Eagle Street Rooftop Farm.

farming, through a USDA Office of Urban Agriculture it created as part of the 2018 farm bill.

Most urban farming nonetheless remains subcommercial in nature. A survey in 2013 found that one-third of urban farms remained not-for-profit, 20 percent were growing all of their products for donation, and 60 percent of the primary operators on these urban farms relied not on market sales for their income, but on fundraising, grant funding, or off-farm work. The commercial for-profit food economy will continue to rely almost entirely on rural farming.

A few prominent for-profit efforts have been made in cities, usually by growers finding space to plant in greenhouses, on rooftops, or inside abandoned industrial buildings. Brooklyn Grange is a for-profit rooftop farm that grows greens and other vegetables for sale through its own CSA plus local farm stands and restaurants. It also earns money by offering training programs for beekeepers ($850 summer tuition) and by renting its garden spaces—which have spectacular views of the Manhattan skyline—for weddings and private dinners. Brooklyn Grange also makes use of labor from "interns" who agree to work without pay.

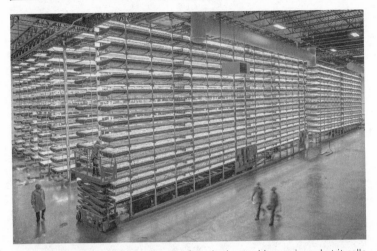

AeroFarms, the largest indoor vertical farm in the world, growing what it calls "Dream Greens" on stacked trays inside a former steel mill in Newark, New Jersey.

Other entrepreneurs have experimented with fully contained growing systems employing hydroponics, aquaponics, or vertically stacked greenhouses. These efforts require high initial investment and continuing energy costs for heating and artificial lighting, and they usually produce only fast-growing, high-value microgreens, winter tomatoes, or herbs. The largest indoor vertical farm in the world is AeroFarms, a seventy-thousand-square-foot operation that started seeding in 2016, located in a former steel mill in Newark, New Jersey. A warehouse operation in Chicago named FarmedHere found the costs were too high and had to close early in 2017. Another high-profile failure was a vertical farm in downtown Vancouver that went bankrupt in 2014, unable to pay $4 million in debts to its creditors. This farm had an innovative design that included stacked growing trays for greens and herbs that moved under automation to maximize natural light exposure. The buyer of the bankrupt property planned to operate it not as a business but as a tourist attraction, to "have something pretty for the city, so we could brag about what we did."

High-profile investors nonetheless remain fascinated by new

designs for fully contained urban food production systems. Kimbal Musk, the younger brother of Elon, the Tesla Motors billionaire, funded ten young entrepreneurs to grow greens and herbs hydroponically in shipping containers in a parking lot in Brooklyn. Musk's ambitious goal is to perfect the system in Brooklyn then roll it out "everywhere." Elon is probably aware of the financial risks, since one of his advisers is the former CEO of FarmedHere, the urban farm that failed in Chicago. One innovator at MIT, Caleb Harper, received millions of dollars in corporate sponsorships to develop fully contained "food computers" that would nurture crops inside precisely controlled environments. In the fall of 2019 MIT shut down the project upon learning that some of the showcase plants supposedly grown inside these structures had actually been bought in stores.

Economic studies of commercial-scale urban farms continue to tell a discouraging story. One study by city planners from Cornell University examined ten farms in New York City. It found these farms were primarily producing leafy greens with only moderate nutritional value, and the greens were being sold at prices only upscale consumers could afford. The few jobs they provided were mostly entry-level and frequently paid less than a living wage. The indoor farms that used LEDs were not as energy efficient as conventional soil-based farms growing similar items outdoors. Total costs were high because urban real estate is expensive in New York. Renting ten thousand square feet for an indoor farm costs more than $300,000 a year.

Some ambitious urban farming schemes never quite get off the drawing board. The "Plantagon," a vertical greenhouse to be built in Linkoping, Sweden, won the "innovator idol" prize for design in 2009, but a decade later construction had yet to begin. The developers were modifying the design to include commercial office space, a more realistic use for expensive urban real estate.

CHAPTER 4

The Panic for Organic

At a recent dinner party, the hostess served me a tasty salad with carrots, raisins, nuts, and baby greens. "It's all organic," she said, expecting my approval. To be polite, I smiled and said nothing, but a voice inside wanted to respond, You paid too much.

Nearly half of all Americans claim to prefer organic food, and the label has spread far beyond food. You can now buy organic lipstick, organic underwear, and even organic water. The 2019 Super Bowl featured ads for organic beer, and health-conscious smokers are able to purchase organic cigarettes. Most farmers, however, have little interest in switching to the more costly and less convenient production methods required for organic certification, so this constrains the supply, making organic food expensive. America's farmers so far have certified less than 1 percent of their cropland for organic production, and fewer than 2 percent of commodities grown in 2017 were organic. Processed and packaged foods can also be organic, but fewer than 6 percent of total retail food purchases are certified organic products. Two decades after federal organic certification began in America, the brand remains a single-digit phenomenon.

Farmers tend to hold back because producing food organically requires more human labor to handle the composted animal manure used for fertilizer, as well as more labor to control weeds without chemicals (sometimes putting down nonbiodegradable plastic mulch instead). It also requires more land for every bushel of production, further driving up costs. Trying to grow all of our food organically today would require farming a much wider area, damaging wildlife habitat. Rachel Carson, the founder of our modern environmental movement, never endorsed organic farming. Her 1962 book *Silent Spring* did condemn synthetic insecticides like DDT, but Carson saw no reason to ban manufactured fertilizers, as the organic standard requires.

The rules for organic farming do deliver some clear benefit in the livestock sector. Producers of organic meat, milk, and eggs are required to provide their animals with more space to move around, an important plus for animal welfare. Also, animal products cannot be labeled organic if the animals were fed or treated with antibiotics, which is good for slowing the emergence of resistant bacterial strains dangerous to human health. Yet even for livestock the organic rule malfunctions, since the animals can only be given feeds grown organically, and organic corn and soy have much lower yields per acre, so more land must be planted and plowed.

Consumers tend to favor organic food because they believe the claims that it is safer and more nutritious to eat, but there is little or no scientific evidence to support these claims. Others buy organic food because they assume it comes from farms that are smaller, more traditional, and more diverse, but this is not a safe assumption either. Most organic food on the market today comes from highly specialized, industrial-scale farms, not so different from those that produce conventional food.

It doesn't usually pay to challenge popular beliefs, even with scientific evidence, but some have felt compelled to do so in the case of organic agriculture. Louise O. Fresco, trained as an agronomist, is the president of Wageningen University in the Netherlands, the world's leading agricultural university. In her 2016 book *Hamburgers in Paradise*, she drew a harsh conclusion: "Organic farming as a whole is a mish-mash of valuable goals and ideals that have either been insufficiently tested or are completely misguided."

Scientists like Fresco view the organic vision as fundamentally misguided because it depends on an ungrounded distinction between materials that come from nature versus those fabricated by human industry. Organic farmers are permitted to treat their crops with the former, but not the latter. The organic rule says we can use nitrogen from animal manure to replace soil nutrients, but not nitrogen synthesized from the atmosphere in a factory. Chemists find no merit in this distinction. No matter what method we use to get a supply of nitrogen for use as fertilizer, it will be the same element within the periodic table, with all the same chemical properties.

Visions that privilege what comes from nature over what is made by people have a mystical appeal, but they malfunction as practical guidance. Nature is often alluring and attractive, yet natural materials can be anything but safe. Arsenic, nickel, and chromium are all dangerous carcinogens, and all come from nature. Many plants that are found in nature contain dangerous poisons, ranging from the deadly ricin found in castor beans (familiar to fans of *Breaking Bad*) to the itch-inducing urushiol in common poison ivy. Microbes from nature have given us malaria, HIV, tuberculosis, botulism, tetanus, and now COVID-19. Mother Nature has also provided us with deadly ice ages, volcanoes, earthquakes, tsunamis, and asteroids.

By focusing on natural versus synthetic, the organic rule loses sight of actual risks. Copper sulfate is permitted as a fungicide because it isn't synthetic, but careless use of this chemical can leave dangerous residues on food and pollute our streams. Animal manure is natural, and an excellent fertilizer when composted, but dangerous bacteria will be introduced into fields and also into groundwater systems if a farmer fails to get the heat in the compost pile up to at least 140 degrees. A close friend with a field of organic blueberries on her hilltop farm in Maine developed serious stomach problems when she located her compost pile too close to the well.

The biggest weakness in the organic rule is *absolutism*. Cutting back on the use of manufactured fertilizer is frequently a good idea, but the idea of cutting back to zero is needlessly rigid and absolute. It becomes a particularly strange quest for purity when it leads to a use of animal manure instead. Quests for purity in food and farming are not as dangerous as they have been in race or religion, but they are just as lacking in scientific justification, and the advocates can be just as exasperating. Calvin Trillin put it nicely: "The price of purity is purists."

Of course, scientific purists can also be exasperating. Michael Specter, in a hard-hitting book critical of science denial, classified organic food as little more than a social fetish. This goes too far. Most who pay more to purchase organic food are not fetishists; they are following a sincere conviction that this food is better for nutrition, better for food safety, or better for the environment. Sincere convictions deserve respect, but in this case they also demand scrutiny.

The conviction that organic food is a better choice did not become widespread in the United States until the 1980s, when national media were calling attention to a number of food safety scares linked to pesticide residues on fresh fruits and vegetables. When consumers learned that organic farming methods did not allow the use of any synthetic pesticides (although naturally occurring poisons could be used), they demanded more organic products, along with a credible national system for certifying and labeling those products in the marketplace. Once this system began to operate in 2002, the farmers who had switched to organic methods could capture sizable price premiums for their goods, and this motivated rapid growth in the sector, but only up to a point.

After two decades of popularity with consumers, the organic share still makes up only a small part of America's national diet. The most popular organic produce choices today are carrots, lettuce, and apples, yet they take up only 14, 12, and 5 percent of total acreage for these crops. Only 3 percent of U.S. dairy cows and just 2 percent of layer hens are certified organic. As for field crops, here the organic share of production is even less significant: In 2016, only six-tenths of 1 percent of total harvested wheat acres in the United States were farmed organically.

Consumers pay considerably more for organic. In 2018, the Food Marketing Institute reported that the average retail price (by volume) for organic produce was 54 percent higher than for conventional produce. One USDA study showed that organic salad mix cost

60 percent more than conventional; organic milk 72 percent more; and organic eggs 82 percent more. Organic corn and soybeans sell for twice as much as conventional. These are high premiums, but not high enough to move most farmers toward organic, because the farming costs required by organic methods can be higher still. The organic market segment remains small because so few commercial farmers convert.

There is nothing novel about producing foods without the use of any synthetic chemicals. Before science first made these chemicals available to farmers early in the twentieth century, all of the foods ever grown worldwide were de facto organic. When synthetic nitrogen first became available for fertilizer, the farmers who began using it saved on labor and enjoyed higher crop yields so uptake spread. The timing for this innovation was fortunate, since the Earth's population was about to increase from two billion up to nearly eight billion today. Vaclav Smil, from the University of Manitoba, has estimated that without nitrogen fertilizer, 40 percent of the increase in food production needed to feed these much larger numbers would never have taken place. For at least a third of humanity in the world's most populous countries, the use of nitrogen fertilizer in the twentieth century made the difference between an adequate diet and malnutrition.

The organic farming idea was launched as a pushback against the use of synthetic nitrogen fertilizer, but as such it never gained wide popular support. That support did not emerge until decades later, following a wave of public concern over synthetic pesticides, and the residues of those pesticides on foods. The original prohibition against synthetic fertilizers remained part of the rule, however, so most farmers were not willing to ride even the second wave. It is a history worth retelling.

Organic farming was born from a mystical heritage, one that it has never quite been able to shed. In 1909, two German chemists, Fritz Haber and Carl Bosch, perfected an industrial method for synthesizing ammonia from the atmosphere, giving farmers a new source of nitrogen to correct soil nutrient deficits. This new approach was rejected by an Austrian philosopher named Rudolf Steiner (1861–1925), who believed the nitrogen used for growing food should come from nature rather than an industrial process. Industrial nitrogen, he argued, would lack a mystical life force.

Steiner was neither a scientist nor a farmer. He began his career as a Goethe scholar, but then developed his own school of thought called anthroposophical spiritual science. He embraced the tradition of "vitalism," a prescientific view which held that life could only be nourished by the products of other living things. This belief, implicitly stipulating the existence of two completely separate spheres of chemistry, was disproven in 1828 when the Wöhler laboratory synthesis successfully created an organic compound from an inorganic compound, but Steiner's thinking was not constrained by laboratory science. Never an empiricist, he was a believer in human reincarnation, the lost world of Atlantis, and also in an earlier lost continent named Lemuria.

Steiner did not want to use synthetic chemical fertilizers in farming because they lacked "biodynamic" force. He explained all this in a series of agricultural lectures in 1924 based on cosmic reference points. The forces from Mars, Jupiter, and Saturn were said to have a silicious nature, with important implications for life on earth, while forces from the Moon, Mercury, and Venus were said to work via their limestone nature. Based on such precepts, Steiner prescribed the best way to improve soil fertility: farmers should infuse cosmic life forces into the soil by placing properly prepared animal manures (prepared, for example, with yarrow flowers and chamomile blossoms) into the horn of a cow, then bury it in the ground. Why the horn of a cow? The explanation is provided in his fourth lecture:

Thus in the horn you have something well adapted by its inherent nature, to ray back the living and astral properties into the inner life. In the horn you have something radiating life—nay, even radiating astrality. It is so indeed: if you could crawl about inside the living body of a cow—if you were there inside the belly of the cow—you would smell how the astral life and the living vitality pours inward from the horns. And so it is also with the hoofs.

Followers inspired by this thinking formed a German "Association of Anthroposophical Farmers" after Steiner's death and created a formal institution called Demeter to certify the farms using genuinely "biodynamic" methods. It was not a large movement, but Germany did claim roughly one thousand biodynamic farms by 1931. As an embarrassing footnote, the movement later received strong backing from a number of top officials in the Nazi Party. A Steiner protégé founded the Reich League for Biodynamic Agriculture in 1933, supported by Nazi functionaries in the German ministry of agriculture. Rudolf Hess, Hitler's deputy führer, even planted a biodynamic garden in his villa, and Berlin's athletic fields for the 1936 summer Olympics were also treated biodynamically. Networks of biodynamic plantations would even be established in German concentration camps.

Germany's party leaders who listened to agricultural experts, and to the chemical industry, fought back against the anthroposophists, accusing them of following "occult doctrines." Biodynamic farming nonetheless had some propaganda value because it was distinctly German, or at least Austrian, and it fit well with the Nazi blood and soil ideology. In more practical terms, some even hoped it could reduce Germany's dependence on imported fertilizer.

The movement spread in a much smaller way to the United States, where the Biodynamic Association (BDA) was founded in 1938, and still survives. The BDA considers itself the oldest sustainable agriculture nonprofit organization on the North American continent and currently claims more than twelve hundred member farmers, gardeners, entrepreneurs, and consumers. In 2016, nearly eight hundred of these members, from forty-six states plus twenty other countries and six continents, gathered for that year's North American Biodynamic Conference in New Mexico.

The idea of avoiding synthetic chemicals in farming also gained early support among England's landed aristocracy. An English translation of Steiner's lectures, titled *The Agricultural Course,* had been published in 1928, while an English agronomist named Albert Howard (1873–1947) was working in India on a parallel track to develop his own case against the new manufactured fertilizers. Howard's more legitimate credentials allowed him eventually to eclipse Steiner as the world's foremost advocate for organic farming.

Howard was raised on a farm, educated at Cambridge, taught agricultural science, and then for twenty-six years was sent out to direct agricultural research centers in colonial India, not returning to England until 1931. Chemical fertilizers were scarcely available in India, so Howard worked to perfect methods for building soil nutrients based on organic waste, including composted manures, human as well as animal. Howard named his composting system the Indore method, and after returning to England he continued to champion this approach, even though most scientists by then were embracing manufactured fertilizers as a better way to correct nitrogen, phosphorus, and potassium deficits in the soil.

Chemical understandings of soil fertility did not appeal to Howard, who focused on biology instead. In part, he viewed synthetic fertilizers as simply unnecessary, since he thought healthy soils, by themselves, could become "factories" for crop nutrients, enough he thought to feed the world. Howard was willing to consider the use of some mineral fertilizers such as pulverized rock, as long as they were sourced from nature, but not "artificial" fertilizers. He gradually became more rigid on these matters and argued for organic compost even when synthetic fertilizers did a better job of correcting specific soil nutrient limitations.

Despite his training and skills as an agricultural scientist, Howard retained a strong mystical attraction to natural systems. In his influential 1943 book *An Agricultural Testament,* he described "Nature's farming" as an ideal:

The main characteristic of Nature's farming can therefore be summed up in a few words. Mother earth never attempts to

> farm without live stock; she always raises mixed crops; great
> pains are taken to preserve the soil and to prevent erosion; the
> mixed vegetable and animal wastes are converted into humus;
> there is no waste; the processes of growth and the processes of
> decay balance one another; ample provision is made to maintain
> large reserves of fertility; the greatest care is taken to store the
> rainfall; both plants and animals are left to protect themselves
> against disease.

Howard viewed nature as an abundant Garden of Eden, one with a harmonious internal balance (assuming we ignore Darwinian competition). Nature can indeed produce abundance on its own, but most natural vegetative growth cannot deliver nutrition through the human stomach. To sustain a burgeoning human population it became necessary, early on, for people to domesticate the plants and animals found in nature and then alter them through selective breeding. None of our staple food crops today, including wheat, rice, and corn, ever existed in their present form in nature. Modern corn was developed beginning about nine thousand years ago from Mexico's wild teosinte grass, which carried an "ear" only one-tenth the size of corn today. Nature's farming thus needed considerable help from humans long before Haber and Bosch gave us synthetic nitrogen.

Disease played an important role in Howard's thinking. He believed that diseases in plants and animals, including humans, were caused by "unhealthy" soils. Disease could only be eradicated by healing the soil through a recycling of organic matter, just like in nature. Howard believed manufactured chemicals were a violation of this natural principle, one that gave us worn-out soils, erosion, and an increase in diseases of all kinds. Howard saw the premodern peasant farmers of Asia as doing a better job of approximating nature's ideal:

> The agricultural practices of the Orient have passed the supreme
> test—they are almost as permanent as those of the primeval for-
> est, of the prairie or of the ocean. The small-holdings of China,

for example, are still maintaining a steady output and there is no loss of fertility after forty centuries of management.

In reality, the farming systems of China or India in Howard's day were falling far short. Colonial India was a land where unimproved farming brought both crushing rural poverty and frequent famine. During Howard's own time, India's food grain production was in steady decline, even as population continued to increase. One reason for India's poor agricultural performance was a depletion of soil nutrients, a problem synthetic nitrogen fertilizers could have helped to address.

Even though Howard's thinking was out of step with modern science, it proved appealing to England's landed gentry. Gerard Wallop (1898–1984), the Ninth Earl of Portsmouth, also known as the Viscount of Lymington, was a Conservative member of Parliament and also a stalwart member of the imperialist India Defence League. Wallop embraced a reactionary "back to the land" philosophy and liked Howard's advice on composting because it would demand more labor on farms, thus keeping workers tethered to the land. Wallop became friends with Howard in 1935 and secured his assistance in writing a 1938 book called *Famine in England*. One critic later provided a telling summary:

> Wallop powerfully combined an angry and at times unpleasant and anti-Semitic critique of British economic policies and their impact on farming and rural life with promotion of a protectionist, nostalgia-driven vision of the future that incorporated adoption of organic techniques to protect and enhance soil fertility. *Famine in England* was a highly successful book, attracting widespread critical praise and discussion.

Another English aristocrat influenced both by Howard and Wallop was Lady Eve Balfour (1898–1990), the niece of a former prime minister and daughter of the Earl of Balfour. In 1946, Balfour cofounded

England's Soil Association, which remains the principal organic farming organization in Great Britain. On her own farm, she began a long-term experiment (the Haughley Experiment, later taken over by the Soil Association) intended to demonstrate the superiority of organic versus chemical-based farming. She also wrote a 1943 book, *The Living Soil,* which reiterated Howard's view that human health was in decline due to a decrease in plant health caused originally by poor soil health. Balfour also embraced extrasensory perception, and under her leadership the Soil Association became known for unconventional spiritualist activities, which is possibly one reason Albert Howard never joined.

The term *organic farming* was coined by yet another book-writing English aristocrat. Walter James, the fourth Baron Northbourne, published *Look to the Land* in 1940, showing himself to be a Steiner devotee by stating that the efficacy of biodynamic methods "may be said to be proved." Baron Northbourne was an unapologetic antimodernist, an active member of a group of thinkers troubled by the demise of traditional forms of knowledge in an increasingly science-based society. England's aristocracy had once made strong contributions to science in the eighteenth century, but by the twentieth century it had become firmly reactionary. To the present day organic farming holds a grip over the English ruling class. Prince Charles converted his own Duchy Home Farm to a completely organic system in 1986.

The organic farming message coming out of England was brought to the United States in the 1940s by an unlikely figure, the son of a Lower East Side grocer named Jerome (J. I.) Rodale (1889–1971), a publisher of popular books and magazines. Rodale came across Albert Howard's work in 1941 and said the message about healthy soil being a source of human health hit him like "a ton of bricks." In 1942 Rodale began publishing a magazine called *Organic Farming and Gardening,* having recruited Howard to be his associate editor. He then wrote a book of his own in 1945 titled *Pay Dirt,* and yet another in 1948 titled *The Organic Front.*

Not just a skeptic on modern agricultural science, Rodale was also suspicious of modern medicine. Not long after starting his *Organic Farming and Gardening* magazine, he launched a second periodical called *Prevention*, which promoted a mistrust of doctors and drugs. In one 1955 article, Rodale even questioned the value of the new polio vaccine, championing dietary cures instead. Preferring both food and medicine to be natural, he argued at one point that drinking artificially softened water could cause cancer. A parallel could be found in Steiner, who had believed that rosemary baths were better for diphtheria than a vaccine. Rodale himself lived a long and productive life but died of a sudden heart attack in 1971 during a taping of the Dick Cavett TV show, despite having just announced he'd never felt better.

Rodale's magazine influenced quite a few home gardeners in his day, but it did nothing to slow the increased use of synthetic fertilizers by commercial farmers. After the Second World War, munitions factories were repurposed to produce fertilizer, so the price of nitrogen dropped, encouraging much greater use. Between 1960 and 1980, inorganic nitrogen use on American farms more than quadrupled. The same thing was happening in England, where average nitrogen fertil-

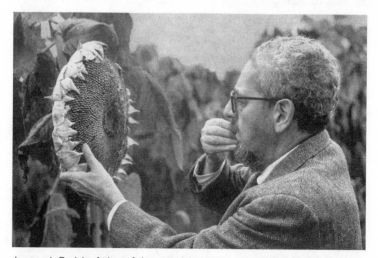

Jerome I. Rodale, father of the organic movement in the United States, sampling a sunflower seed.

izer dressings for winter wheat more than tripled between 1950 and 1980.

Rodale dismissed this as "chemical farming," but the charge was never entirely fair since in addition to using manufactured fertilizers, commercial farmers continued to rotate crops, plant cover crops, and spread animal manure. No American crop farm in the 1960s was complete without a mechanical manure spreader, and even now commercial farmers continue to rotate crops. In the American Midwest, well more than a third of all fields growing corn in one year will have grown some other crop—often soybeans, a legume that fixes nitrogen into the soil naturally—in the previous year. This use of multiple tools, known as integrated soil fertility management, is what works best.

The rigid organic standard, which allowed no synthetic chemicals at all, became even less advantageous once plant breeders began developing new crop varieties capable of using nitrogen with greater efficiency, which brought a still larger payoff from fertilizer use. In 1940, the average corn yield in the United States had been thirty bushels an acre, but by 1960 it had increased to fifty-five bushels, and by 1980 to ninety-one bushels. John Nidlinger now gets more than two hundred bushels. For farmers experiencing gains like these, a reversion to nineteenth-century soil management techniques held little appeal. Organic farming was also a nonstarter for most commercial farms because of its high labor requirement at a time when the population on farms was falling from thirty million in 1940 down to less than five million by 1990.

Organic farming even failed to catch on during the period of environmental activism launched in the United States following Rachel Carson's 1962 book *Silent Spring*. This seems surprising, since the popular book argued strongly against the imprudent use of synthetic chemicals on farms. But *Silent Spring* was not focused on chemical fertilizers; it targeted the synthetic chemical pesticides then being used to kill insects and weeds.

Rachel Carson was an extremely private person, yet on one occasion she did allow an interviewer to ask, "What do you eat?" Her

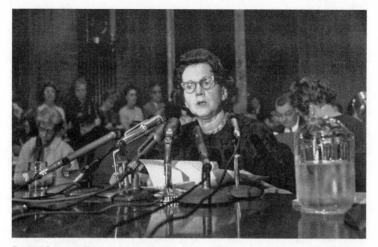

Rachel Carson offering congressional testimony in June 1963. She told a Senate committee, "I think chemicals do have a place."

sardonic answer: "Chlorinated hydrocarbons like everyone else." She was referring to a family of pesticides that included DDT, widely used at the time for insect control. These chemicals became pervasive in the environment and to varying degrees entered the human food supply. Her book highlighted their many risks to human health as well as the natural environment.

Carson was not a purist. Even for synthetic pesticides, she advocated a selective and restrained use, not complete disuse as the organic standard would require. In *Silent Spring* she said, "The ultimate answer is to use less toxic chemicals so that the public hazard from their misuse is greatly reduced." When Carson later testified before Congress in 1963, she said straight out, "I think chemicals do have a place."

When Carson's book became a sensational bestseller, advocates for organic farming were torn over how to respond. J. I. Rodale was jealous of Carson's celebrity, since he had criticized DDT two decades earlier but gotten little notice. He also faulted Carson for leaving synthetic fertilizers out of her argument. Rodale's son Robert, who by 1962 was editing their magazine, realized Carson was not on board with the strict organic rule, but he couldn't resist trying to depict her as a supporter. He hailed her book as a "masterpiece," and said it presented "the organic point of view."

Carson resisted this embrace, distancing herself from organic advocates. She refused to speak before organic advocacy groups and on one occasion even canceled out of an event after learning that J. I. Rodale had been booked on the same panel without her approval. Carson viewed Rodale as lacking scientific credentials and she had branded him "an eccentric." Carson did correspond with some Rudolf Steiner followers while researching her book on DDT, but opted not to acknowledge these contacts.

Carson tragically died of cancer just eighteen months after her book was published. When we look back on her legacy, she was on solid environmental grounds not to endorse organic farming, given the much larger land footprint organic methods would require. USDA data show that output on organic farms in the United States is on average one-fifth lower per acre than on conventional farms. From this difference, crop biologist Steven Savage calculated that replacing conventional production with organically grown crops would require cultivating an additional 109 million acres of land, an area equal to all parklands and wildlands combined in the lower forty-eight states. The resulting destruction of wildlife habitat would bring on a silent spring of a different kind.

For Carson and other early environmentalists, the enemy was pesticides, not fertilizers. *Silent Spring* had seventeen chapters, all on pesticides and none on fertilizers. Insecticides like DDT and herbicides like 2,4-D (an ancestor of Agent Orange) had become widely available to farmers after the Second World War, and between 1945 and 1972 pesticide use in the United States increased tenfold. This dangerous growth was put to an end by Carson's book, which triggered passage of the Environmental Protection Act in 1970, creating the new federal Environmental Protection Agency (EPA), which banned the agricultural use of DDT in 1972.

Other pesticides remained in use, yet human exposure to these chemicals has steadily fallen, thanks in part to increased federal regulation. In the 1950s and 1960s, regulations were put in place to set maximum allowable residue levels on foods while denying official registration to products deemed unsafe. In the 1970s, the EPA removed not just DDT but a number of other persistent pesticides from the market. In 1996 the Food Quality Protection Act set stricter standards and required a new review of allowable residue levels. In response to federal requirements such as these, the chemical industry worked to develop synthetic products less toxic to farmworkers and less persistent in the environment.

Pesticide risks have also been diminished thanks to integrated pest management (IPM), a crop protection technique that advises spraying only when monitored pest damage threatens a commercial loss, and only after nonchemical control options (for example, using good bugs to kill bad bugs) are no longer working. In this system, a judicious use of chemicals is nonetheless permitted, something the organic rule does not allow. New varieties of crops with better genetic defenses of their own against insects have also reduced insecticide use in America, and "smart" sprayers now apply chemicals at optimal rates and with far greater precision.

Thanks to all these things in combination, farmers in the United States have reduced pesticide use significantly since the 1970s. The total pounds of herbicide and insecticide ingredients applied to crops declined by 18 percent between 1980 and 2008, even as total crop production increased 46 percent. For insecticides specifically, total use peaked in 1972, and has now fallen more than 80 percent below that peak. All these gains were achieved without any significant switch to organic farming methods.

Pesticide use remains a contentious issue in the United States, partly because new concerns have arisen. One is a suspected risk to honeybees and other nontarget insects from a class of insecticides called neonicotinoids, known as neonics. These chemicals are less toxic to humans and other mammals, but they have been identified since 2006 as one possible contributing factor to a "colony collapse disorder" affecting honeybees, which, apart from their honey, are commercially vital to farmers as pollinators. The issue is complicated because there are other contributing factors to the disorder, including invasive varroa mites, changes to the habitat where bees forage, and the stress bees experience being transported to multiple locations.

New controversies have also emerged around glyphosate, an herbicide with the trade name Roundup. The first problem was an emergence of weeds that evolved a resistance to the chemical, which was predictable following decades of heavy use. This forced some farmers to switch to other herbicides. The second glyphosate problem was a finding in 2015 from the International Agency for Research on Cancer (IARC) that the chemical was "probably carcinogenic to humans." The IARC methodology did not take into account different levels of human exposure to glyphosate, normally a critical component of chemical risk analysis, so the finding was widely challenged. The EPA took a second look, but restated its earlier conclusion that glyphosate was "not likely to be carcinogenic to humans." This more benign conclusion was also reached by official bodies in the EU, Canada, Germany, Australia, New Zealand, and Japan.

The IARC finding nonetheless triggered an aggressive move by personal-injury law firms who put up television ads seeking former Roundup users who had cancer and wanted to join in lawsuits. In one resulting case a California jury awarded the plaintiffs $2 billion in punitive damages, to be paid by Bayer, which had inherited responsibility for Roundup when it bought out the original maker of glyphosate, the Monsanto Company. These punitive damages were reduced to $69 million in 2019 by a California judge, but thousands of other cases awaited trial. Worries such as these focus on pesticides, so they are far distant from the original organic aversion to manufactured fertilizers. Yet they always get wide play from modern advocates for the organic standard.

While commercial farmers and mainstream environmentalists continued to reject the organic approach in the 1960s and 1970s, it did take hold within a new subculture of "back-to-the-land" hippie farmers. The food studies historian Warren Belasco estimated that between 1965 and 1970 the number of rural communes in America increased fivefold, reaching more than three thousand. According to another estimate, by the 1970s nearly a million Americans had experienced living on a commune, attempting to grow their own food. They learned how from publications such as *Mother Earth News*, which promoted organic methods, and Rodale's *Organic Gardening and Farming*, which saw its circulation increase 40 percent between 1970 and 1971 alone.

This new back-to-the-land movement rejected modernity itself. As Belasco explained, the rusticators wanted to avoid "anything complex, anything you can't pronounce, anything chemical, synthetic, or plastic." Eleanor Agnew, author of *Back from the Land*, summarized the outlook of the new rural dwellers: "Fed up with capitalism, TV, Washington politics, and 9-to-5 jobs, they took up residence in log cabins, A-frames, tents, old schoolhouses, and run-down farmhouses; grew their own crops; hauled water from wells; avoided doctors in favor of natural cures; and renounced energy-guzzling appliances."

Jonathan Kauffman, the author of *Hippie Food*, has shown that this countercultural interlude did have some lasting impact on diets in America, by creating a greater awareness of benefits from low-meat diets, nuts, and other unprocessed foods, but not all were impressed. Alice Waters, who lived through the era, said she "didn't want anything to do with the hippies' style of health food cooking," since it meant too much stale, dry brown bread. While most of the rural communes failed, some individual rusticators did stick it out, remaining true to the organic small farm ideal. Many provide leadership for that ideal up to the present day, including Representative Chellie Pingree of Maine, author of the 2013 Local Farms, Food, and Jobs Act in Congress. As a teenager in 1971, Pingree lived on a back-to-the-land organic farm.

This countercultural embrace of organic farming in the United States was never commercially significant, in part because most of the growers disliked the very idea of commerce. Organic food was for sale at the time mostly through small local farmers markets, roadside stands, consumer cooperatives, or health food stores. Because the early growers lacked a credible certification system, they could not consistently receive a higher price for their goods. As late as 1979, only one out of five organic growers in the United States received any price premium at all.

Organic farming even failed to spread following a fresh wave of concern about environmental sustainability triggered by a 1972 book titled *The Limits to Growth*. This book caused a sensation by purporting to show that exponential growth rates in population, manufacturing, and food production were destined—perhaps soon—to exhaust the Earth's finite supply of natural resources. This message brought a new search for ways to farm with fewer inputs, including fewer chemical inputs. In 1976, Wes Jackson, a proponent of switching from monocultures of annual crops to polycultures of perennial crops, called this approach "sustainable agriculture." The USDA disliked the implication that conventional farming was somehow unsustainable, but finally in 1985 it did agree to launch a new federal program to promote what it called Low-Input Sustainable Agriculture, or LISA. Most commercial farmers suspected that LISA actually stood for low-*income* sustainable agriculture.

Organic farming was not promoted even within LISA, because of damning conclusions reached in a 1980 USDA study titled "Report and Recommendations on Organic Farming." This report found that even a modest 30 percent shift to organic methods in U.S. corn and soybean acreage would be enough to drive up prices by 28 and 53 percent, respectively. By implication a complete shift to organic would be disastrous for consumers as well as farmers. Such calculations reinforced the mainstream rejection of organic. Kenneth Beeson, a soil scientist at Cornell University, argued that the "extremists" promoting organic farming were flirting with a future of widespread malnutrition, and Professor Jean Mayer, a leading nutritionist at the Harvard School of Public Health, said he saw no reason to follow proponents of organic food "back to the stone age."

More recent assessments have revived such concerns. In 2019, a study published in *Nature Communications* calculated that if England and Wales made a switch to 100 percent organic farming, average national crop yields would fall by roughly 40 percent. Wheat and barley production would be cut in half. Since there is limited potential to plow up more land, these production shortfalls would have to be made up through increased imports. Total land use requirements would increase, and total greenhouse gas emissions would rise by 21 percent.

O rganic food finally became commercially significant in America for reasons that had nothing to do with greenhouse gas emissions, fertilizers, soils, going back to the land, or running out of resources. The cause was a series of media-led cancer scares linked to pesticide residues on foods. The climax came in 1989 with a report on *60 Minutes* (then viewed by eighteen million households) describing the chemical Alar, used on apples, as "the most potent cancer-causing agent in the food supply today." This headline-making report opened with a sensational skull and crossbones image superimposed on a red apple. The content was largely based on materials provided by the Natural Resources Defense Council (NRDC), an environmental advocacy organization that campaigned against chemicals.

Four years earlier an EPA report had asserted that consuming the Alar residues found on food over an entire lifetime would bring a risk of one more cancer death per ten thousand people. Yet the finding was challenged as invalid by the EPA's own scientific advisers, and the director of the National Cancer Institute's cancer etiology division characterized the cancer risks from eating Alar-treated apples as nonexistent. The EPA never did ban the chemical, but when growers voluntarily stopped using it due to consumer fears, this was taken as evidence that the threat must be real. Apple sales in the United States dropped by 30 percent, leading some nutritionists to worry that the panic would harm public health by reducing fresh fruit consumption.

Consumer fears of pesticide residues on food persist to the present day. In poor countries these risks can be real, because sales and applications of pesticides tend to be poorly regulated, and because foods are often sold unwashed. In the United States since the 1970s, however, increased regulation plus reduced spraying have brought risks under control.

In 2003, when the FDA analyzed several thousand food samples from the marketplace, it found less than one half of 1 percent had chemical residues exceeding regulatory tolerance levels. Those tolerance levels, in turn, were set conservatively at only one one-hundredth of an exposure level that still did not cause toxicity in laboratory animals. Ninety-nine percent of products tested by the USDA also have residue levels that are below, often significantly below, EPA tolerance levels. Food scientists at the University of California, Davis, have concluded, "The marginal benefits of reducing human exposure to pesticides in the diet through increased consumption of organic produce appear to be insignificant."

New scares often arise, but most are traceable to faulty research designs. In 2018 an observational study published in *JAMA Internal Medicine* appeared to show that the participants who consumed organic food had slightly lower breast cancer risks over a five-year follow-up period, but an accompanying editorial in the same journal, from a trio of researchers at Harvard's Chan School of Public Health, faulted this study for not taking socioeconomic factors or the other health behaviors of the participants into account. They cited the Million Women Study from Great Britain that found organic food consumption was actually linked to slightly higher breast cancer risks.

Advocacy organizations nonetheless continue to promote residue fears. The Environmental Working Group (EWG) produces an annual "Dirty Dozen" report, listing fruits and vegetables with the highest pesticide residue levels. Strawberries and spinach were at the top of the list in 2018. The name given to this list is deceptive, since in any examination of multiple products, one will have to be the "dirtiest" even if all are essentially clean. It's a bit like warning swimmers about the deepest part of a wading pool, or telling climbers to avoid the tallest mountain in Florida. One paper published in 2011 looked at average pesticide exposures on that year's EWG "Dirty Dozen" products. All were well below the EPA reference dose, and the vast majority were at less than 0.01 percent of the reference dose. Consumers who allow themselves to be influenced by the "Dirty Dozen" list may needlessly avoid some of our most healthful foods, including both strawberries and spinach.

Advocates for organic foods also like to claim nutrition benefits, yet once again independent experts have not been convinced. In 2012, a review of data from 237 studies conducted through the Center for Health Policy at Stanford University and published in the *Annals of Internal Medicine,* concluded there were no convincing differences between organic and conventional foods in nutrient content or health benefit.

The Organic Center, a pro-organic institution founded in 2002, has argued to the contrary. It published a study of its own in 2008 claiming that plant-based organic foods have more vitamin C and vitamin E, as well as a higher concentration of polyphenols like flavonoids. Conventional nutritionists rejected these claims as either not peer reviewed or insignificant for consumer health. For example, organic milk may indeed have 50 percent more beta-carotene, but there is so little beta-carotene in conventional milk that the resulting gain is insignificant for consumer health. From each quart of milk it amounts to less than 1 percent of what would be found in a single baked sweet potato. If all fruit and vegetable production in the United States suddenly became organic, the nutrition benefit would actually be negative since the price of fruits and vegetables would go up, causing the consumption of these healthy products to go down.

Although dubious on its merits, the 1989 Alar scare created what *Newsweek* magazine called a "panic for organic." Lynn Coody, a founding member of a West Coast organic farmers' organization, remembered this as the moment when organic foods caught hold in the marketplace. "When Alar happened," she said, "the organic industry started going ballistic. We suddenly had to ramp up supply. . . . And we realized then that the writing was on the wall. There was going to be a federal law, and we better be involved in the process of making it workable."

Coody was right. In 1990, Congress passed the Organic Foods

Production Act to create a uniform understanding of the practices that would disqualify a farm from organic certification. The strongest push for this new law came not from the small countercultural farmers who pioneered the movement, since they mostly mistrusted the USDA and did not want the government involved. The push instead came from large-scale commercial organic growers, especially in California, plus consumer groups, some environmental organizations, and animal welfare advocates.

The new uniform standard that emerged blocked all synthetic chemical use, including manufactured fertilizers as well as pesticides. Yet it did nothing to limit the size or specialization permitted on organic farms, and it even created an expandable list of synthetic materials that *would* be permitted in the processing of certified organic foods. These features left open a wide path for industrial-scale organic farming and food manufacturing.

When the new National Organic Program came into full effect in 2002, commercial production and sales began to increase rapidly. Food stores specializing in organic products, such as Whole Foods and Wild Oats, expanded their operations by building new retail outlets and buying up or consolidating existing organic and natural food stores. Like all supermarkets, these retailers sought out suppliers who could deliver a steady volume of high-quality products on time, at a consistent grade and uniformly packaged. Small, diverse organic farms could not meet these requirements, so it was the highly specialized, industrial-scale operations that expanded to take over. Earthbound Farm in California started out with just 2.5 acres of organic raspberries in 1984, but now it manages fifty thousand acres and has taken over more than half of the national market for organic packaged salad greens.

In 2007, a *Time* magazine cover story noted this trend, explaining that Big Organic had taken over by adopting "the same industrial-size farming and long-distance-shipping methods as conventional agribusiness." Organic today usually does not mean local, since 38 percent of all organic sales originate from California. America's leading source of organic tea and ginger is actually China. Retail chains do

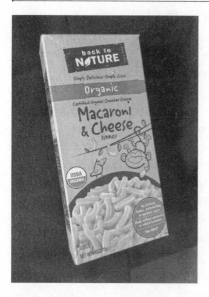

Back to Nature's good-tasting Macaroni & Cheese dinners carry the USDA organic seal, but a one-cup serving delivers 330 calories plus 520 mg of sodium, so the product earns zero Guiding Stars.

sometimes source small batches of organic food from independent local growers, but often just as window dressing.

Organic foods today have also become processed foods. By 2003, more than four-fifths of all organic sales in the United States were being made under brands owned by corporate conglomerates like ConAgra, H. J. Heinz, and Kellogg. The biggest retailers of organic foods now are Walmart, Costco, and Kroger. By 2014, only 8 percent of organic sales in the United States were made directly from small farmers to consumers at farmers markets or through CSAs.

Most organic egg production today resembles nonorganic egg production. I sometimes take students to a Pete and Gerry's organic egg farm in New Hampshire, so they can see what the mainstream organic sector looks like. This is a well-managed operation, but it consists of a single long structure housing twenty thousand tightly packed birds. The building has open bays that provide access to a fenced area outside, so it can be certified organic.

Some organic egg operations stray even further from the small farm ideal. At Herbruck's organic egg farm in Saranac, Michigan, each rectangular building holds about 180,000 birds, with three hens for each square foot of floor space. The "outside" area required for organic certification is only a roofed-over screened porch. Katherine Paul of the Organic Consumers Association complains that this is "not at all what consumers expect of an organic farm." She says consumers ought to wonder, "Why the hell am I paying more for this?"

By going industrial, organic farming has been able to enjoy two decades of rapid growth, but not rapid enough to take over much of the market. Even with the price premiums and the permissive rules, in 2017 only 1.8 percent of farm commodities produced in the United States were organic, and in 2018 certified organic products made up just 5.7 percent of all food sold through retail channels. The organic share of America's diet is even smaller than this, since the high retail price for organic means the tonnage share is smaller than the dollar share. The retail sales figures also do not take restaurant eating into account, and half of all food spending in the United States has taken place in restaurants. Organic menu items are still a rarity in most mainstream establishments.

The USDA makes formal organic certification optional for restaurants, so some chains have promoted their offerings as organic with a minimum of accountability. In 2017, a New York City chain named Bareburger claimed it was selling "organic grass-fed burgers," and it flaunted the word *organic* on its awnings, windows, and menus. One suspicious Manhattan resident, a strong organic advocate, did a stakeout and saw no organic seals on the products being delivered to the restaurant. He lodged a complaint, the National Organic Program investigated, and Bareburger was found not to be in compliance with the Organic Foods Production Act, yet no fine was levied. The Cornucopia Institute, an organic watchdog group, was disappointed: "It would have been entirely appropriate to levy a fine on the ill-gotten gains by this one chain. We need strict enforcement and penalties to act as a deterrent for other potential scofflaws in the organic industry."

Some of the biggest organic scofflaws are the foreign exporters selling faux organic animal feed to livestock producers in the United States. America's organic milk, meat, and egg sector must use feeds grown organically, and the nation's farms don't produce enough of these, so imports become necessary, including from suspect countries like Romania and Ukraine. In 2019, the USDA decertified 60 percent of the organic farms in the Black Sea region. Organic products imported from China also raise suspicion. One German company testing Chinese products for organic certification found significant pesticide residues on more than one-third of the 232 samples tested.

The organic sector would be much larger today if synthetic fertilizers were allowed and only synthetic pesticides were prohibited. This would satisfy most public expectations, since insecticides and herbicides have always been the biggest consumer concern. If the organic standard had emerged as a move against chemical pesticides following Rachel Carson's *Silent Spring*, rather than as a mystical rejection of nitrogen fertilizers half a century earlier, many more farmers would be ready to participate. A synthetic pesticide prohibition would still impose costs on farms, but there are naturally occurring biocides available that help to reduce these costs—like spinosad, Bt, and horticultural oils. The organic livestock sector also would be much larger today if the restriction against growing feed with synthetic fertilizer

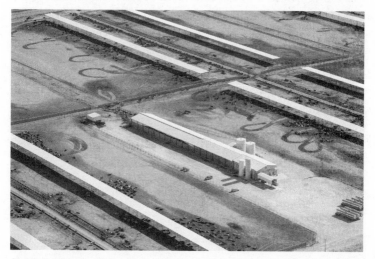

Aerial view of a certified organic dairy farm with 18,000 cows in Stratford, Texas. A half dozen such farms in Texas produce more milk than over 450 smaller organic dairy farms in Wisconsin.

were dropped. Organic traditionalists have no interest in making such changes, however. When I asked Andrew Rodgers at Clark Farm if he thought it would be a good idea, he said no.

Today the fight is between industrial-scale organic farms represented by the Organic Trade Association and the smaller, more diverse organic farms represented by the Cornucopia Institute. The Cornucopia Institute defends the original organic vision by running campaigns against "factory milk" from organic dairy farms with thousands of nonpastured cows, and by trying to block organic certification for things like hydroponic tomatoes grown without any soil.

Assuming the rules do not change, a continued expansion of the organic sector will most likely come from investments by big corporate players who stay just barely within the rules by devising technical workarounds. They control against crop pests by growing indoors hydroponically; they control weeds with gas-powered flamethrowers instead of chemicals, or with "mulch" carpets made of black plastic. Some organic farms in Pennsylvania, Georgia, and Florida are spreading plastic over thousands of acres, even though each acre farmed this way generates more than one hundred pounds of nonbiodegradable plastic waste that must be loaded into dumpsters, then taken to a landfill. Conventional farmers also use plastic mulch, but not as much, and the plastic they use is biodegradable, so it does not go to a landfill. The National Organic Program does not allow organic farmers to use most biodegradable plastic mulches because they contain petroleum-based materials. Purity comes with a price, once again.

CHAPTER 5

Should Peasants Stay Poor?

Africa is a special place, the original home to us all, but most Africans today remain cut off from modern material comforts. A majority are still traditional farmers or animal herdsmen, and they remain poor because they lack the things that have been used by farmers everywhere else to escape poverty: improved rural roads, rural electricity, powered machines, irrigation pumps, improved seeds, chemical fertilizers, and veterinary medicine for their animals. As a result, four out of ten Africans remain poor today, and two out of ten are chronically undernourished.

Concerned outsiders should be looking for ways to upgrade farm technology in Africa, but instead some are proposing solutions that require no access to the essentials of modern, productive farming. These outsiders benefit from modernity themselves, but they advise African farmers to look for solutions that do not require significant investments in modern farming assets.

On one of my first research trips to Africa, I visited an international institute in Nigeria promoting a tantalizing shortcut known as "alley cropping." Poor farmers who could not afford nitrogen fertilizer were told to plant strips of small leguminous trees capable of fixing nitrogen into the soil with their roots. Food crops planted in the alleys between the trees would then be naturally fertilized. This scheme had worked on test plots at the research station, but I asked if the method had been adopted anywhere by poor farmers on their own land. I was told there had been some spontaneous adoptions at one site in the neighboring country of Benin, so I decided to go see for myself. When I got there, I found that the local farmers were indeed planting strips of trees, but not nitrogen-fixing leguminous trees. They had tried those, but the leaves cast too much shade on the crops and had to be constantly pruned. They decided to replace them with palm trees, since these needed no pruning and could be tapped to make palm wine. This left the food crops still struggling without fertilizer.

The alley cropping idea was an early effort to promote "agroecology," a method of growing food that is meant to imitate nature, parallel to what Albert Howard had called "Nature's farming." For example, it intermingles different crops in the same field (intercropping) to take advantage of beneficial interactions between crops, and between crops and animals. Agroecologists believe they can cut the need for purchased fertilizer if they rely on biodiverse mixes of crops and animals that recycle nutrients internally. They can control crop pests by planting polycultures instead of monocultures, and by supplying habitat for the natural enemies of crop pests. The dream of agroecologists is to let nature itself do most of the work.

Agroecological production methods have been developed and promoted for decades now by many highly capable innovators. The concepts are sound and produce results in experimental settings, but farmers have shown little interest because the labor requirements are too time-consuming and complex, as with alley cropping. Whether it is pruning the trees, carrying in the mulch, rebuilding the raised beds, composting the manure, tending the animals, or hand-harvesting the crop, agroecological methods often cost too much in terms of both time and physical effort. This is work Nature will not do. Farmers around the world know this, so once they gain access to things like manufactured fertilizers, irrigation pumps, and powered machinery, they are happy to leave behind the laborious hand-tending of complex garden-like systems. They let modern science do more of the work.

A decade ago I had a conversation with a prominent agroecology activist at a university seminar. I asked if she could think of a country that had used agroecology with success either to feed its people or to lift its farmers out of poverty. She thought for a moment then said, "Bhutan." Bhutan, a tiny mountain kingdom, does still rely on hand labor in farming, but there is little to show for it. Bhutan depends on imports for half its total food consumption, and even with these imports up to one-third of its children are stunted from malnutrition.

Olivier de Schutter, a former UN Special Rapporteur on the Right to Food, has said that agroecology is superior to conventional farming because it means "embracing the complexity of nature." Successful farming, however, usually requires not an embrace of nature but keeping nature at bay. Weeds from nature compete with crops and must be removed. Drought must be corrected with irrigation, and insect pests and crop diseases that come from nature must be beaten back, not admired for their complexity and "embraced." But, in a happy paradox, if modern farming is done properly, nature will be better protected in the end, since securing higher crop yields per acre in a well-managed farm field will reduce the need to clear and plow still more acres.

Some environmental leaders have understood all this. In May 2002, James Lovelock, the creator of Gaia Theory, and Patrick Moore, the cofounder of Greenpeace, signed the "Declaration in Support of Protecting Nature with High Yield Farming and Forestry." This declaration explained that high-yield farming was not just the best way to produce an adequate supply of food; it simultaneously delivered a "preservation of the natural environment and its biodiversity through the conservation of wild areas and natural habitat." By asking poor farmers to imitate nature, today's advocates for agroecology are not only asking too much of farmers; without knowing it, they are putting nature itself at risk.

The modern idea of agroecology gained strength as a pushback against something called the "green revolution." This was the rapid upgrade in farm technology that swept through much of the countryside in Latin America and Asia in the 1960s and 1970s. In Asia, it brought a welcome escape from a widespread fear of famine. In 1967, William and Paul Paddock, a former agronomist and a former State Department official, had written a bestselling book titled *Famine 1975!*, which predicted India would never be able to feed its fast-growing population. The Paddocks even advised against giving food aid to India, since that would keep people alive just long enough to produce more children, increasing the ultimate famine toll. In 1968, an American entomologist named Paul R. Ehrlich published his own bestseller titled *The Population Bomb,* an even more fatalistic book that predicted hundreds of millions would die in the 1970s, since food production in Asia could never hope to keep up with population growth. His book opened with a memorable first sentence: "The battle to feed all of humanity is over."

One impetus behind both books was a devastating two-year drought that hit India in 1965 and 1966. The monsoon rains failed, causing India's food grain production to fall by a disastrous 19 percent in the first year, and then by nearly as much in the second. Impoverished villagers streamed into towns and cities to beg for food. An actual famine was avoided thanks to a tripling of United States wheat exports to India in 1965 and 1966, a massive food aid effort of the kind the Paddocks said would be futile. In 1966, the United States shipped roughly one fifth of its entire wheat harvest to India, some six hundred shiploads in all, nearly two a day leaving the docks.

I was in India myself in 1967, as a new college graduate on the way to visit my older brother, who was serving as a Peace Corps volunteer in Nepal. The drought had ended by then, but many who earlier fled their villages were still in Calcutta, homeless beggars sleeping on the sidewalks in long rows, making it difficult to walk. From the window of my bus coming in from the airport I made out block after block of dimly visible human figures, wrapped head to foot in white cotton, almost as though awaiting burial. To my impressionable young eyes, it looked like the Paddocks' grim projection of an Indian famine was about to come true.

I did not know it at the time, but an escape from India's dangerous food deficits had already been found. A team of crop scientists in Mexico, supported by the Rockefeller Foundation, had developed new varieties of wheat that could deliver yields twice as high as India's traditional varieties, assuming they were provided with irrigation water and adequate fertilizer. The Indian government had made a bold decision to begin importing these new seeds in 1964, and by 1967 they were already spreading rapidly into wheat-growing areas. In a parallel fashion, plant breeders in the Philippines had successfully developed improved rice varieties that were also capable of giving much higher yields, and these seeds as well were soon to reach India's small farmers.

These new "green revolution" seeds predated genetic engineering, so they were not GMOs. Developed through simple crossbreeding, they were not even hybrid seeds, so their desirable traits were not lost when farmers saved seeds from their harvest and replanted. Crop scientists had secured this breakthrough by patiently screening seeds from all over the world, finding wheat and rice varieties with unique "dwarfing" traits they could crossbreed into the crops grown by farmers in tropical climates. The dwarfed wheat and rice plants were an improvement because they devoted less of their growth energy to producing leaves and straw and more to producing grain, and because the short, stiff straws could hold a much heavier weight of grain without falling over in the wind or rain.

When the new dwarf wheats were first given to farmers in Mexico in 1961, they doubled yields. Farmers began planting the new wheat varieties in India in 1964, and by 1970 total production had nearly doubled, ending the fear of famine. In 1970, the American scientist who led the original wheat-breeding effort in Mexico, Norman Borlaug, was awarded the Nobel Peace Prize. When India brought in the new rice varieties from the Philippines, rice production in Punjab and Haryana nearly doubled between 1971 and 1976. By 1973, India had become a small net exporter of rice, and by 1978 a net exporter of wheat as well.

All this added grain production brought down food prices, so India's poor could afford to purchase and consume more. Studying one district in southern India in the 1980s, economists Per Pinstrup-

Andersen and Mauricio Jaramillo calculated that one-third of all consumption gains there could be attributed to the increased rice production made possible by the new seeds. The original goal was simply to produce larger quantities of wheat and rice, but numerous collateral benefits were soon noted, including increased income for poor farmers, increased working opportunities and wages for landless rural laborers (because more grain now had to be harvested), and also more off-farm jobs in activities like grain storage, processing, and transport.

India was not the only country to benefit from the green revolution. By 1998, more than four-fifths of the entire crop area in Asia, including China, was planted with these modern varieties. The improved rice varieties that were originally developed by the International Rice Research Institute in the Philippines eventually spread to more than seventy countries, and by the 1980s improved varieties of maize, sorghum, millet, barley, and cassava had also been developed. Overall, more than eight thousand new seed varieties were introduced for at least eleven different crops. In South Asia specifically, between 1965 and 2000 the percentage of harvested rice area under modern green revolution varieties increased from zero to 71 percent, and the share of wheat area increased to 95 percent. In East and Southeast Asia, modern variety coverage for rice by 2000 was more than 80 percent, and for wheat nearly 90 percent.

This nearly universal planting of the new seeds showed that small as well as large farms were participating. In one study of thirty rice-growing villages in Asia between 1966 and 1972, the farms classified as "small" (less than one hectare, or 2.2 acres) had actually taken up the new seeds more quickly than those classified as "large" (above three hectares). More than nine-tenths of both small and large farms had adopted the modern rice varieties within a decade after they became available.

Small farms were able to participate because the new seeds could be planted, grown, and harvested without expensive machinery. If a farmer had irrigation water and could get credit to purchase fertilizer, the seeds paid off even on small, nonmechanized plots. Appreciating this fact, national governments promoted the uptake of the seeds with new investments in irrigation, fertilizer subsidies, credits, and extension training. In 1972, the government of India spent more than one-fifth of its entire public budget on agricultural improvements to support the spread of green revolution seeds and methods.

The environmental benefits of the green revolution were harder to notice but important as well. In 1964, before the green revolution, India produced twelve million tons of wheat on fourteen million hectares of land. Thirty years later it was producing fifty-seven million tons of wheat on twenty-four million hectares. To produce that much with the old seeds would have required sixty million hectares, so thirty-six million hectares were being saved from the plow, exactly the environmental benefit from high-yield farming that James Lovelock and Patrick Moore endorsed in their 2002 statement.

The nutrition benefits over time were sizable. One calculation by Yale economist Robert Evenson found that if the modern seed varieties had not been introduced, annual crop production in the developing world as a whole in the year 2000 would have been almost one-fifth lower than it actually was, pushing food prices higher by one-third to two-thirds. With prices at this higher level, an added 6 to 8 percent of children in the developing world would have been malnourished.

India's green revolution is still rightly celebrated by advocates for science-based farming. In 2018, Bill and Melinda Gates pointed out that "Indian farmers get almost four times the amount of wheat from the same piece of land as they did 50 years ago." Hoping to extend this success, the Bill and Melinda Gates Foundation has sponsored a follow-on Alliance for a Green Revolution in Africa, the continent today where farming methods remain least improved.

But the green revolution inevitably attracted critics. In 2018, Charles Mann wrote a book titled *The Wizard and the Prophet,* profiling Norman Borlaug as the prototypical man of science, the wizard. The purpose of Mann's book was to explore recurring conflicts between

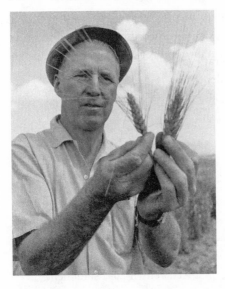

In a research field in Mexico, Norman Borlaug compares wheat varieties. Photo taken in 1970, the year Borlaug won the Nobel Peace Prize.

those (like Borlaug) who think modern science can be a salvation versus those who view modern science as a Faustian bargain, destined to bring us down in the end. Borlaug became a hero among the first group, but his green revolution continues to be vilified by those mistrustful of science-based change.

In Borlaug's 2009 obituary, the *Guardian* recounted the viewpoint of one of these critics, Vandana Shiva, an Indian environmental activist. Shiva, according to the *Guardian*, saw the green revolution as having led to "rural impoverishment, increased debt, social inequality and the displacement of vast numbers of peasant farmers." A few of Borlaug's critics went even further. In 2007 the political journalist Alexander Cockburn said, "Aside from Kissinger, probably the biggest killer of all to have got the peace prize was Norman Borlaug, whose 'green revolution' wheat strains led to the death of peasants by the million."

Borlaug had grown up on a small farm in Iowa and felt a strong kinship with peasant farmers, so charges such as these were personally wounding. But he had a combative side (having been a wrestling star at the University of Minnesota) and fought back hard against his critics, dismissing them as elitists who had never missed a meal in their life. I came to know Borlaug in the 1990s, when we served together on the board of an agricultural development organization in Arkansas. At every board meeting at least once, Norm would let loose with a tirade against the opponents of agricultural science, cranking his voice up to a near shout while pounding his fist on the table. He had used such outbursts to advantage in persuading timid governments to adopt his new seeds. Norm's friends said there were three different ways to persuade: dialogue, monologue, and the most extreme form of monologue, which they called "Borolaug."

Serious environmental problems did emerge from the green revolution, including excessive water and chemical use, but these resulted from unwise government policies used to promote the new seeds, not from the seeds themselves. In Punjab in northwest India, excessive groundwater extraction was caused by a government policy that subsidized nearly nine-tenths of the electric bill for pumping, which of course encouraged too much pumping. Excessive insecticide spraying in Indonesia in the 1970s became a problem because the government subsidized chemical purchases by as much as 85 percent. Indonesia finally removed the subsidy and banned the use of fifty-seven different insecticides for rice, ending the problem. In making these corrections, Indonesia knew better than to stop using the improved seeds themselves.

Vandana Shiva, the single most prominent critic of the green revolution, does blame the seeds themselves for environmental damage. Shiva, who was identified by *Forbes* magazine as one of the seven most powerful women on the globe, is a spellbinding speaker, able to weave together scientific terminology with moral indignation and a deep mistrust of western-led industrial development. Shiva originally studied physics but then went on to earn a Ph.D. in philosophy from the University of Western Ontario. In 1991, she wrote a book-length polemic titled *The Violence of the Green Revolution: Third World Agriculture, Ecology, and Politics,* which accused the green revolution of introducing a dangerous new farming model:

> It was based not on the intensification of nature's processes, but on the intensification of credit and purchased inputs like chemical fertilizers and pesticides. It was based not on self-reliance, but dependence. It was based not on diversity but uniformity. Advisors and experts came from America to shift India's agricultural research and agricultural policy from an indigenous and ecological model to an exogenous, and high input one.

Shiva predicted this green revolution model would fail in India because it was replacing "the diverse knowledge of local cultivators and plant breeders" with what she called "uniformity and vulnerability." The diversity of indigenous agriculture was being "replaced by a narrow genetic base and monocultures." This reduction in genetic diversity was taking place at two levels:

> Firstly, mixtures and rotations of diverse crops like wheat, maize, millets, pulses, and oil seeds were replaced by monocultures of wheat and rice. Secondly, the introduced wheat and rice varieties reproduced over large-scale monocultures came from a very narrow genetic base, compared to the high genetic variability in the populations of traditional wheat and rice plants. . . . The destruction of diversity and the creation of uniformity simultaneously involves the destruction of stability and the creation of vulnerability. . . . On this narrow and alien genetic base, are the food supplies of millions precariously perched.

Shiva's critique was factually mistaken in several respects. The new seeds did *not* require more inputs like water and fertilizer; each wheat and rice plant yielded so much more grain that the use of water and fertilizer actually declined relative to output. The United Nations Food and Agricultural Organization (FAO) later confirmed that the green revolution rice varieties increased water productivity threefold compared to traditional varieties. As for fertilizer, the new green revolution varieties produced more than twenty pounds of added grain for each added pound of nitrogen, while the traditional rice and wheat varieties produced only ten, so the need for fertilizer fell roughly in half for each pound of grain produced.

Crop scientists have long been frustrated by Shiva's unjustified assertions of increased water and chemical dependence. Sir Gordon Conway, a pioneering agricultural ecologist and former president of the Royal Geographical Society, has said, "It is absolutely remarkable to me how Vandana Shiva is able to get away with saying whatever people want to hear."

Shiva's warning about increased crop vulnerability due to less diversity was also off target. According to a 2019 study published in *Global Change Biology*, crop diversity in India—measured both in terms of numbers of different crops grown and the dispersion of those different crops across cultivated area—has actually shown a "remarkable increase" since the 1960s. Green revolution farming may have reduced the diversity of crop varieties in individual fields, but this did not necessarily narrow the genetic base of those crops. Plant breeders value *pedigree complexity*, which is the number of different crop selections originally bred into a variety of wheat or rice. One of the green revolution rice varieties (IR 66) actually had forty-two different pre–green revolution selections in its parentage, so it had multiple sources of resistance to pests and diseases. As Professor Thomas R. DeGregori at the University of Houston has pointed out, a field planted with a monoculture of green revolution seeds can actually be more diverse genetically than a polyculture of traditional varieties. In 1996, Melinda Smale and Tim McBride reported from the International Wheat and Maize Improvement Center in Mexico that "yield stability, resistance to rusts, pedigree complexity, and the number of modern cultivars in farmers' fields have all increased since the early years of the Green Revolution." Biodiversity in nature has also been better protected, thanks to the wildlife habitat spared due to higher yields.

It has now been more than a quarter century since Shiva branded the green revolution in India unsustainable, yet crop yields have continued to increase. Data from the FAO show that average wheat yields in India in 2014 were 38 percent higher than when Shiva wrote in 1991, and 244 percent higher than when the green revolution began in 1965. For rice, yields were 36 percent higher and 177 percent higher. Trends in fertilizer use show that these yield gains did not come from abandoning the green revolution in favor of agroecology, as nitrogenous fertilizer use in South Asia continued to increase on a tonnage basis.

The green revolution seeds delivered a less positive outcome in Central and South America, where colonization by Spain and Portugal had created highly inequitable patterns of landownership, and where governments have remained far more beholden to large landowners as opposed to small farms and the landless rural poor.

Large landowners controlling the fertile valley lands that were easy to irrigate in Latin America took up the new green revolution seeds and fertilizers quickly, and with great success. Agricultural production increased at an average annual rate of 3 percent between 1955 and 1974, which helped boost the dollar value of agricultural exports threefold. To speed the new technology uptake, governments offered the large commercial growers subsidized credits, extension assistance, new irrigation canals, and subsidies for fertilizer and pesticides.

The majority of the rural poor, owning little or no land, were left behind. Landownership in Latin America has long been badly skewed. At one point, just 4 percent of all property owners in Brazil controlled 63 percent of total landholdings. Things were even worse in Chile, where just 3 percent controlled 79 percent of the land. Impoverished peasants and socially marginalized indigenous communities were left planting subsistence crops on sloping hillsides, on drylands, or on lands newly cleared from the forest, which often brought serious environmental damage. In Mexico, where roughly half of all farmers tried to subsist on only 10 percent of the nation's farmland, more than one-third of total forested area was lost between 1961 and 1990 alone. The failure of Norman Borlaug's new wheat seeds to protect either the rural poor or the rural environment in Latin America made them an easy target for attack.

Mexico, the starting point of the original green revolution, fittingly became home to some of its harshest critics, including a number of American academics working there. Among these was a University of California plant ecologist named Stephen R. Gliessman, who became a convert to agroecology in 1976 while teaching at Mexico's College of Tropical Agriculture (CSAT) in the state of Tabasco. CSAT's primary mission at the time was to spread the green revolution, but Gliessman came to believe some of the traditional methods used by local farmers were actually superior, since they were more firmly grounded in ecological principles. He noticed, for example, that traditional Mexican farmers would often tolerate "weeds." Instead of being eradicated, extraneous plants in the field were managed for their beneficial traits, such as shading and cooling the soil.

For Gliessman and others, the local knowledge embedded in traditional cropping systems was a storehouse of value dating back many centuries to pre-Hispanic times. Hundreds of years before Columbus arrived, farming in Mesoamerica had been productive enough to sustain sizable urban populations in cities like Teotihuacan, with more than twenty thousand inhabitants, or Tikal, with ninety thousand. The farming systems of the day somehow managed this without any use of chemical fertilizers, powered machinery, or plow-pulling oxen or horses, and some of the success appeared traceable to a harmonious integration with nature.

For example, the Mayan and Aztec people constructed raised planting beds (*chinampas*) on the margins of wetlands that were naturally subject to shallow flooding. Canals were maintained between these raised beds to provide irrigation water, access for canoes, muck for fertilizer, and habitat for fish. Instead of draining the wetlands, which became the Spanish approach, these indigenous people produced an abundant supply of food by adapting to a natural marshland ecology.

The raised bed system merits admiration, but it could only operate on topographies subject to periodic flooding and it required intensive hand labor for constructing and maintaining the beds, as well as for planting and harvesting. Even its advocates concede that this system depended on a "large amount of individual care given to each plant in the chinampa." Mobilizing this labor was not a problem for the ruling kings and priests of Mesoamerica, but in modern times the coercion required would not be acceptable.

In the end, these early farming systems may also have lacked environmental sustainability. Between the eighth and ninth centuries, the classic Mayan civilization collapsed and its cities were abandoned. The reasons are still debated, but one factor may have been soil erosion, which silted up the canals. *Chinampas,* in any case, play no significant role at all in providing Mexico with food today. They operate here and there only for show, at protected World Heritage Sites.

An even earlier raised bed and canal system, called *waru-waru,* was developed three thousand years ago in the Peruvian Andes. Advocates for agroecology have tried valiantly to revive these systems, but the labor costs are again too high. The Peruvian raised beds needed hand planting, hand weeding, hand harvest, regular maintenance, and a

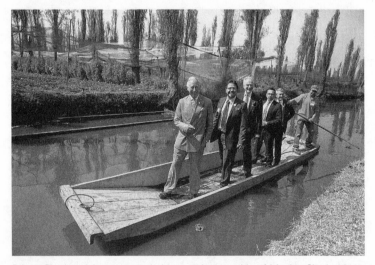

Prince Charles visits a restored *chinampa* just outside of Mexico City in 2014.

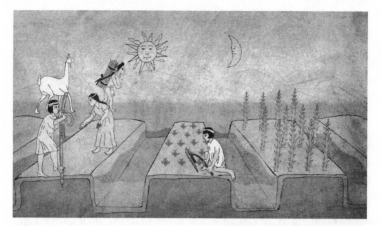

An idealized vision of *waru-waru* farming three thousand years ago in the Andes.

complete rebuilding every ten years. Miguel A. Altieri, a Chilean-born agronomist and a leading agroecology promoter, admitted in 1999 that for potato production these systems required 270 person-days per hectare every year. A report from the Organization of American States on *waru-waru* farming in Peru showed that the total production costs came to $1,460 per hectare, working out to $480 for each twenty-five pounds of potatoes. This report said, "The technology produces economic benefits during the first three years following construction, but shortly thereafter reconstruction becomes necessary to maintain the productivity of the system." Such results might have discouraged further efforts, but the Global Environment Facility, the FAO, and various local governments have all continued to sponsor *waru-waru* demonstration projects as part of a Globally Important Agricultural Heritage System.

Another pre-Columbian farming practice is *milpa* farming in dense tropical forests, a technique more commonly known as slash and burn. Forest dwellers clear a small patch of land with a machete or an ax, then they burn the trees in place. The exposed soil is loosened with a hand hoe to sift in the ash, providing a fertile bed for a mixed planting of corn, beans, and squash, crops that work well in combination. The low growing squash plants between the corn help maintain soil cover and prevent weed growth. After a few seasons the soil nutrients are exhausted, so the cultivators move on to clear a new patch of land, allowing the forest to regrow on the old patch, not to be cleared again for a decade or more.

These methods were environmentally sustainable when the human population in Central America was sparse enough to permit extended fallow times, but as the population grew the fallows had to be shortened, preventing an adequate grow-back. Wildlife habitat could not recover, and the fragile tropical soils eroded in the rain or baked hard like a parking lot in the sun. Rather than working with nature, this kind of *milpa* farming ended up destroying nature. Even when sustainably managed, these forest systems offer little escape from poverty, which is why Mayan youth in the Yucatán today continue to abandon *milpa* farms to look for work around tourist resorts in Cancún and Tulum.

Efforts have been made by organizations like the Nature Conservancy and USAID to transform *milpa* farming into something more rewarding. Knowing that traditional forest farming won't succeed without becoming more like modern conventional farming, these organizations have brought in irrigation, gas-powered garden tillers, and fertilizer. Advocates for traditional Mayan forest gardens resist, seeing this as tampering with an ancient, proven practice.

Hoping to preserve the ancient ways, an organization named Exploring Solutions Past has created the El Pilar Forest Garden Network in Belize, with more than seven hundred acres of land maintained in the traditional manner by modern-day Mayans. This site, complete with authentic Mayan ruins, does not produce a great deal of food, but it attracts visits from students, university interns, and environmental educators. The California-based archaeologist who created this project intended it to be "a living museum and laboratory, drawing from what can be learned about ancient cultural practices to create a conservation model for the future of our own civilization."

At the project level, agroecology has produced some apparent gains. One report prepared in 1999 by Miguel Altieri surveyed projects led by non-governmental organizations (NGOs) in nine different Latin American countries and reported success claims that ranged from "yield increases" of 20 percent in one intercropping and agroforestry project in Peru, all the way up to 250 percent for projects using green manures—fast-growing plants dug into the soil to provide nutrients—in Guatemala and Honduras. The added labor requirements needed to get these results were not carefully accounted for. Also, some of the higher yield claims were a comparison to completely unimproved peasant farming systems, so they told us little about the even greater improvements a green revolution approach might have delivered.

Trends in fertilizer use in Latin America confirm that most farmers in this region, just like in Asia, continue to choose the green revolution over agroecology. UN data show that between 1980 and 2002 the use of urea fertilizer in South America increased 60 percent, and the use of nitrogenous fertilizers increased 139 percent. Then between 2002 and 2014 in Latin America and the Caribbean overall, total fertilizer consumption per hectare of arable land increased by another 43 percent.

The green revolution came up short for the rural poor in Latin America, but a return to premodern, labor-intensive farming systems would make things worse. A better approach is to address the social and landowning inequities that explain so much rural injustice in the region. Equalizing access to good agricultural land is an obvious place to start, but this would mean attacking rural injustice at its strongest point of resistance. A second-best approach is to create more rural jobs off the farm, reduce racial discrimination against citizens of non-European descent, improve public education for the poor, and end the second-class status of women and girls. Ills such as these remain the real source of poverty in Latin America's countryside, not improved seeds, fertilizers, and monocultures.

. . .

Agroecology advocates continue to look for success stories. One they have claimed is Cuba, a country where farmers were forced to abandon modern methods when highly subsidized imports of fuel and chemicals disappeared after the Soviet Union collapsed in 1989. When these supports for modern farming were taken away, the nation's per capita agricultural production dropped by almost half between 1990 and 1994. At this point, simply from necessity, farmers retreated to preindustrial techniques. They replaced tractors with oxen and hand hoes, fertilizers with animal manure, and chemical pest controls with biological controls and intercropping. Cuba's National Association of Small Farmers launched an official Farmer to Farmer Agroecology Movement.

Advocates for agroecology have tried to hail the results as a vindication for their cause. Peter Rosset, an agricultural ecologist and green revolution critic, praised the "rapid and successful" spread of agroecology methods that he saw under way on the island. Miguel Altieri and Fernando Funes-Monzote, writing in the *Monthly Review* in 2012, said Cuba's embrace of agroecology was one reason that nation had managed what they depicted as the best food production performance in all of Latin America and the Caribbean between 1996 and 2005. Altieri and Funes-Monzote said, "No other country in the world has achieved this level of success with a form of agriculture that uses the ecological services of biodiversity and reduces food miles, energy use, and effectively closes local production and consumption cycles." An NGO named La Via Campesina went even further: "In just over a decade, the campesino family which practices agroecology has attained the greatest levels of productivity and sustainability in Cuba. Agroecology has achieved what the conventional model has never accomplished in Cuba or any other country: more production from less."

Partly in response to such reviews, the United Nations began to promote agroecology in Cuba as "an example on a global level," but a less positive story is told by the UN's own official data. Several decades into Cuba's forced experiment with agroecology, data from the FAO show that in 2014, Cuba's official net per capita food production index was still 37 percent lower than it was in 1990. The dollar value of food production per capita has also continued to lag. In 2016 it was more than one-third lower than it had been fifteen years earlier. A persistence of serious food shortages obliged the Cuban government in 2019 to begin widespread rationing of chicken, eggs, rice, and beans.

To deal with such problems, the Cuban government today is not counting on agroecology. Instead it has been trying to revive conventional farming by boosting the use of synthetic chemicals and by rebuilding its inventory of large-scale machinery, such as center-pivot irrigation rigs. Rather than going organic, Cuba increased mineral fertilizer use by one-third between 2002 and 2012, and it has even pursued research on genetically engineered crops. In the meantime, Cuba feeds its population mostly on imports. Between 1995 and 2013, with Cuba's own per capita food production stuck at a low level, its agricultural imports grew by more than half. In February 2007, a Cuban vice minister admitted that more than four-fifths of the items in the nation's basic food basket were being imported.

Ordinary farmers may show little interest, but agroecology has nonetheless come to be endorsed by multiple agencies inside the UN system, including the United Nations Environment Programme and the United Nations Development Programme. Even the FAO, once a strong supporter of green revolution farming, has switched much of its allegiance to agroecology. I saw the extent of this switch firsthand when I was asked to chair a 2009 panel on agricultural technology at an FAO event in Rome titled "Feed the World 2050."

The opening speaker on my panel, a distinguished plant breeder from India, spent most of his time praising Norman Borlaug, who had died at age ninety-five one month before. This fit my expectations for an FAO event. The next four invited speakers took the panel in a completely different direction. The first was an international consultant on agroecology, the second was the executive director of an international organization promoting organic farming, the third a community organizer who worked with indigenous people in the Philippines, and the fourth an advocate who said scientists should be learning from farmers instead of the other way around. So much for science, so much for plant breeders, and so much for Borlaug and his green revolution.

The FAO was backing away from its long-held pro-science position on agricultural technology because of intense criticism from international civil society networks that opposed the green revolution. At an FAO World Food Summit in Rome in 1996, twelve hundred NGOs from eighty different countries had convened their own parallel forum to criticize the FAO's traditional support for what they called "industrialized agriculture," and to endorse instead organic farming and agroecology. In an effort to appease such critics, the United Nations began allowing civil society organizations to gain formal "consultative status" inside the special agency system, and more than two thousand NGOs soon gained that status, but this did nothing to dissuade them from attacking green revolution farming. At yet another Food Summit in Rome in 2002, an independent NGO forum blamed the green revolution for what it described as a rise in world hunger. This made little sense, since the only region where hunger was actually rising was Africa, and this was the only region not to have experienced a green revolution. Two years later, however, a coalition of 670 separate NGOs once again attacked the green revolution, this time branding it a "tragedy."

These green revolution critics, now on the inside, also helped to author a lengthy 2008 report, jointly issued by the United Nations and the World Bank, that was called the *International Assessment of Agricultural Science and Technology for Development*. This was not so much a scientific assessment as it was a crowdsourced assemblage of viewpoints (the report claimed to have "400 authors") from organizations that included Greenpeace, Friends of the Earth, and the Pesticide Action Network. The report briefly paid tribute to the green revolution, but then said "business as usual is no longer an option" due to emerging environmental challenges, and it went on to endorse organic farming and agroecology.

Agroecology has continued to win official endorsement inside the UN system. In 2010, the UN Special Rapporteur on the Right to Food, Olivier De Schutter, pointed to agroecology as the best way to guarantee the human right to food. In 2013, the United Nations Conference on Trade and Development also endorsed agroecology in calling for a "fundamental transformation of agriculture" based on "agro-ecological production methods." The FAO convened an International Symposium on Agroecology in 2014, followed by a second such symposium in 2018 that attracted seven hundred government participants as well as more than three hundred different nonstate actors, launching a new "Scaling Up Agroecology Initiative." The ten-year targets for this new initiative included an increased knowledge base for agroecology in fifty countries and technical support for the agroecological transition process in twenty countries.

Since agroecology has only limited attraction for farmers, these UN efforts are likely to have limited practical impact. Declarations made by UN functionaries and civil society organizations in Rome seldom shape government policies or private investments. National governments do far more to shape food and farming, and even in the case of Cuba these governments have tended to favor scientific knowledge over traditional knowledge, monocultures over intercropping, fertilizer use over a recycling of animal waste, and powered machinery over hand labor. A 2016 review in the journal *Horticulturae* summed it up nicely: "Despite the call for alternative methods of production over the years, the paradigm of industrial or conventional agriculture still dominates and permeates most mainstream academic and policy discussions about the future of agriculture."

The legitimate environmental concerns surrounding the green revolution can be addressed in the meantime without abandoning its gains. In 1997, Gordon Conway published a book calling for a "Doubly Green Revolution," one that would be kinder to the environment by combining animal manure with synthetic fertilizer use and using biological controls along with synthetic pesticides. As Conway explained, "I believe we should draw on all technical tools available to us for food production: conventional technologies such as fertilizers and pesticides, but used with precision; intermediate technologies such as improved treadle pumps; traditional technologies such as rainwater harvesting techniques; and new platforms for innovation based on scientific advances such as genetically modified crops for drought, pest and disease resilience."

This results-oriented, evidence-based integrated approach is also advanced under the banner of Sustainable Agricultural Intensification (SAI), promoted by Jules Pretty, a biologist and professor of environment and society at the University of Essex. SAI does not try to imitate nature; instead it seeks to protect nature by using inputs with greater precision, and minimizing land use with continued yield gains. Agroecology purists accuse Conway and Pretty of proposing something that looks too much like "business as usual," yet both are offering a marked improvement because they make environmental sustainability an explicit objective, not just a hoped-for side benefit from productivity gains.

The integrated methods Conway and Pretty propose are also something farmers can actually agree to adopt. In 2018, Pretty published the results of a study estimating that various SAI techniques—including IPM, micro-irrigation, and reduced tillage farming—were already in use on 453 million acres around the world, nearly one-tenth of agricultural land worldwide. Methods with potential to scale are the methods to favor.

Several years ago I was in Ottawa, seated in a convention center ballroom waiting my turn to speak at a conference on Canada's national food policy. At the podium was someone from an organization named Food Secure Canada who was saying Canada's food policy should be based on the concept of "food sovereignty." A big-shouldered farm equipment dealer from Saskatoon, sitting immediately to my right, leaned over and asked, "What's food sovereignty?" I wanted to tell him it was a concept that would terminate most of Canada's wheat and canola exports, making it harder for him to sell farm equipment. Food sovereignty is, however, an idea even less likely to scale up than agroecology. If it ever did come to pass, the intended beneficiaries—poor farmers in the developing world—would be harmed even more than tractor salesmen in Saskatoon.

The lead organization promoting food sovereignty is La Via Campesina (LVC), translated as "the peasant's way." This is a global network of 182 separate local peasant organizations in 81 countries claiming to have at least two hundred million members. This last claim is suspect since the network was not originally created by peasants. LVC was initially led by antiglobalization activists in Europe and funded by European donors and foundations. LVC has always tended to promote an outsider's vision of what peasants in poor countries ought to do and want.

Like so many other food movement visions, the food sovereignty idea began as pushback against something new. Local food was a pushback against supermarkets, organic food a pushback against nitrogen fertilizer, and agroecology a pushback against the green revolution. Food sovereignty was originally a pushback against corporate-led globalization, advanced in the 1980s by Prime Minister Margaret Thatcher and President Ronald Reagan, along with international institutions such as the World Trade Organization (WTO), the International Monetary Fund (IMF), and the World Bank. Leaders in Europe felt threatened by globalization, since opening up to international markets would subject their heavily protected farmers to stronger foreign competition—for example, from American farmers. Farmers in Europe mobilized to resist, and created LVC as an allied "peasant" network to support their fight.

Economic globalization was indeed a threat to European farmers, just as it threatened some factory workers in the United States, but more open markets for trade and investment have delivered substantial gains in the developing world. China opened its market to foreign investment beginning in the 1980s, and by 2010 subsidiaries or joint ventures with multinational firms were providing 30 percent of China's resulting growth in industrial output. In China, globalization created factory jobs instead of destroying them. Income surged in India as well when that country reduced its trade barriers and opened up to foreign firms after 1991. By 2011, India's GDP had quadrupled, its exports had increased tenfold, and its foreign exchange reserves had increased almost fiftyfold.

European industries, like farmers, had long been given protection from foreign competition, so factory workers joined to resist market opening. Large street protests were staged in Berlin in 1988 during the annual meetings of the IMF. In Paris in 1989, ten thousand demonstrators gathered to protest globalization at a meeting of the Group of Seven (G7). In Madrid in 1994, an ad hoc coalition of antiglobalization protesters demonstrated on the fiftieth anniversary of the IMF and World Bank. Then in June 1999, in dozens of cities from London to North America, protesters staged what they called a "Carnival Against Capital."

One of the European organizations that had emerged to oppose a lowering of farm trade barriers was the European Peasants' Coordination, known as CPE. In December 1990, this organization brought twenty thousand European farmers into the streets of Brussels to march in protest. Eighteen months later, thirty thousand farmers gathered outside both the European Parliament and the American Embassy in Strasbourg to protest agricultural reforms. Despite the protests, the United States and the EU reached a new agreement later in 1992—the Blair House Agreement—to begin reducing trade protections for Europe's farmers.

This was when the embattled CPE joined with a Dutch NGO named the Paulo Freire Foundation to co-organize a network that became La Via Campesina. It held its first meeting in Mons, Belgium, in 1993, with fifty-five farm or peasant organizations from thirty-six different countries represented. LVC presented itself as "a grassroots mass movement" representing poor peasants, yet its first coordinator was a farmer-activist from Spain.

In 1996, LVC moved its administrative headquarters from Europe to a new International Operational Secretariat in Honduras, where the office was headed by an activist with a law degree named Rafael Algeria. Some LVC affiliates did have genuine grassroots credentials, but the network was funded by European NGOs, particularly three from the Netherlands: the Inter-Church Organization for Development Cooperation, Oxfam-Novib, and Friends of the Earth International. Added support came from the Food First Information and Action Network based in Germany. LVC specialized in issuing bold proclamations at international gatherings and getting press attention by organizing street demonstrations.

The European origins of LVC left the network tone-deaf to most of the real problems faced by poor peasants around the world, problems that had little to do with free trade or multinational corporations. In Latin America, it was unequal land holdings, originally created by the Spanish and the Portuguese, that had done the most to keep peasants poor. These original colonizers from Europe did not bring free markets or private enterprise to the region; instead they brought in deadly disease, state-controlled mercantilism, feudalism, racism, human slaves, and naked plunder.

LVC first gained international prominence by presenting its Food Sovereignty manifesto to a forum of more than a thousand NGOs in Rome in 1996. Added attention was gained in November 1999 when antiglobalization protesters successfully disrupted the WTO ministerial meeting in Seattle, amid clashes with riot police that left thousands injured and six hundred under arrest. Central American activists from La Via Campesina were in the middle of the street action, wearing colorful green ball caps and bandannas and demanding food sovereignty. LVC had an early gift for street theater; at the 1996 Rome meeting the organization brought truckloads of earth into the city to create a farm field, where supporters engaged in a symbolic planting of seeds. In Seattle, LVC distributed Roquefort cheese sandwiches to people in the streets, to dramatize their solidarity with European "peasants" seeking to block the import of farm products from the United States.

LVC's food sovereignty vision has evolved over the years toward something increasingly utopian and abstract. In 2007, the Declaration of Nyeleni (named for a village in Mali) proclaimed that food sovereignty now meant "new social relations free of oppression and inequality between men and women, peoples, racial groups, social and economic classes and generations." It also said food sovereignty meant fighting for dignity, a living wage, and respect for different languages and cultures, plus opposition to imperialism, neoliberalism, neocolonialism, and patriarchy. LVC called as well for a rejection of privatization, because it led to the "commodification" of food, basic public services, knowledge, land, water, seeds, livestock, and nature.

LVC grabs headlines with pronouncements and demonstrations, but it lacks a practical strategy for altering the policies of the institutions it complains about the most, such as the World Trade Organization or the World Bank. The network refuses to negotiate with the WTO, or even engage in a dialogue. LVC claims to want more farmland distributed to poor peasants, but then it spurns working with the World Bank on projects that actually distribute land, because it sees giving land titles to individual farmers as a "bourgeois" approach. The network endorses instead communal ownership systems (such as the *ejido* system in Mexico), because they do not turn land and food into commodities to be bought and sold.

LVC's narrative is fundamentally ahistorical. It imagines that peasants around the world were living in contentment within their own traditional communities right up to the moment neoliberal trade and investment policies began exposing them to exploitation by global capital. Today's international companies, rather than the original colonizers, are blamed for grabbing up communal lands, imposing privatization, forcing peasant farmers to produce for export, taking away their traditional food sovereignty, and leaving them impoverished and miserable. LVC depicts transnational corporations as "the worst enemy of peasants and farmers," and asserts that global capitalism is "the ultimate source of the problems facing the rural world."

Consider how far this narrative strays from reality on the continent of Africa. Poor smallholder farmers and herdsmen there do face acute hardships, but these problems are largely unrelated to international trade, transnational corporations, or foreign direct investment. International agribusiness companies take little interest in Africa's farmers, because most are too poor to produce a marketable surplus or to purchase seeds, chemicals, or farm equipment. While more than three out of five Africans still work in the agricultural sector, only 5 percent of foreign investments in Africa go into any kind of agriculture, and these investments are small to begin with. Foreign investments in all the economic sectors in Africa add up to just 4 percent of total global investment flows.

Africa's considerable isolation from global capital is partly self-imposed, brought on by border policies that place high barriers in the path of both foreign investments and imports. International companies also tend to stay away due to burdensome and unpredictable regulations, often linked to pervasive official corruption. When the World Bank reported on the least business-friendly countries around the world in 2019, eleven out of the bottom twenty were found in Africa.

Beyond the off-putting regulations, African governments also keep international agribusiness companies away by investing too little in rural roads, rural electric power, and physical security. These are the public goods that private firms normally require before they put in their own money. African governments also make few investments of their own in farmers. In 2003, Africa's heads of government pledged to be spending at least 10 percent of their public budgets on agriculture by 2008, yet nearly all missed this target, and currently most governments on the continent devote only about 5 percent of their public spending to the agricultural sector. India, during its green revolution, was at one point spending more than 20 percent.

Partly because of official neglect, farm-to-market roads in rural Africa are so sparse and poorly maintained that more than two-thirds of farmers live five hours or more from the nearest market town. This by itself is enough to cut them off from most global investment and commerce. High transport costs make it extremely difficult to bring in fertilizer or get a surplus out to the market. Isolated as they are from global markets, African farmers are twice as likely as Asian farmers to be living on less than $1.25 a day.

Consider the experience of Ethiopia, where the average rural household still lives 10.9 kilometers from the nearest weekly market, and thus depends on subsistence production for nearly 60 percent of its food. This looks a lot like food sovereignty, but the price is food deprivation. Out of 125 countries, Ethiopia scored lowest on a food quality index created in 2014 by Oxfam. Ten percent of all Ethiopians are wasted (too thin) or acutely malnourished. These food outcomes primarily reflect Ethiopia's distance from the global economy, not its deep integration. In fact, Ethiopia, was never colonized by Europeans (only occupied briefly by Italy 1936–41), and has had scant exposure to global capitalism. In 1974, the country went straight from feudalism to being ruled by a self-described Marxist-Leninist. A recovery from this difficult history is at last underway, but it is one that should be based on closer ties to the outside world, not more food sovereignty.

Neither agroecology nor food sovereignty has put the interests of poor peasants first. Agroecologists prioritize hand labor and the imitation of natural ecosystems over productivity, while food sovereignty prioritizes an ideological struggle against global capital. No wonder most governments and farmers in the developing world continue to prefer the green revolution approach.

Occasionally governments do endorse both agroecology and food sovereignty, but with discouraging results. In Venezuela from 1999 to 2013, the government of President Hugo Chavez endorsed food sovereignty and partnered with La Via Campesina to create a new international university designed to teach both agroecology and activist organizing skills. Even if these were just token endorsements, they didn't do Venezuela's food economy any good. When oil prices collapsed, inflationary policies by the successor government of Nicolás Maduro left the food economy in ruins. By March 2017 it took four times the monthly minimum wage to purchase a basket of basic grocery items such as eggs, milk, and fruit. Food eventually disappeared completely from supermarket shelves, and Venezuelan children took to begging in the street or searching through piles of garbage. When some ordinary Venezuelans out of desperation tried growing their own food, advocates for food sovereignty claimed this was consistent with their vision of self-reliance.

Despite such setbacks in the developing world, the food sovereignty concept continues to find supporters in rich countries, as an academic enterprise or a belief system expressing solidarity with the poor, even if the poor may not be participants. In Europe, gatherings to support food sovereignty can sometimes resemble New Age weekend retreats, featuring song-led name-spelling games followed by a sharing of personal experiences, or group discussions on how to integrate the physical and the personal into an intellectual whole. The United States has its own food sovereignty movement, one that is organized around an online "alliance" of thirty-six separate organizations with names like Live Real, Soul Fire Farm, and Movement Generation. In 2019 this alliance awarded its annual Food Sovereignty Prize to a socialist organization in Venezuela named Plan Pueblo a Pueblo (Plan People to People).

In academic circles, an increasingly abstract body of scholarship has now sprung up around food sovereignty. In 2013 and 2014, Yale University and the International Institute of Social Studies in the Netherlands hosted two international conferences on food sovereignty, sponsored by the *Journal of Peasant Studies,* which featured more than ninety different papers or presentations. The second of these conferences had a mostly academic purpose: "exploring whether the subject of food sovereignty has an 'intellectual future' in critical agrarian studies and, if so, on what terms." One of the published papers offered a murky conclusion: "This is thus an investigation into food sovereignty construction, meaning how food sovereignty is being articulated and attempted, as well as contested—including resisted, refracted, or reversed—in a given setting." An interesting new challenge for scholars, perhaps, but distant from the practical needs of poor peasants.

CHAPTER 6

Rejecting Biotech Food

M ark Lynas, a young environmental activist in Britain, was an early opponent of genetically engineered foods. In the 1990s he joined others invading crop research facilities at two o'clock in the morning, ripping genetically engineered crops (known as GMOs) out of the ground. In response to such protest actions, supermarkets in Europe stopped stocking GMO foods, farmers stopped growing them, and European Union authorities eventually placed them under a thick blanket of stifling regulations. Lynas and his fellow activists had won a stunning victory.

GMO regulations in the United States are not as stifling, so farmers have gone ahead to plant genetically engineered varieties of corn, soybeans, and cotton over wide areas. John Nidlinger, the Indiana farmer we met earlier, is a committed GMO corn and soy producer. Yet these crops are mostly grown for animal feed and transport fuel (ethanol), or for industrial use in textiles, not for human food. Staple food crops like wheat, rice, potato, and nearly all fruits and vegetables in the United States have remained strictly non-GMO, even without regulatory blockage. Seed companies have voluntarily agreed not to put such crops on the market and farmers have voluntarily agreed not to plant them knowing there would be consumer resistance, or at least resistance from activists. As a result, nowhere in the world are farmers planting genetically engineered varieties of wheat, rice, or potato for food, even though the seeds for such crops were developed more than two decades ago.

It is rare to see a useful new technology rejected in this way. In the food world, one parallel example might be the radiation technique that makes food safe by eliminating harmful bacteria, insects, and parasites. This is a well-tested method and approved by the FDA, yet it is seldom used by private food companies because consumers fear the word *radiation*.

We might expect a new technology to be rejected if it has failed to deliver a promised benefit or brought a significant new risk, but GMO crops have performed as advertised on farms, and so far no new direct risk has been confirmed either to human health or to the environment. National academies of science all over the world, including throughout Europe, have endorsed this conclusion. These official safety assessments did not persuade most activists to drop their opposition to GMOs, but Mark Lynas became one prominent exception. In 2013, Lynas acknowledged the official scientific consensus and offered a public apology for his own earlier actions. He

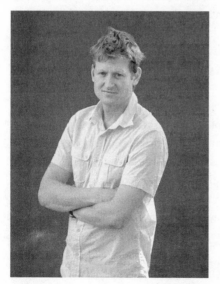

Mark Lynas, the British environmental activist and early opponent of GMO crops who later changed his position, when he saw a new scientific consensus emerge.

said he now believed GMO crops were "an important technological option which can be used to benefit the environment." By that time, however, most governments around the world had already put blocking regulations in place. Lynas ruefully acknowledged that his original anti-GMO activism was "the most successful campaign I have ever been involved with."

Local food has not replaced supermarket food, organic food has not replaced food grown with nitrogen fertilizers, and agroecology has not replaced green revolution farming, but activist opposition to GMO food crops has widely prevailed. In fact, the opponents of GMO foods are now trying to extend this victory to cover a more recent crop improvement method, a genome-editing technique known as CRISPR. Much will be at stake in this new political struggle because CRISPR is an even more powerful laboratory tool.

My own personal interest in crop biotechnology was originally spurred by an expert on African agriculture, Montague Yudelman. Monty was famous for his breadth of professional experience and his technical knowledge of farming, but he had a colorful personal history as well. Born in rural South Africa, he earned a Distinguished Flying Cross fighting fascism in the Second World War, then worked his way to the United States by signing up as a carpenter's mate on a cargo vessel. He made it to Berkeley, where he earned an undergraduate, master's, and then a doctoral degree in agricultural economics, all in just six years.

I first met Monty when he was serving as the director for rural and agricultural development at the World Bank. One day in 1998 we were having lunch when I mentioned that I needed a new research project for my upcoming sabbatical leave from teaching. Without hesitation, Monty said I should study the intensifying regulatory struggle between Europe and the United States over GMOs, including the implications for farmers in the developing world. "I promise you," he said, "this conflict will be with us for a while." He certainly got that right.

Working with a grant from the International Food Policy Research Institute, I made four separate trips to Kenya, Brazil, India, and China in 1999 to speak with local regulators and scientists about the actions they were taking on GMO crops. All these were countries that had welcomed the earlier green revolution, and all the crop scientists I spoke to wanted to work with GMOs as well, but government officials uniformly wanted to go slow, or not go at all. Kenya, Brazil, and India had not approved any GMO crops for planting at that time, and China had only approved GMO cotton, an industrial crop. Chinese scientists had successfully developed their own GMO rice and maize seeds by 1998, but an official approval for planting these crops had not been given—nor has it been given to the present day.

Countries that had earlier welcomed new seed varieties were saying no to GMOs, and no to GMO food crops in particular. I did not know at the time that two decades later there would still be no GMO varieties of staple food crops grown with official approval in any of these countries. Along with most, I was underestimating the ability of private advocacy networks to redirect global biotechnology policy. Their success came through a two-step strategy. Organizations like Greenpeace and Friends of the Earth, both based in Amsterdam, were first able to turn European consumers and politicians against GMO foods, then they leveraged Europe's rejection to launch and win follow-on battles in Asia, Africa, and Latin America. European policy choices carried great influence in the developing world, thanks to Europe's foreign assistance programs, its influence within the UN system, its close cultural ties to urban elites in former colonies, and also thanks to its market power as a big importer of food. Developing countries don't want to plant something European importers might refuse to buy.

The organizations opposing GMOs framed their struggle as a David versus Goliath fight, pitting ordinary people against the greed of monopolistic American biotechnology companies, especially Monsanto, which was redubbed Mon-Satan. Since GMO crops carried genes introduced from unrelated species they were called "Frankenfoods," dangerous creations of a new science gone mad. These scare tactics worked. Biotechnology companies including Monsanto, Dupont, and Syngenta, which had spent hundreds of millions of

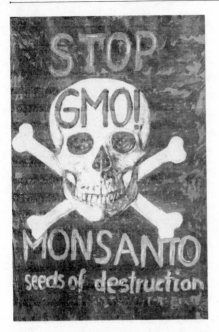

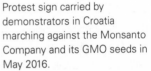

Protest sign carried by demonstrators in Croatia marching against the Monsanto Company and its GMO seeds in May 2016.

dollars to develop GMO varieties of wheat, rice, and potato, were stymied when one country after another made it illegal for farmers to plant these seeds. Just like in the original tale, David had found a way to topple Goliath.

To keep Goliath on his back, David will now have to go after a new breakthrough in crop biotechnology: genome editing, a technique first accomplished in the laboratory in 2012. Biologists have begun using this new method to engineer a wide range of more precise changes into the genetics of plants and animals, without relying on the older recombinant DNA (rDNA) method that inserted genetic material from unrelated species. Because of this difference, scientists originally hoped gene editing would encounter less social resistance, but the same advocacy organizations that earlier blocked GMOs have decided to oppose gene-edited crops as well, labeling them "GMO 2.0." The opposition first arose, once again, in Europe.

The United States, Canada, Sweden, and even Japan originally decided not to treat gene-edited crops like GMOs, but the European

Union chose a different path. In 2018, advocates led by Friends of the Earth secured a judgment from the European Court of Justice that gene-edited crops should be regulated like GMOs. Unless this judgment is reversed, government authorities in the developing world will face a difficult choice between following America or once again copying Europe.

When it comes to reassuring consumers about food safety, scientific findings often carry little weight, as noted earlier in the case of pesticide residue risks. Most European consumers today continue to reject GMOs even though the Royal Society in London, the British Medical Association, the French Academy of Sciences, and the German Academies of Science and Humanities have all said, in writing, they find no convincing evidence of any new risks to human health or to the environment from any of the GMO crops developed for commercial use so far. The International Council for Science, the Organization for Economic Co-operation and Development in Paris, the World Health Organization, and the Food and Agriculture Organization of the United Nations have reached this same benign conclusion.

Even scientists in the European Commission have gone along with this view. In 2010, the Research Directorate of the European Union conducted an analysis of more than 150 projects funded by the EU (not corporate-funded) over two decades and concluded: "Biotechnology, and in particular GMOs, are not per se more risky than e.g., conventional plant breeding technologies." Official scientific bodies in the United States have agreed as well. In 2016 a study committee at the National Academies of Science examined more than nine hundred research studies and stated the following: "The committee carefully searched all available research studies for persuasive evidence of adverse health effects directly attributable to consumption of foods derived from GE crops but found none."

This was the growing scientific consensus that eventually persuaded Mark Lynas to change his mind and make a public apology. He explained it this way in 2018:

How could I so forcefully endorse the scientific consensus on climate change while simultaneously denying the scientific consensus on GMOs? . . . I have often been attacked, especially by my onetime activist friends, for changing my mind on GMOs. But what was the alternative? To stick to a position that I knew to be false in order to avoid losing reputation? Environmentalism, perhaps more than any other philosophy, requires science. And science means that you must change your mind when the evidence changes, however inconvenient that might be.

Given the novelty of transgenic GMO crops, some of the early precaution was fully understandable. The new GMO corn and cotton plants had been engineered to contain in their tissues a protein that some insects could not digest. These were called Bt crops, named for the transgenic trait that had been brought in from a naturally occurring soil bacterium. The new soybean plants had been engineered, also with a bacterial gene, to resist the herbicide glyphosate. They were called Roundup Ready crops, based on Monsanto's trade name for the chemical. Laboratory tests with rodents had indicated no new health risks from eating these crops, but it was more difficult to test for all the hypothetical risks to the environment that might emerge once these crops were grown in open fields. Suspicions were heightened because Monsanto was selling both the patented soybean seeds and also the patented Roundup herbicide to be used with the seeds, so it looked like a sinister attempt at market control.

On top of all this, Monsanto's GMO soybeans began arriving in Europe at exactly the moment a traumatic food safety scandal came to light. In March 1996, European officials had finally acknowledged that eating meat from animals contaminated with BSE (mad cow disease) was dangerous, and possibly even deadly. These were the same officials who earlier said the meat was perfectly safe to eat. They now were saying it was perfectly safe to eat GMO soybeans, but maybe they were again wrong, thought the critics. Given this combination of circumstances, opposition was easy to rally. Ordinary citizens joined activists in the streets and even on the docks, attempting to obstruct the unloading of ships bringing GMO soybeans into Europe. European supermarkets, not wishing to become the next target for demonstrators, began rejecting products with GMO ingredients.

Public fears spread, and in hopes of restoring calm the EU announced in June 1997 that any foods with GMO ingredients would have to carry an identifying label. This move drove such products out of the stores completely, convincing European farmers it would be safer not to plant the seeds. Rather than calming consumer fears, the new labeling requirement was greeted by the public as evidence that GMO foods must indeed be dangerous. By 1998, anxieties were so high that EU regulators placed an informal moratorium on any new approvals of GMO crops.

European regulators did not lift this moratorium until 2004, but by then they had set impossibly stringent requirements in place. In addition to labeling, the EU would now require continuous record keeping. All operators in the marketplace would have to maintain for five years a record of every single GMO they handled, where it came from, and where it went. This burdensome tracing requirement discouraged European companies from investing in the development and sale of GMOs and led European food companies to reformulate their products completely away from any remaining GMO ingredients, including oil from American soybeans and starch from American corn.

It is noteworthy that the same Europeans who recoiled in response to GMO foods had no objections to GMO medical drugs. Genetic engineering had been widely used in commercial medicine since 1982, when the FDA in the United States first approved a recombinant form of human insulin that was created by inserting the appropriate human gene into a bacterium, which then manufactured insulin as it multiplied. European drug companies began using similar genetic engineering techniques, and they also met no citizen objections. By 2006 the European Medicines Agency had approved eighty-seven recombinant therapeutic proteins for use in medicine.

What made genetically engineered drugs more acceptable was the direct benefit they could provide to so many average citizens. The drugs, like GMO food crops, were patented and sold by large American multinational corporations, and they were anything but risk free. The multiple new risks discovered during clinical trials had to be spelled out on the label. These genetically engineered medical drugs were welcomed in Europe not because risks were absent, but because a clear and direct benefit was delivered to the final consumer.

The GMO crops introduced in the 1990s were different. They delivered valuable benefits to farmers by making it cheaper and easier to protect against insects and control weeds, but there were no direct benefits to the final consumer. Compared to conventional corn and soy, the GMO varieties didn't look or taste any better, they didn't have better cooking properties, they weren't any more nutritious, and once they were mixed into packaged food products they were not noticeably cheaper. Because consumers did not see any clear benefit from consuming these products, even an unconfirmed allegation of risk became enough to trigger rejection.

Opponents of GMOs publicized multiple risk allegations. Critics claimed to have found allergic reactions to corn chips, or tumors in lab rats, or dead monarch butterfly caterpillars, but when public agencies and science academies reviewed these studies all were found to be flawed and unconvincing. As one example, a 2012 study published in the journal *Food and Chemical Toxicology* claimed to find tumors in rats that had eaten GMO corn, but the study had used Sprague-Dawley rats known for their high incidence of tumors. This study was formally dismissed by the European Food Safety Agency (EFSA) as well as by Germany's Federal Institute for Risk Assessment, and the journal retracted the paper.

One of the most easily refuted allegations against GMO crops was the bogus assertion that they contained "terminator genes" that made the seeds sterile. The fact that Brazilian farmers for several years had been saving and successfully replanting GMO soybean seeds that they had smuggled in from Argentina (because they couldn't yet legally buy them in Brazil) should have put this allegation to rest, but the idea lived on.

Regulators in the United States were more permissive toward

GMOs than their European counterparts, but most ordinary American consumers, when asked, expressed anxieties. One 2003 survey by the Food Policy Institute at Rutgers University found that fewer than half of Americans felt it was safe to consume GMO foods, and more than half believed "serious accidents involving GMO foods are bound to happen." The technology encountered less regulatory blockage in the United States in part because America's politically powerful farmers found the new seeds useful and wanted them to remain available; Europe also had politically powerful farmers, but few planted corn, soybeans, or cotton, so the political backing for these seeds was far less strong.

Consumers in the United States had few objections to GMO corn, soy, and cotton seeds in particular because these crops were used mostly for animal feed, fuel, or industrial purposes. American farmers had decided voluntarily not to plant any GMO wheat or rice seeds, knowing that consumers both at home and abroad might reject these products. Some United States growers did plant GMO potatoes and tomatoes for a time after 1998, but stopped once retailers and fast-food chains began turning these foods away.

Many processed food products in the United States do contain oils, starches, and sweeteners from GMO maize, soybeans, and sugar beets, but nearly all unprocessed foods in America's supermarkets today are non-GMO. The exceptions are papaya from Hawaii, some summer squash, and a bit of sweet corn. In other words, GMO food crops have been driven out of the marketplace in the United States almost as much as in Europe.

Food consumers in Europe and the United States can easily accept this outcome, since GMO food crops never gave them any direct benefit. Even American farmers will find the outcome acceptable, so long as they can keep planting GMO corn, soy, and cotton seeds. These three crops together occupy more than 70 percent of the nation's total harvested area. So long as GMO seeds aren't taken away for these crops, most American farmers won't complain.

Doing without GMO varieties of basic food crops will be a bigger sacrifice for farmers and consumers in Africa and Asia, because animal feed and industrial crops are less important there. For small farmers in these regions, some of the GMO technologies currently available would be delivering a significant benefit already if national governments would only make it legal to plant the seeds.

For example, farmers in Africa struggle every year against stalk borer insects that reduce their maize yields. If it were legal for them to plant Bt maize, the insect damage could be contained without chemical sprays, but planting Bt maize is not yet legal anywhere in sub-Saharan Africa other than in the Republic of South Africa. On most of the continent, simply doing research on GMO maize can violate the rules. In Tanzania in 2018, even an officially approved confined research trial for drought-tolerant Bt maize became embroiled in political controversy and was terminated, with the planting materials ordered destroyed.

Advocates for GMO crops in Africa—scientists, for the most part—have recently seen a few signs of policy change. In 2018, Ethiopia and Nigeria finally approved Bt cotton for commercial planting, and Nigeria also gave technical approval to an insect-resistant Bt cowpea. But technical approval is not the same thing as final commercial approval. Ghana gave technical approval to the cowpea as well, but then the agricultural minister undercut this move by saying his country didn't really need the technology, adding that many of his countrymen were staunchly opposed to GMOs. Late in 2019, the Kenyan cabinet passed a resolution to approve Bt cotton, but an Environmental Impact Assessment for the cotton still had to be completed and an earlier official ban on GMO *foods* in Kenya technically remained in place.

Advocates for GMO seeds were initially baffled when so many countries in Africa with persistent farm production deficits opted not to allow their use. Following my own four-country research travel in 1999, I was asked to share my findings with the Rockefeller Foundation in New York, an organization that supported GMOs and had initially expected high demand. The experts at Rockefeller originally assumed Asia and Africa would want the seeds, and worried only that the patents would get in the way. This worry was addressed when most of the patent holders agreed to donate their technology for use in the developing world on a royalty-free basis. What kept the seeds out of Asia and Africa instead was the decision of so many governments there to adopt European-style regulations. When I reported this conclusion to the senior leadership at Rockefeller in New York late one afternoon, nobody in the room yet realized how far the opponents of this new technology would be prepared to go.

This became clear in 2002, a year when southern Africa was struck by a severe drought that left fifteen million people across seven different countries in need of international food aid. Yellow corn from the United States, which happened to be GMO, had until then been welcomed in Africa as food aid, but in August 2002 the government of Zambia turned it down. Zambia's president, Levy Mwanawasa, later explained his decision: "Simply because my people are hungry, that is no justification to give them poison, to give them food that is intrinsically dangerous to their health."

Official hostility toward GMOs in Zambia had partly been stoked through an assistance relationship with Norway's Institute for Gene Ecology, but opposition also came from a Jesuit agricultural training center that worked closely with Agriflora, a company growing organic produce for export to Europe. The center's slogan was "Organic Farming: Keep Zambia GMO Free." Other civil society groups also joined to oppose the American food aid. At one open meeting, the most impassioned public speaker was a local NGO leader named Emily Sikazwe, who told her fellow Zambians, "Yes, we are starving, but we are saying no to the food the Americans are forcing on our throats." Sikazwe's organization received its funding from the Swedish embassy in Lusaka, the Norwegian embassy, and the Danish foreign assistance agency DANIDA.

By the time President Mwanawasa decided to reject America's food aid, some of the corn had already been delivered, but he ordered these stocks removed despite the continuing drought emergency. Ordinary Zambians were puzzled, with one saying, "They have said that the food is not good for us, but we don't know . . . they don't explain." In one town outside the capital an angry mob overpowered an armed guard at a warehouse and looted several thousand bags of the food before it could be taken away.

As this spectacle unfolded, American officials sought to reassure the Zambians by inviting a government delegation on a fact-finding visit to the United States, but the Zambians had also been invited to visit Europe. There they met with groups hostile to GMOs, including Greenpeace, Friends of the Earth, the UK Soil Association, Norway's Institute for Gene Ecology, and an organization named Genetic Food Alert. Greenpeace warned the visiting Zambians that organic food sales to Europe would collapse if the nation opened itself up to GMOs, and Genetic Food Alert warned of the "unknown and unassessed implications" of eating GMO foods. An organization from the United Kingdom named Farming and Livestock Concern warned the Zambians that GMO maize might introduce a retrovirus similar to HIV. Upon returning home, a spokesperson for the Zambian delegation said the trip had confirmed his negative view of GMOs.

This 2002 advocacy campaign against GMOs in Africa subsequently shifted its focus to a highly publicized UN event in Johannesburg, the World Summit on Sustainable Development. At this meeting Friends of the Earth and several other anti-GMO groups persuaded 140 local African organizations to sign an open letter protesting all shipments of GMO food aid. The letter was circulated widely on the Internet, and it listed a number of frightening but undocumented charges: "GM food can potentially give rise to a range of health problems, including: food allergies; chronic toxic effects; infections from bacteria that have developed resistance to antibiotics, rendering these infections untreatable; and possible ailments including cancers."

Advocacy groups in Johannesburg also managed to ventriloquize their message into the mouths of local African farmers. An organization named Participatory Ecological Land Use Management (PELUM), with funding from NGOs in Belgium, Germany, and the Netherlands, organized what it called a "Small Farmers' Convergence" that culminated in a four-day trek from Lusaka to Johannesburg by 120 farmers. At a press conference at the end of their walk the farmers announced, "We say NO to genetically modified foods." PELUM's chief African organizer for the march, who was not a farmer himself, told interviewers he didn't like GMOs because he had learned that, if eaten, they would change the genetic composition of the human body (there is no scientific basis for such a claim). Even the wildest charges were taken seriously. One African minister in Johannesburg, from a Muslim country, asked USAID administrator Andrew Natsios "if it was true" that GM maize contained pig genes.

Policymaking elites in Africa can be influenced by campaigns launched from Europe due to a lingering postcolonial sense of deference. As one local Kenyan leader said in 2006, "Europe has more knowledge, education. So why are they refusing [GM foods]? That is the question everyone is asking." The fact that Europe's own science academies had found no evidence of any new risks from GMOs was something the Africans were seldom told. The smallholder farmers in Africa who could have been benefiting from the technology had little or no political voice because most were poor, female, and physically remote from the capital city. Typically, the only farmers well enough organized to express a view in Africa are those growing specialty crops for export to Europe, and they are usually against the technology due to fears that exports will be rejected.

Activist campaigns in Asia stopped GMO food crops there as well. In India in 2010, anti-GMO advocates blocked the commercial planting of a GMO variety of eggplant (brinjal), even though the benefits would have included fewer pesticide sprays, lowering chemical exposure risks to farmers as well as consumers. India's environment minister intervened at the last minute to stop this technology due to a firestorm of protest actions led by international NGOs. India's prime minister, Manmohan Singh, later expressed regret about this foreign interference: "Biotechnology has enormous potential, and in due course of time we must make use of genetic engineering technologies to increase the productivity of our agriculture. But there are controversies. There are NGOs, often funded from the US and Scandinavian countries, which aren't fully appreciative of the developmental challenges our country faces."

When controversies of this kind arise, scientists normally keep their heads down, but one plant geneticist at the University of California, Davis, named Pamela Ronald has been willing to speak out publicly against the ill-informed critics of GMO crops. She has the scientific credentials and professional independence needed to survive the blowback. For the past twenty-five years her research has been funded only by government institutes such as the NIH, NSF, and USDA, or by nonprofit philanthropies like the Rockefeller Foundation, not by private industry. This is not so unusual among university-based agricultural scientists. UC Davis is America's top university for agricultural research, yet it gets less than 0.1 percent of its research funding from Monsanto.

Pam Ronald's own lab has worked to develop varieties of rice able to survive flooding and resist crop disease, ongoing problems facing smallholder farmers in tropical countries. Pam manages to play several different roles. She is both a locked-down bench scientist and also an energetic public advocate for science, including GMO science. At Davis in 2014 she founded the Institute for Food and Agricultural Literacy, which runs "boot camps" designed to break down cultural barriers between scientists and nonscientists. This can be a frustrating task in the area of crop biotechnology, but Ronald persists, relying on her signature cheer and optimism.

Pam Ronald originally fell in love with plants while hiking in the Sierras with her family as a youngster, staying in a tiny cabin her father hand-built from a kit. One summer when she was fifteen, she encountered a man and a woman on the trail using a book to identify plants. A wild idea popped into her head: "Gosh, I could have a job looking at plants." She does not fit the science nerd stereotype. Pam went to Reed College, shopped at health food stores, stopped eating meat after reading Frances Moore Lappé's 1971 book *Diet for a Small*

Planet, and eventually married an organic farmer. Then a strong pull from science brought her to Berkeley for a Ph.D., followed by Cornell for a postdoc. While at Cornell she decided to work on rice, a crop that was then feeding half the world's people.

Pam learned about the controversy surrounding genetic engineering early because her Berkeley lab in 1987 was directly across from a facility preparing to conduct the world's first nonconfined GMO field test. This was not for a crop, but instead for "ice minus," a modified version of a common bacterium that could be sprayed on strawberry plants as protection against frost damage. The planned test triggered vigorous opposition from Earth First, an organization that warned about "corporations invading my body with new bacteria that hadn't existed on the planet before." The fields for the experiment were raided and damaged the night before the test, a protest technique later perfected by Mark Lynas and his friends in Britain.

Pam Ronald supports GMO crop improvement methods because they can do things conventional breeding cannot, such as introducing beta-carotene into rice to counter vitamin A deficiencies, or adding Bt genes to help corn and cotton self-protect against insects. In her own lab, the crop improvement method she uses most often is known as marker-assisted selection (MAS), an advanced non-GMO (non-rDNA) breeding method. In one particularly successful project, she managed to isolate a gene that could protect rice plants against damage from flooding, then she partnered with scientists in the Philippines to move this gene into commercial rice varieties using MAS. The resulting flood-tolerant rice is now in use by six million farmers, with disproportionate benefits going to the poor because they are often relegated to the most flood-prone lands.

Pam is known for her readiness to defend GMO science in public in front of skeptical audiences. In 2010 she coauthored, with her husband Raoul Adamchak (the organic farmer), an award-winning book titled *Tomorrow's Table,* which explained GMO crop improvement methods to nonspecialists. The book was endorsed by Bill Gates, and in 2015 she gave a TED Talk on the subject that received nearly two million views online. Early in 2017 she spoke to fifty-five thousand attendees at a San Francisco "March for Science" rally, pushing back against the new Trump administration's policies on science.

Like Mark Lynas, Pam is frustrated by critics who invoke scientific consensus when it comes to climate risks, but then deny what she sees as an equally strong scientific consensus on the safety of GMO crops. Pam recalls once attending a forum on "trust in science" where she met a prominent climate scientist who was complaining about the frequent attacks he endured from climate denialists. Sensing an opportunity to bond, she described her own encounters with critics who were ignoring the scientific consensus on GMOs. When she suggested crop scientists and climate scientists were facing a similar problem, he answered, "Oh, no, no. It's completely different, you all work for Monsanto."

Organizations critical of GMOs often accuse scientists like Pam Ronald of being shills for private industry. Beginning in January 2015, an organization calling itself USRTK (U.S. Right to Know) used the Freedom of Information Act to oblige public universities to collect and hand over all email messages, going back several years, between a list of eight university scientists and fourteen different agribusiness firms. UC Davis was one of the universities, and Pam Ronald was on the list of targeted scientists.

USRTK was founded in 2014 to promote the mandatory labeling of GMO foods, and it was originally funded by the Organic Consumers Association, so it was hardly a neutral referee. The head of the organization, Gary Ruskin, characterized what he was doing as "citizens reviewing what our government does, to see what corporate influence lies within," but in the end nothing nefarious was found in the emails, and the *New York Times* concluded that no academic work had been compromised. The scientists knew they were simply being harassed because they had spoken out publicly in favor of GMOs.

A gricultural biotechnology is now moving into a new zone of controversy, thanks to a recently discovered technique known as genome editing. In its simplest form, this technique cuts the strands

of an organism's DNA at specific locations to "knock out" an unde-
sired genetic trait. First mastered in 2012, gene editing should have
been less controversial than transgenic work because it more closely
resembled the natural process of genetic mutation, and because it
did not rely on bringing in "foreign genes" from unrelated species.

Gene editing nonetheless met social and regulatory resistance,
beginning once again in Europe. In 2018 the European Court concluded that gene-edited organisms should fall under the same regulatory requirements earlier imposed on GMOs, including mandatory
case-by-case review prior to approval for new plants, strict segre-
gation in the field from conventional plants, and the labeling and
tracing of all the derived food products in the marketplace. These
are the regulations that drove GMOs out of supermarkets and farm
fields in Europe, so they could now do the same to gene-edited foods
and crops. If other governments around the world decide to follow
Europe's regulatory lead on gene-edited food crops, another potentially useful advance could be stillborn.

The official EU definition of a GMO is an organism in which "the
genetic material has been altered in a way that does not occur naturally by mating and/or natural recombination." This definition might
seem to encompass plants altered through exposure to chemicals or
radiation for the purpose of inducing mutations, but the EU has always exempted such mutagenesis crops from the GMO regulations.
European scientists originally expected gene-edited crops would be
exempted as well, since the technique was not recombinant or transgenic, and it produced outcomes similar to a natural mutation.

The DNA within living cells often breaks apart naturally, and is
repaired naturally as well by cellular enzymes. Gene editing brings
this common process under human control, by creating a break at
an intended location using a repeat DNA sequence called CRISPR,
originally discovered in a naturally occurring salt-tolerant microbe
in Spain in 1993. CRISPR stands for Clustered Regularly Interspaced
Short Palindromic Repeats. These repeat sequences had evolved
in nature to allow microbes like the one found in Spain to defend
themselves by cutting the DNA of invading viruses. These molecu-

lar CRISPR scissors were made useful when scientists finally learned
how to direct them to precise locations. It took a decade, but diverse
teams of scientists working in Spain, France, Lithuania, Holland,
Canada, Sweden, Austria, California, and Massachusetts eventually
devised something called a Cas9 nuclease to accomplish this task.
The most common label for this kind of gene editing thus became
CRISPR-Cas9.

CRISPR was named runner-up Breakthrough of the Year by *Science* magazine two years in a row, then in 2015 it won the award outright. Large numbers of scientists were in a position to begin using
this new method almost immediately because it was relatively simple
and surprisingly inexpensive; novices could purchase a CRISPR toolkit for less than fifty dollars. Potential benefits for human medicine
quickly emerged when researchers at the University of Texas in 2014
showed that CRISPR could correct human mutations associated with
muscular dystrophy, and then when a biotech company named Editas
made progress pursuing a CRISPR correction for inherited childhood
blindness. The anticipated applications for crop and animal improvement ranged from tastier tomatoes and high-fiber wheat to crops
better able to survive drought and animals better able to resist disease.

In 2015 a plant biologist at Penn State named Yinong Yang used
CRISPR to modify an edible white mushroom so it would not turn
brown on the shelf. Uncertain how his new mushroom would be
regulated, Yang sent a letter to the Animal and Plant Health Inspection Service (APHIS) at the USDA to ask if it would be regulated like
a GMO, and APHIS replied it would not. The Canadian government
reached a similar regulatory judgment, as did Sweden, where a scientist named Stefan Jansson made news in 2016 by serving a meal with
a gene-edited head of cabbage he had grown on the Umea University
campus. He facetiously described his meal as "tagliatelle with CRIS-
PRy fried vegetables."

It did not take CRISPR long to deliver proof-of-concept results
for nearly twenty different crops, including each of the world's most
important food crops—rice, wheat, maize, and potato. Edited food
animals also began to appear. Gene-edited hogs were produced that

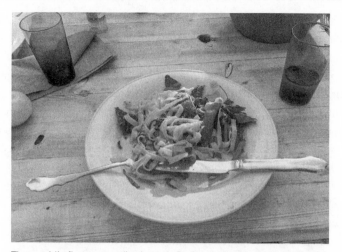

The world's first gene-edited meal: Stefan Jansson's 2016 pasta dish with his own CRISPR-Cas9 cabbage.

could resist porcine reproductive and respiratory syndrome, an illness that costs the industry hundreds of millions of dollars every year. Researchers in the United Kingdom found a way, with gene editing, to prevent the spread of a bird virus in chickens, a serious disease threat that forced a culling of millions of birds in the United States in 2014.

The USDA subsequently restated its decision not to require a premarket review of gene-edited crop plants unless they were a potential plant pest or a noxious weed threat, and President Trump reinforced this policy in June 2019 when he instructed the USDA, EPA, and FDA to use their existing powers to "exempt low-risk products of agriculture biotechnology from undue regulation." The EPA indicated it would exempt low-risk plants from a premarket review, and the FDA said nothing about a mandatory premarket review for gene-edited plants, though it did impose tight control over gene-edited animals by classifying them—curiously—as similar to new animal drugs. The first product from a gene-edited plant reached the market in the United States in 2019, a restaurant frying oil from a gene-edited soybean, produced by a Minnesota company named Calyxt. It had no trans fats and a longer shelf life than other soybean oils. A

Maryland company named Intrexon also began commercial trials of non-browning, gene-edited lettuce.

While CRISPR plants were getting a regulatory green light in the United States and elsewhere, a threatening legal challenge began making its way through the courts in Europe. An affiliate of Friends of the Earth, together with a French organization representing small farms (Confederation Paysanne), had challenged French regulations concerning CRISPR, and the French government asked the European Court of Justice for a ruling. The EU advocate general at first offered his nonbinding opinion that CRISPR crops should be exempt from its GMO Directive, similar to mutagenesis crops, but in July 2018 the European Court ignored this advice and ruled that CRISPR crops would not be exempt. They would be regulated like GMOs.

The court explained that gene-editing methods differed from mutation breeding because they lacked a long history of safe use. It then went on to speculate that new risks from CRISPR "might prove similar" to those associated with transgenic crops, a curious statement that ignored the 2010 conclusion from the EU Commission's Research Directorate that no new risks had been found from transgenic GMOs.

This 2018 court ruling hit European crop scientists hard. One researcher at the Heinrich Heine University in Germany predicted it would be "the death blow for plant biotech in Europe." Reacting to the judgment, the chief scientific advisers to the EU Commission recommended that the GMO Directive be revised "to reflect current knowledge . . . on gene editing," and the Commission itself scrambled for a way to undo the ruling through a revision of the Directive. The European Academies Science Advisory Council (EASAC), representing the science academies of all twenty-eight EU member states, called the decision a "setback for cutting-edge science and innovation in the EU" and predicted troubling consequences in the wider world of food and farming: "EASAC reaffirms that breakthroughs in plant breeding technologies, such as genome editing, remain crucial for food and nutrition security globally. It remains to be seen what implications this decision may have outside of the EU, particularly in developing countries who stand to benefit most from crops that better withstand the devastating effects of climate change."

Later in 2018, this view was seconded by the World Resources Institute in Washington, D.C., which noted the "far greater potential" for CRISPR crops to "combat environmental challenges" in the years ahead, even compared to GMO crops. In July 2019, researchers at 120 institutes across Europe begged the European Parliament and Commission for new legislation to undo the damage.

Researchers in Africa who had already been working on gene-edited varieties of maize, sweet potato, and cassava have reason to worry. If African governments decide to copy the new European policy, CRISPR crops will become just as hard to commercialize as GMOs. Stefan Jansson, the CRISPRy cabbage scientist from Sweden, merely said, "This proves how stupid the European system is for regulating GMOs."

Critics of gene editing moved quickly to consolidate their new advantage after the court decision. The EU organic farming movement denounced CRISPR techniques as "not compatible with organic farming" and called on the European Commission to immediately develop detection methods to prevent gene-edited crops from "contaminating" organic and GMO-free food. Greenpeace called on the United Kingdom to halt earlier approved field trials of a gene-edited variety of camelina oilseed that was high in omega-3 oils. Similar demands were made to end CRISPR crop trials underway in Belgium, Sweden, and Finland.

The European Court opinion assumed, implicitly, that CRISPR crops would be more likely to introduce new risks than traditional mutation-developed crops. This ignored evidence that nothing, in fact, is more risk-prone than mutation breeding, since it exposes crop seeds to ionizing radiation and toxic chemicals that cause DNA breaks in numerous locations in a completely random fashion. Most of these breaks are so harmful to the health of the plant that the results must be discarded. When the United States National Research Council (NRC) examined twelve different methods of breeding new plant varieties in 2004, it concluded that "induced mutagenesis is the most genetically disruptive and, consequently, most likely to display unintended effects." This NRC report ranked mutation breeding as more likely than transgenic methods (GMO) to produce unintended effects, yet the EU was deciding to rank both GMOs and CRISPR crops, somehow, as more risky than mutation breeding.

Gene-editing methods are significantly more precise than GMO methods. When transgenic GMO techniques are used, foreign materials are added to a plant's genome, often by bombarding its cells with microparticles covered with the transgenic DNA molecules. It is impossible to control where the foreign DNA will land in the genome of the target plant. Gene editing, by contrast, can delete genetic material at precisely targeted locations. If this highly precise gene-editing technique had emerged before GMOs, crop biotechnology might have encountered far less organized resistance. By the time CRISPR arrived, however, social opposition to crop biotechnology had already been mobilized. The European organizations that originally formed to block GMOs welcomed gene-editing as a fresh new target.

Some groups in the United States, including the organic community plus organizations like USRTK, also wanted CRISPR crops to be treated like GMOs. The fact that the Monsanto Company, before being taken over by Bayer, invested $125 million in a gene-editing start-up named Pairwise raised an alarm for such groups. The National Organic Standards Board voted in 2016 to exclude gene-edited crops from organic certification, and the Non-GMO Project, a private certification system, also refused to accept gene-edited crops. Fighting on the other side was an industry-supported organization named the Center for Food Integrity (CFI), which formed a Coalition for Responsible Gene Editing in Agriculture in 2016, offering communications training, toolkits, fact sheets, and infographics to demonstrate the safety and benefits of gene editing.

If gene-edited foods do come to be labeled and regulated just like GMOs, a significant opportunity for crop and animal improvement will be lost. One preliminary 2017 inventory of gene-editing advances included wheat varieties resistant to powdery mildew, maize plants with higher yields under drought conditions, rice plants resistant to a fungal pathogen called rice blast, herbicide-tolerant soybean plants, grapefruit trees resistant to citrus canker, and tomatoes with anthocyanin (the compound found in blueberries that reduces cardiovascular and cancer risks).

G ene-edited animals are likely to encounter even more resistance than gene-edited plants. Together with transgenic (GMO) animals, they will fall under the regulatory authority of the Food and Drug Administration, which for legal purposes views both as similar to new veterinary drugs. So far, only one GMO animal has been approved for food consumption by FDA, a fast-growing AquAdvantage salmon that reaches a market size in just eighteen months, half the normal time for farmed salmon. The formal approval process for this animal dragged on for twelve years, and the salmon is still not being sold commercially due to retailer anxieties. Kroger, Safeway, Target, Trader Joe's, Whole Foods, and Walmart all pledged not to sell it, and uncertainties have lingered over federal labeling and disclosure requirements.

Gene editing has considerable potential to improve farm animals. It could give us meatier pigs, cashmere goats with longer hair, or cows better able to survive in tropical climates. In 2018 the *Washington Post* reported that more than three hundred pigs, cows, sheep, and goats had already been created with gene-editing tools. None of these gene-edited farm animals has yet been approved by the FDA for food consumption, a particular frustration to pork producers who want to start raising disease-resistant gene-edited pigs. The fact that the FDA regulates gene-edited animals like drugs seems nonsensical to impatient farmers and scientists. Alison Van Eenennaam, an animal geneticist at Davis who has used gene editing to produce dairy cows without horns—an alteration that might save millions of animals from the painful process of dehorning—complains that "my cows are not drugs. They're cows."

CRISPR-altered farm animals encounter resistance in part because they bring us one biological step closer to gene-editing humans, something already done by a renegade scientist in China. In 2018, a researcher in Shenzhen named He Jiankui gene-edited human embryos using CRISPR-Cas9, resulting in the birth of twin baby girls with immunity to HIV. Despite the intent of the scientist to do something beneficial, the initial response in China was widespread revulsion followed by official censure. Gene-editing humans for resistance to COVID-19 is probably off the table as well.

No less controversial will be the gene editing of insects to improve disease control. The most dangerous animals on earth today are the Anopheles mosquitoes that transmit malaria, killing more than four hundred thousand people every year, mostly in Africa, and most often children under age five. Gene-edited versions of these mosquitoes released into the wild might eliminate the vector for the disease without doing any harm to the three thousand other species of mosquitoes that do not feed on people. This, too, has already been done, at least in the laboratory. Scientists at Imperial College London in 2018 used CRISPR-Cas9 to alter the "doublesex" gene of *Anopheles gambiae* mosquitoes, a step that created a "gene drive" that ensured nearly all of the progeny of the altered mosquitoes would also be altered. One hundred fifty altered males were then introduced into a cage with three hundred normal female mosquitoes, plus one hundred fifty normal males. The altered males produced female offspring that were nearly all unable to bite or lay eggs, along with male offspring that continued to spread the mutation. Within seven to eleven generations the mutation had spread throughout the population, egg production fell to zero, and soon all the mosquitoes were gone. Here is a genuine terminator technology, but for insects instead of plants.

The Gates Foundation and the Indian Tata Group have now invested more than $140 million to research gene-drive technologies of this kind, with applications that might include agricultural pest control as well as disease vector control. When a gene drive is used, insect populations that are invasive or resistant to chemicals could simply be eliminated. Austin Burt, coauthor of the paper that reported the mosquito experiment, is enthusiastic about these methods. "If there are no unexpected technical or regulatory delays," he said, "it's possible to envisage that gene-drive mosquitoes, in combination with other approaches, could have eliminated malaria in significant parts of Africa in fifteen years."

Yet regulatory delays, for good reason, are highly likely. The National Academy of Sciences in 2016 called for extensive testing plus public consultation before any gene drive is released. Public consultation will be a challenge. A national survey by the Food Marketing Institute in 2020 revealed that more than half of consumers had never heard of gene editing. Prior to field tests of gene-drive mosquitoes there should also be broad international consultation and agreement, since even a small release of altered insects on the continent of Africa might spread rapidly across international borders. Africans continue to reject GMO foods as something of an experiment *on them,* so they can be expected to view gene-drive insects with even greater suspicion, whatever the possible public health benefit. Nnimmo Bassey, director of the Health of Mother Earth Foundation in Nigeria, says the mosquito scientists are "trying to use Africa as a big laboratory to test risky technologies."

Corporate mischief is also a risk. We can imagine agribusiness companies wanting to alter insect populations that are currently resistant to their chemicals to be vulnerable once again, in order to sell more chemicals. The regulation problems will be challenging in part because the science is so accessible. Constructing a new gene-drive organism might require only a few months and perhaps just a thousand dollars' worth of consumables. If an unregulated competition emerges to edit the genomes of all the insects farmers currently find undesirable, potentially dangerous and irreversible ecosystem changes might result.

To discourage this, techniques are being developed to disperse gene-edited insects without gene drives, for example by making the altered males sterile. A newly developed "precision guided sterile insect technique," or pgSIT for short, uses targeted introductions of CRISPR-edited eggs from which only adult sterile males emerge, a method intended to suppress local populations without passing on the alteration.

In a way all this is nothing new. For thousands of years, humans have employed simple but slow controlled breeding methods to introduce surprising alterations into the genetics of crops and animals. Consider Mexican hairless dogs. It was even acceptable up to a century ago to consider controlled breeding of people. The nightmare of Hitler's Germany put this idea to rest, and made genetic tampering of any kind more controversial. The use of advanced laboratory techniques to alter genetics is particularly fraught today because these modern methods can do so much more, and far more quickly.

The highly precautionary response to crop and farm animal biotechnology we have seen so far suggests we do not yet trust ourselves to use this new power responsibly. Yet it could also suggest something less commendable. It may partly reflect the fact that today's wealthy societies, who make the global rules, feel no urgent need to develop novel varieties of food crops or food animals, because their own farmers are already prosperous and their own consumers are already well fed, indeed overfed. Perhaps if the rural poor in Africa were making the rules, we would see outcomes less timid.

CHAPTER 7

The Fate of Farm Animals

❧

Would most egg-laying hens be better off dead? This grim possibility was raised by an agricultural economist at Oklahoma State University, Bailey Norwood, in a 2011 book titled *Compassion by the Pound*. Based on results from a mathematical welfare model for hens named FOWEL, plus his own judgment, Norwood concluded that hens in cages had a welfare score of negative eight (on a scale from negative ten to positive ten). Some of the birds' physical and behavioral needs were being met, but "the negative emotions experienced outweigh the positive, and the animal is better off euthanized."

Some of these miserable hens are now being moved into bigger cages, or taken out of cages entirely, thanks to vigorous animal welfare advocacy. In 2018, voters in California passed Proposition 12, a measure that will make egg production in that state essentially cage free. The measure also blocks the sale of pork if sows are held in small crates, plus veal from tightly confined calves. Prop 12 was promoted by the Humane Society of the United States (HSUS) and it passed by a 61 percent majority, so it looked like a significant victory for the animals, but for some groups in California the measure did not go far enough. People for the Ethical Treatment of Animals (PETA) led three other California groups in condemning Prop 12 as a fraud, and a "capitulation to the egg industry." Welcome to the conflicted, emotion-laden debate over the welfare of farm animals.

Most of us have at least some experience taking care of animals.

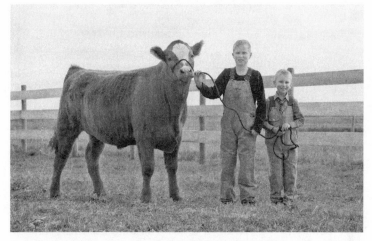

Honoring tradition, a young boy hand-trains his 4-H calf. The modern livestock industry has brought an end to traditional husbandry.

Over the years for me this has included two dogs and three parakeets as a child, and now a total of ten different cats in my adult life. All these animals have been marvelous companions, even the parakeets. My job was simply to protect them and tend to their various needs until the end of their natural lives. When the end inevitably came, I felt I had done my best for them.

Youngsters who grow up on farms must navigate quite a different path with their animals. Many join the local 4-H club to raise a calf or a pig they will show with pride at the county fair, knowing that the animal will then be sold and slaughtered in its prime, for meat. The young club members are told from the start that their animals must come to the fair at a market weight, ready for processing. Each exhibitor is required to sign an "intent to sell" form before weigh-in day. If the animal wins a blue or a red ribbon, the club member must personally lead it into the auction ring, then continue to care for it right up to the moment it leaves the fairgrounds.

The final parting is usually an emotional experience, since 4-H members bond deeply with their animals through the lavish daily care they provide. Hours are spent hand-feeding, grooming, then training the animal to walk on a halter. Before being shown, beef cattle will be washed, trimmed, clipped, and the hooves are even polished. Pigs are hand-washed with mild soapy water several times in the two weeks before the show and brushed frequently to improve the appearance of their coat, which is made still more glossy by applying a small amount of transparent mineral oil.

When these animals are finally sent off for processing, tears will be shed. Katie Pratt, who is now a corn and soybean farmer in northern Illinois, sold her first market calf when she was eight years old. "He was my best friend," she later told a journalist. "We went to the fair and I got a blue ribbon. When the reality of the fact that he had to go to market hit, it was just awful." But then Pratt's realism kicks in. "I hate to sound crass or blunt, but you get over it."

These 4-H rituals teach important lessons about the final destiny of food animals, but they no longer reveal much about the methods used to raise those animals by the livestock industry. Modern commercial practices are a world away from the antiquated 4-H program. For example, 4-H exhibitors are advised to provide their pigs with at least three hundred square feet of space per animal, inside covered pens with a southern opening to the sun and the outdoors. In commercial hog operations in the United States today, pigs are often confined with only eight square feet of space per animal, and no opening at all to the outside.

Modern livestock systems have been pushed to this extreme through a merciless competition in the marketplace to reduce production costs. This is identical to the competition that has also reduced production costs for crops, but plants are not sentient beings, deserving of humane treatment.

On traditional farms a century ago, working animals such as oxen, mules, and horses, were also sometimes mistreated, but powered machines eventually solved that problem by making these animals unnecessary. The arrival of tractors and trucks meant overworked horses and mules no longer had to pull heavy plows and wagons.

America's mule and horse population, which stood at twenty-six million in 1915, fell to just three million by 1960. Not having to pasture or produce feed for all these draft animals also brought a land-saving benefit.

Food animals have not fared as well under the forces of market competition. As industrial development and urbanization began moving workers off of the farm, the large labor supply needed to perform traditional animal husbandry practices began to decline. Traditionally, farmers had to feed and water their animals by hand every day, milk the cows several times a day, gather eggs by hand, clean out the stalls in the barn and the hog shed by hand, spread the manure, and move the animals back and forth from pasture to barn. By the middle years of the twentieth century, a labor exodus to the city plus smaller farm families left too few workers to perform these traditional chores. The logical solution was for crop farms to grow crops only while moving the animals to separate indoor production facilities where they would be easier to control, and where the feeding, watering, and cleanup could eventually become automated. I once asked an Alabama cotton farmer why her operation didn't include any animals. She said her father originally decided to do without the animals "because they move around."

The labor-saving benefits that came from confining farm animals were enormous. As previously noted, the hours of human labor required to produce milk eventually fell by 94 percent, and to produce chicken meat by 99 percent. Moving everything indoors also gave the animals better protection from temperature extremes, wild predators, and parasitic disease, allowing more to survive for a commercial sale. This transition to indoor confinement took place over the second half of the twentieth century, beginning with hens and broiler chickens then followed by pigs and dairy cows. Only beef cattle have continued to live mostly outside.

Commercial egg producers went first. When kept inside temperature-controlled buildings, hens can produce at an optimal rate all year long, no matter how hot or cold it might be outside. Once the birds are indoors, cages can be used to protect timid ones from their more aggressive flock mates and reduce competition for feed and water. If raised off the ground, the cages will also reduce contact with waste and create new options for labor-saving feed and water automation. By the 1960s, conveyor belts were in place to collect the eggs as soon as they were laid, taking them to automated washers.

Hens were then bred to suit this kind of confinement. They went from being multipurpose birds used for meat as well as eggs to being specialized egg layers. Better genetics plus high-energy feed rations increased egg production per hen from 150 eggs a year in the early twentieth century to roughly 250 per year today. Total egg production in America increased from thirty-five billion to more than one hundred billion. The structure of the industry was also transformed. Millions of very small flocks kept on separate farms were replaced by a few thousand specialized layer operations with "flocks" of one hundred thousand hens or more. Today, nearly nine out of ten eggs produced in America come from just sixty-three egg-producing companies, each with more than one million hens.

Raising meat chickens—called "broilers"—emerged as a separate industry, but also one based on indoor confinement and genetic specialization. Cornish Cross breeds became dominant because they offered more white meat. Broiler chickens are now raised in climate-controlled confinement houses, each holding tens of thousands of individual birds. Production expanded rapidly after the 1970s, as consumers began seeking alternatives to red meat, and still more in the 1980s after McDonald's restaurants introduced Chicken McNuggets as a popular menu item. Between 1960 and 2018, the annual slaughter of broiler chickens in the United States increased from fewer than two billion birds to almost nine billion.

Pork production began moving indoors in the 1960s, once slatted floors were devised to reduce the labor required for indoor waste removal. The new pig barns were quickly automated, with self-feeders and self-watering, wall-mounted ventilation to remove moisture and control odor, and temperature-triggered misting systems to prevent heat stress. Feed use was optimized through split-sex feeding and segregated early weaning. Disease was controlled by power-washing and disinfecting the facility after the removal of each group of pigs, plus strict showering protocols for the workforce. Biosecurity in a modern pig barn is reminiscent of a hospital ward. Pig confinement systems became so productive by 1980 that small and part-time producers mostly disappeared from the marketplace. By 2012, more than eight out of ten pigs in the United States were raised by large operations with more than five thousand animals each.

Milk production also moved in the direction of year-round confinement. In summer months dairy cows were traditionally fed on pasture in the United States, but beginning in the late 1950s farmers began to experiment with no pasturing at all. They confined the cows either in free-stall barns or on unpaved and partially shaded drylots, where specialized feeds (a combination of forages, grains, protein feeds, minerals, vitamins, and feed additives) could be delivered to large numbers of animals by powered machines with far less human labor required. In the western and southwestern regions of the country these operations expanded rapidly, and by 2012 half of all dairy cows in the country were producing milk in herds of one thousand cows or more.

Small, traditional dairy farms in Wisconsin and the Northeast have continued to disappear, along with pasturing. Currently fewer than one out of three U.S. cows has access to pasture even during the growing season. Production has meanwhile become more concentrated. Between 1987 and 2007, the total number of dairy farms in the United States decreased by two-thirds, even though total milk production was increasing by more than half.

Beef cattle production is less concentrated in the United States, and the animals remain far less confined. Calves are born on separate cow/calf farms and ranches, and there are seven hundred thousand of these in all, with most keeping relatively small average herd sizes of only forty head. The calves are raised traditionally on mother's milk and pasture, then after weaning they are sold to stockers who will keep them on grass or other forage until they are twelve to sixteen months of age. Only at this point do they enter a confined outdoor feedlot for four to six more months, gaining weight by eating mostly a grain-based diet. Only about 6 percent of beef sold in the United States today is raised and finished entirely on grass.

In feedlots the cattle will typically be grouped into pens holding roughly one hundred head each. Some feedlots are relatively small, with fewer than a thousand head overall, but eight out of ten cattle fed today are on the 5 percent of operations with more than a thousand head each. Feedlot finishing is a proven weight-gain strategy; it has more than doubled America's average beef production per animal since 1950.

If the animals were not sentient beings, this twentieth-century revolution in livestock production might be seen as a marvelous achievement. Between 1948 and 1996 total output grew annually by 2 percent, even as labor costs were falling rapidly. For dairy, each million pounds of milk production now requires not just less labor, but also 90 percent less land, two-thirds less feed and water, and—most surprising of all—79 percent fewer animals. For pork since the nineties, average feed requirements for every added pound of weight have fallen by almost half. For chickens since 1950, average feed requirements per pound of live-weight broilers declined more than one-third. In beef since the seventies, every pound of meat production now requires 12 percent less water, 19 percent less feed, 30 percent fewer animals, and 33 percent less land, while generating 18 percent less manure.

These huge gains in productivity brought down prices, saving money for consumers. The price of hogs at the farm fell by half in the twentieth century in real dollars, while the retail price of eggs fell nearly 80 percent. One social benefit has been more equitable access to animal products. Lower-income families can now afford a bacon and eggs breakfast along with the middle class.

Thanks to today's livestock industry practices, greenhouse gas emissions have also been reduced for every pound of meat produced. According to UN data, livestock production in the United States has more than doubled since 1961, yet direct greenhouse gas emissions from livestock have declined 11 percent. Methane emissions are also down, because the total number of cattle needed to produce today's meat and milk supply is down. In 1950 the United States had twenty-five million dairy cows; now the number is nine million, even though milk production is 60 percent higher.

Frank Mitloehner, a professor of animal science and an air quality specialist at the University of California, Davis, looks at these numbers and concludes that the climate burden of a single glass of milk in the United States today is two-thirds smaller than it was seventy years ago. Mitloehner points out that the United States has the lowest greenhouse gas emissions per unit of milk production of any country in the world. In Mexico it takes up to five cows to produce the same amount of milk as one U.S. cow, while in India it takes up to twenty cows to do that.

Animal confinement thus looks like a great achievement, so long as we ignore the welfare of the animals. To a sorry extent, that is exactly what we did.

D omesticated farm animals are no longer able to survive in nature, so they must depend entirely on the care they receive from people. We took them out of nature, so we must assume ethical responsibility for their humane treatment. If we care for them properly they can have a good life, better in some ways than the lives of their wild ancestors. The world of nature, for all its majesty, can be exceptionally harsh. The evolutionary biologist Richard Dawkins explained it this way in his 1995 book *River Out of Eden:*

> The total amount of suffering per year in the natural world is beyond all decent contemplation. During the minute that it takes me to compose this sentence, thousands of animals are being eaten alive, many others are running for their lives, whimpering with fear, others are slowly being devoured from within by rasping parasites, thousands of all kinds are dying of starvation, thirst, and disease. It must be so. If there ever is a time of plenty, this very fact will automatically lead to an increase in the population until the natural state of starvation and misery is restored.

Most of this animal suffering in the wild takes place out of human sight. The doe with her spotted fawn, seen by us in the meadow on a warm summer morning, appears to be enjoying an idyllic life, but many fawns will be killed and eaten by coyotes, and in the coming winter still more will face an even greater test of survival. White-tailed deer spending the winter in the wild North Woods find little to eat, so they often lose 25–30 percent of their body weight, and a number of the fawns born the previous spring will starve to death. They will still be undersized and may be unable to get up if they founder in deep snow. A slow death by starvation then follows, typically in the last week of February or the first week of March.

Wild animals can also be cruel toward each other, including not just their prey but even their own siblings and offspring. In the Gala-pagos Islands, masked boobies lay two eggs. On the day after the second egg hatches, the older chick will force its younger sibling out of the nest, where it dies from the heat or succumbs to predators, like patrolling mockingbirds. As this takes place, the parent birds position themselves to give the attacking chick more room to maneuver.

Domesticated food animals in the United States seldom have to worry about starvation, since rapid weight gain is the fate we have designed for them. They will experience a premature death in a slaughterhouse, but in most cases the end is mercifully unanticipated and nearly instantaneous. The welfare of food animals today is none-theless compromised in several ways. Overbreeding leaves some in a diseased state and with physical impairments, while extreme con-finement for others causes boredom, emotional depression, and even mental derangement. Important physical comforts are denied to the animals in tight confinement, and instinctive social and exploratory behaviors are continuously frustrated. These are lapses that go beyond human ignorance, or even carelessness. The livestock industry car-ries a heavy responsibility for these outcomes because it turned to overbreeding and excessive confinement for its own commercial gain.

The magnitude of this responsibility has grown globally, since the number of animals we raise for food has grown. Counting up all of the domestic buffalo, camels, cattle, goats, pigs, sheep, ducks, rabbits, turkeys, geese, and chickens that people now use for meat, milk, and eggs, this number has more than tripled since 1970. The Earth now holds more than three times as many domesticated food animals as people. A surprising 73 percent of these animals are chickens raised for meat or eggs, including the caged hens so poorly treated on America's farms that they might be better off euthanized.

If confining hens in cages too small for perching or wing flapping is an ethical failure, what would an ideal management system look like? One tempting approach is to think about moving the animals back outside, returning to the pasture and barnyard systems that were commonplace a century ago. This would provide a more familiar fit to the biology of the animals since it mimics what their bodies and brains evolved to expect while living for several thousand years under human care. It might also be a better fit with the evolved instincts of the humans. People who see farm animals in tight confinement for the first time are nearly always uncomfortable. Humans instinctively prefer a more traditional bond between the animals and their individual handlers, something closer to the 4-H club ideal.

The appeal of pasture and barnyard systems is something I notice every time I take students to visit Clark Farm, with its pastured chickens and pigs, lightly fenced but otherwise roaming about outdoors. An even more famous outdoor grazing system is the one developed by Joel Salatin at Polyface Farm in Virginia's Shenandoah Valley, a farm profiled by Michael Pollan in *The Omnivore's Dilemma*. Salatin raises beef, pork, broilers, hens, seasonal turkeys, and forage-based rabbits. His system is not entirely pastured, since the poultry and pigs eat corn, soy, and oats purchased from off the farm, but the animals walk about outdoors, recycling nutrients into the soil through their waste.

A pastured life might seem ideal, but it can be a mixed blessing for the animals, since lambs and chickens outdoors are sometimes killed by predators. They also become more vulnerable to endoparasitic infestations. For birds, the spread of disease worsens outdoors, especially when mosquitoes are active under wet and rainy conditions. Even birds that are mostly raised indoors but are "free range," with some access to the outside, can experience mortality rates three times as high as caged birds.

Salatin's pasturing system is better for animal welfare than tight confinement, but it cannot meet consumer expectations for convenience and affordability. Polyface depends on sales to upscale restaurants, plus "buying clubs" whose members are willing to meet deliveries at specified times and locations, mostly in northern Virginia, Maryland, or Washington, D.C. This clientele can afford Salatin's boneless skinless chicken breasts for fourteen dollars a pound, roughly five times the Stop & Shop price. Labor costs keep the price high, since taking care of outdoor birds under changing weather conditions requires intensive management. Salatin's fully pastured beef system also requires much more land. Agricultural specialists at Michigan State University calculated in 2013 that Salatin's system required roughly 43 percent more total land per pound of meat produced, compared to conventional systems that start the animals on grass then finish them on grain in a feedlot. All this explains why Salatin's livestock production system is admired and sometimes imitated, but not widely adopted.

For veterinarians and animal scientists who want to protect animals from temperature extremes, predators, and disease, a pasture and barnyard system creates too many risks. It might seem "natural" to accept these risks, since they resemble the risks all animals endure in the wild, but we took them out of the wild and must assume responsibility for their ethical treatment. Bringing the animals inside to reduce their exposure to peril is ethical, *so long as adequate protections are provided against physical discomfort and emotional stress.*

Beyond the industrialized world, food animals are still being raised outdoors in large number, without any enclosed barns, feedlots, or even fences. In much of Africa, pastoralist communities continue to depend for their livelihood on cattle and goats that live under minimal confinement. Do these animals enjoy a high quality of life, higher than a food animal in much tighter confinement in the United States? Delia Grace, an Irish epidemiologist and veterinarian, currently works in Kenya, at the International Livestock Research Institute (ILRI) in Nairobi, and has done research on animal health and welfare issues since 1995. In 2014 the British Veterinary Association recognized her with the Trevor Blackburn Award, for her "multiple outstanding contributions," including voluntary service in rural Bangladesh, work on community-based animal health systems in East Africa, and on trypanosomiasis control in West Africa. Delia is deeply familiar with traditional livestock systems in Africa, including the pastoralist cattle-grazing systems that operate in rural Kenya.

For Delia Grace, raising animals for food makes perfect sense in Africa, because there is often too little rainfall to grow crops. In dry grassland areas it would be impossible to support a significant human population without ruminant animals like cattle and goats. The animals eat the grass that our human stomachs cannot digest, then the humans eat the meat and drink the milk provided by the animals. When it comes to killing the animals, Delia has a straightforward ethical code. She was a vegetarian for fifteen years but now believes it is acceptable to take an animal's life for food so long as it was continuously well treated before meeting a quick and unanticipated death. The goal is to avoid any suffering, and even Peter Singer, the vegetarian philosopher who authored *Animal Liberation* in 1975, has agreed that "the slaughter of an animal with no comprehension of death need not entail suffering." Based on this, Delia draws her firm conclusion: "If an animal is treated well and happy, and then has a good clean death, no problem."

Delia knows that food animals can experience such a death even in low-income countries. She points to the way some traditional African communities kill their domestic pigs. The pig about to be killed wanders about freely in a pen, unsuspecting of any danger. A handler will enter the pen, select his pig, and then with a sudden and well-practiced move, bang a spear directly and precisely into its heart. "The pig will just fall over," explains Delia. "One moment the pig was walking around with its friends and the next moment it was dead."

Delia approves of this method not only because the death is completely unanticipated and quick, but also because the animal was never removed from the comfort of its familiar surroundings. It did not have to undergo the trauma of being hauled in a noisy truck, and then the terror of being held in a strange space for several days before eventually being guided onto a killing floor to be "humanely" stunned and slaughtered.

When she compares the treatment of cattle in Africa to ranching in the United States, Delia points to important differences, both good and bad. On the bad side, African cattle suffer almost continual hunger due to dry-season weight loss, and there is a constant plague of gastrointestinal parasites and infectious diseases carried by ticks. In addition, the young animals experience trauma and pain when they are all at once weaned, hot-iron branded, castrated, then dehorned. African herdsmen nonetheless know how to use close and continuous supervision to calm their cattle, to reduce their fear and distress. African cattle have a low "flight distance" from approaching strangers, indicating higher levels of trust and comfort.

African farmers name their cattle. Bulls will often be named after a nation's president. The Maasai, who sometimes engage in cattle raids, may name their stolen cows to commemorate the fight, calling them "fear me" or "nobody slept." The Maasai use cattle for everything from food and drink to awarding damages and settling debts. Their unique respect for these animals is expressed in a sardonic proverb: "Save an old cow, but do not save an old man."

On traditional small farms in the United States, dogs, horses, and milk cows were named, but not the meat animals. Animals raised for wool sometimes also merit individual names. One time driving in Spain, south of Toledo, my spouse and I were brought to a stop by a shepherd on foot leading his several dozen sheep across the narrow country road. Hoping to learn the Spanish word for sheep, I waved my hand toward the animals and asked, "What name do you give to these animals?" The shepherd was happy to tell me. Pointing with his stick he began to name each one: "Mateo, Alejandro, Sophia, Luciana . . ."

Herdsmen in Africa tend their animals closely and with great care, but they are also capable of casual abuse. "They love their animals, they seek help for their animals, but they also beat them," says Delia. "It's not easy for privileged Europeans or Americans today to understand. It isn't like Walt Disney." In Disney cartoons, because the animals all speak—conveniently, in English—we always know what they are thinking and whether they are happy. Delia is comfortable using words like *happy* when talking about food animals, particularly if they are mammals like us, since she knows they have social and emotional lives somewhat parallel to human experience.

While measuring farm animal happiness can be difficult, illness and stress can readily be seen. Scientists are able to measure stress in farm animals by monitoring levels of hormones like cortisol. Stressed animals also can be identified at the time of slaughter, since the muscle cells in their meat will have lost some capacity to retain moisture. When stressed animals are butchered, the meat drips wetness and may not taste as good. Scientists—and even nonscientists—can also identify emotionally damaged farm animals if they see repetitive stereotypic behaviors like pacing back and forth, or chewing the metal bars of a pen.

Farm animals cannot speak to us, but we can learn a great deal about their preferences by giving them a structured choice. Using this method, says Delia, we have learned that farm animals do not like being out in nature all that much.

> We know that if farm animals have a choice between outdoors and indoors, they will prefer indoors; if given a choice between harassment by predators and safety from predators, they will prefer safety. But once they are safe indoors, they also want comfort. Given a choice between a pen with slats and one with hay, they will always prefer hay. If you ever see cattle on deep straw bedding, they are so happy, they love it. They will always choose to go to that straw bedding. So why can't we give them that? It doesn't cost a lot. We're very rich people, with many resources.

Because Delia knows it is possible for indoor systems to provide this kind of comfort for the animals, she is unforgiving toward livestock producers who give chickens too little room to perch or flap their wings, and pigs too little room to turn around. Such systems, she says, are "very wicked" and "need to be stopped."

Broiler chickens may not be mammals, but nine billion are raised and killed for food every year in America so our treatment of them deserves scrutiny. Since 1960 in the United States, the average weight of a meat chicken has nearly doubled and the time required to gain each pound has fallen by more than half. Broiler chickens can now reach a "harvest" weight of more than three and a half pounds after only thirty-three days of life. Each pound of weight gain requires less than half as much feed compared to the 1930s, so these fast-growing birds are highly profitable. Unfortunately, the fast growth has brought serious health and welfare problems for the birds.

The broiler chicken industry in the United States is distinctly structured, with individual producers providing the climate-controlled

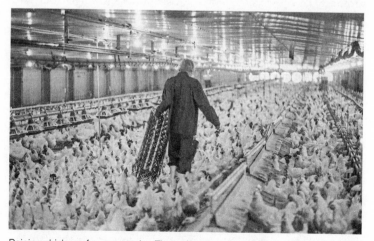

Raising chickens for meat today. These fast-growing birds are ready for market in less than two months' time.

confinement houses that raise the birds, often tens of thousands in a single building. Poultry companies supply these producers with the chicks and feed and then manage the final slaughter and packaging process, paying by the bird, with feed and heating costs factored in. Four big integrating companies—Tyson Foods, Pilgrim's Corporation, Perdue Farms, and Koch Foods—supply more than half the total market.

Because broiler chickens can walk about freely on the floor of their confinement house, rather than being caged, Bailey Norwood gives them a low but positive welfare score of +3, far better than the −8 score he gave to caged egg-laying hens. The score is nonetheless low, in part because the birds have been bred to gain weight so quickly. The Humane Society says if human babies grew at a similar rate to broiler chickens, they would weigh more than six hundred pounds after just two months. Rapid early growth is a common trait in all birds (songbirds can fly within just three weeks of being hatched), but broiler chickens today develop skeletons and muscles so quickly that the metabolism of their body has trouble keeping up.

One resulting problem is an avian variant of sudden death syndrome (SDS) known as "flip-over disease." Birds showing no outward sign of disease will suddenly extend their necks, gasp or squawk, flap their wings, then flip over dead. Up to 4 percent of birds in a healthy broiler flock may succumb. The cause is believed to be a metabolic disease linked to rapid growth from high carbohydrate intake. Another problem is ascites, a disease linked to the disproportionately underdeveloped cardiorespiratory systems of modern broilers, leading to low blood oxygen and death. Both SDS and ascites can be mitigated by slowing the growth of the birds.

An expert who knows these issues well is Bruce Webster, professor of poultry science at the University of Georgia in Athens, about an hour and a half east of Atlanta. Georgia, for decades, has led the United States in broiler production; broiler chickens, together with egg-laying hens, generate more than $5 billion a year in the state. As a researcher, Bruce has served on several of the standing committees set up by companies like Tyson, Perdue Farms, and Wayne Farms to advise on animal welfare issues. His own research covers topics such as fear-related behavior in chickens, the enrichment of cages for laying hens, assessments of the walking abilities of broiler chickens, and humane slaughter methods.

Bruce is not afraid to speak up against industry practices. At one public meeting he described a preslaughter method then widely in use for broilers (hanging chickens by their legs and electrocuting them in a tank of water to induce paralysis) as a "dinosaur." After PETA cited his comment in a legal action against Kentucky Fried Chicken, people in the poultry industry started "calling for my head," he says.

Slaughter methods get attention, but the poultry industry must also be faulted for its breeding practices. The companies pushed so hard for genetic specialization between meat birds and egg birds that both lost the health balance earlier found in general purpose breeds. The metabolic problems found in broilers, including SDS and ascites, first emerged about two decades ago. Corrections are finally being made by the industry, because both these problems have had bottom-line implications. "The primary breeders are now building into their genetic indices things that will reduce these risks," Bruce says. "And

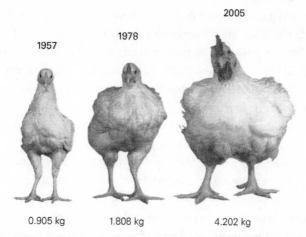

These dramatic size differences show what poultry breeders have done since 1957 to alter the genetics of broiler chickens. All these birds are an identical fifty-six days old.

they've had some success. Ascites is nowhere near the problem it used to be." Since rapid weight gain also brings a reduction in meat quality, companies like Wendy's have been switching their purchases to smaller birds. Yet some in the industry continue to resist change. The National Chicken Council tries to defend current practice by warning that slower-growing birds will require more feed per pound of production, more land to grow the feed, and could generate billions of added pounds of manure.

Companies that purchase chicken meat, including Whole Foods, Bon Appétit, Aramark, Panera Bread, Starbucks, Chipotle, and Subway, have now pledged to move toward slower-growing birds. The Global Animal Partnership, or GAP, a group founded in partnership with Whole Foods Market, announced that beginning in 2024 it will give its certification only to farms that raise slower-growing chickens, a move that sends signals to more than six hundred GAP-certified farms. The GAP welfare standards also include access to natural light, enrichments like perches and bales of straw in chicken houses, and new slaughtering practices to replace electrical stunning.

Other countries have used certification systems of this kind to good advantage. In France since the 1960s, the government has sponsored a Label Rouge certification process that requires slower-growing heritage breeds for broiler chickens, lower-density houses, and access to pasture. The meat is nearly twice as expensive as conventional chicken, but French shoppers have a strong preference for the traditional quality and taste, so Label Rouge birds have captured a quarter of the market.

Perdue Farms, which has pledged to meet the GAP standards, is now conducting trials with slow-growing birds that take about 25 percent longer to mature compared to conventional broilers. Tyson Foods so far has lagged behind. Tyson, when it announced a new animal welfare plan in 2017, stopped short of promising better breeds, improved housing, or more humane slaughter methods. Its hands were full at the time responding to charges of outright cruelty in its processing plants, accusations backed by video evidence collected and distributed through an organization named Mercy for Animals.

After the damning videos surfaced, Tyson fired ten workers, ended its contract with one farmer, and hired an outside company to monitor video streams from cameras in all thirty-three of its processing plants, hoping this would convince critics the cruelty had stopped. The Humane Society welcomed this as a first step but still wanted stronger core animal welfare commitments from Tyson. Big chicken buyers like Burger King, Popeye's, Subway, Sodexo, and Aramark are beginning to require such commitments, so Tyson soon may be forced to shape up.

The best known of America's twenty thousand animal protection groups, and also the biggest, is the Humane Society. In addition to farm animal welfare, HSUS takes on the fur trade, blood sports, animal experimentation, puppy mills, and wildlife abuse. The organization gets results by staying away from polarizing stunts and simple protests, and by avoiding extreme demands such as ending the use of animals for food altogether. Some HSUS staff would no doubt like the world to become entirely meat-free and egg-free, but for now the organization is willing to focus more on making livestock production cruelty-free. Enacting new state laws to end the tight confinement of hens and pregnant sows has been a central goal.

HSUS has learned to outmaneuver industry-dominated state legislatures by relying on citizen-initiated ballot procedures. Wayne Pacelle, the CEO and president of HSUS between 2004 and 2018, saw such ballot campaigns as a nearly failure-proof tactic. When successful, they put legal protections in place, but even if the vote falls short the effort will raise awareness and create popular support for an eventual reform.

To build its reputation for success, HSUS often begins its campaigns in states not heavily dependent on livestock production. In 2002 it won an early victory to end the confinement of pregnant sows in metal-bar stalls, called gestation "crates" by the critics, by starting in Florida. This was an easy entry point because the pig industry in Florida was small, with only two farms using gestation crates at that time. Four years later HSUS won a similar victory in Arizona, which was only slightly more of a pork state than Florida, but this second victory built momentum, and liberal state legislatures in Oregon and Colorado soon passed laws of their own banning gestation crates.

With these victories in hand, HSUS was ready to promote a landmark law in California, Proposition 2, requiring more space not just for pregnant sows but also for egg-laying hens and veal calves. On Election Day in 2008, Prop 2 was approved by two-thirds of California voters. To get the eight hundred thousand signatures needed to put Prop 2 on the ballot, HSUS waged a yearlong campaign, and to ensure the win on Election Day it used a mix of effective strategies, such as persuading *The Oprah Winfrey Show* to dedicate an entire program to the issue. It also produced a creative animated video that went viral online, showing farm animals singing a parody version of the Stevie Wonder song "Superstition." ("This place is like a factory, it ain't a farm at all . . .") In addition, an undercover video was aired just before the November vote showing a worker from a major West Coast egg producer stomping on a sick hen.

Two years after the victory, California's state legislature went on to widen the reach of Prop 2 by enacting a measure applying the new standards not just to eggs produced in California but also to those brought in from other states. The goal was to protect California's producers against a flood of cheaper eggs from states with lax regulations, but this measure was met by a legal challenge from industries in a dozen states. The challenge was initially beaten back in federal circuit court, but the other states are still hoping the Supreme Court will step in to nullify Prop 2's extended reach.

To date, HSUS has secured sow gestation crate bans in Arizona, California, Colorado, Florida, Maine, Massachusetts, Michigan, Ohio, and Rhode Island, plus battery cage bans for hens in California, Massachusetts, Michigan, Ohio, Oregon, and Washington. As a supplementary benefit, these campaigns have inspired a growing consumer demand in the marketplace for higher standards leading to pledges from corporate meat buyers to require such standards. By 2016, more than sixty companies—including McDonald's, Burger King, Oscar

Mayer, Costco, and Kroger—had promised soon to sell only crate-free pork, and Whole Foods Market and Chipotle were already doing so.

A second successful HSUS ballot effort in California in 2018, mentioned earlier, requires even more space for hens and sows. This measure now requires at least twenty-four square feet of usable floor space per sow, and one and a half square feet of usable space per hen, plus freedom to move around. This new measure will also extend to eggs brought into the state, so by 2022 all eggs eaten in California will essentially be cage-free. Only about 17 percent of egg production nationwide was cage-free in 2019, so California is taking a strong lead.

California's Prop 12 campaign met far less industry opposition, because egg and pork producers in the state knew they were going to have to move away from cages and crates sooner or later, in response to growing demands from meat companies, retailers, and restaurant chains. Companies like Nestlé, Mondelez, PepsiCo, Sodexo, and McDonald's were pledging to move to fully cage-free sourcing in the years ahead. Surprisingly, the most vocal opposition to Prop 12 came from animal welfare groups in California, who said it did not go far enough. Some thought it should have included a ban on antibiotic use, while others wanted to halt raising animals for food altogether. These more militant groups worried that Prop 12 would be used by the livestock industry as a cover, to buttress a claim that it was now producing "happy meat."

HSUS had made itself suspect in the eyes of these other animal welfare groups when it agreed in 2011 to cooperate with the United Egg Producers, negotiating a national definition for cage-free egg production. The industry by then preferred a single definition nationwide to a patchwork of different guidelines set state by state. HSUS went along with this strategy, agreeing at a joint press conference to cooperate. The proposed national guidelines that emerged were introduced as legislation in Congress two years in a row but not enacted due to opposition from beef and pork producers, who feared it would be a precedent for federal meddling with their own practices. When HSUS decided in 2018 to incorporate aspects of these UEP-approved guidelines into the language of Prop 12, rival animal welfare advocates viewed it as a concession to industry preferences, and then decried Prop 12 as a hollow victory when it passed.

Jennifer Fearing knows this history well. Now the president of a Sacramento-based lobbying firm named Fearless Advocacy, she led the successful Prop 2 campaign in California working for HSUS, but she did not work on Prop 12, having by that time left the organization. She was trained as an economist, earned a graduate degree in public policy, then found work in the private sector. Her interests turned to animal welfare after she and a friend in Sacramento found a stray dog in obvious need of help. When they took the animal to a shelter, Jennifer was dismayed by the conditions at the shelter and began working there as a volunteer, to make things better. She became a committed vegetarian, started lobbying the city council for progressive changes in shelter rules, then formed her own nonprofit, and eventually took a position with a disaster relief organization that rescued animals.

Jennifer's interests soon shifted from animal rescue to animal protection, and her talents were noticed by HSUS, which hired her to work at their national headquarters as chief economist. I had a chance to ask Jennifer why HSUS needed an economist. "All animal use is financial," she explained. "The worst things that happen to animals are because there is money to be made at their expense."

Jennifer welcomed the chance to return to California in 2008 to run the HSUS Prop 2 campaign, although the she knew building popular support for chickens was going to be harder than for pandas or puppies. After winning her campaign, she leveraged the victory into a new opening line she uses when lobbying the legislature: "If seventy percent of the people in your district just voted to give *chickens* more space, they are definitely going to support . . ." Jennifer believes the Prop 2 victory launched the most significant period of legislative activity on behalf of animals ever seen in California.

Jennifer had left HSUS by 2018, but faulted the Prop 12 effort as not ambitious enough. As a strong environmentalist, she wishes plant-based protein could replace animal-based foods in the diet, and worries that a move toward slightly more humane confinement stan-

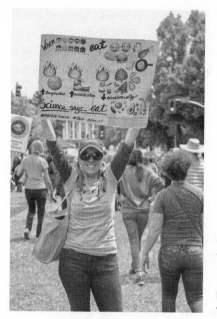

Animal welfare lobbyist Jennifer Fearing, marching in Sacramento on Earth Day, 2017. Her poster depicts the link between animal foods, global warming, and biodiversity loss.

dards might actually encourage consumers to increase their meat consumption. The lack of serious industry opposition to Prop 12, she says, "should make us wonder if we got all that we could." Costly ballot efforts like Prop 2 and Prop 12 can be made only once every decade or so by animal welfare advocates in California, and Jennifer thinks HSUS missed a chance with Prop 12 to seek progress on more than just confinement. She would have wanted to see something on antibiotic use at least, and possibly dehorning. A ballot victory can feel good, but gains for the animals are what matter most. "The animals need you to do well, not just mean well. Your emotions are the gas in the tank, but your brains should be driving the car."

Europe raises twice as many pigs as the United States, mostly indoors just like in America, but with better protection for the welfare of the animals. Consider the experience of the Netherlands, a small country crowded not just with people but also with four thousand pig farms. The Noordman farm, in Lemelerveld, is one of them. It is larger than most, featuring a dozen perfectly aligned barns, plus a single taller structure standing off to one side with an atrium-style triple-rounded translucent roof. The dozen conventional barns house four thousand pigs being fattened ("finished," in the language of the industry) for the market, soon to be trucked to a local slaughterhouse. This is a successful operation that puts money in the bank for the hardworking Noordman family, consisting of Herbert, Annemarie, his wife, and their four children.

The Noordman farm raises only pigs, and all are confined indoors just like in the United States, yet the animals are offered a better experience thanks to new regulations set in place by the Dutch government beginning in the 1990s. It started with tougher environmental regulations, designed to combat waste smells in the densely populated southern province of Noord-Brabant, where almost half of all Dutch pig farms are located. These smells became less of a problem as more of the pigs were moved indoors, but that only set up follow-on concerns for the health and welfare of the confined animals.

A crisis moment arrived during an extreme outbreak of swine fever in 1998, an event that brought a precautionary slaughter of countless healthy piglets on farms adjoining outbreak locations. For the animal-loving Dutch this became traumatic, with the eight o'clock evening news showing shocking images of dead animals being hauled and shoveled about. Citizen groups with names like Pigs in Distress and Animal Awake began to demand radical livestock industry reforms. A new political party was formed, the Party for the Animals, which quickly won two seats in the Dutch Parliament.

By then parallel livestock reform campaigns were also underway in Britain and in the Scandinavian countries, and in 1999 these likeminded nations pushed through the Treaty of Amsterdam, a progressive new measure to improve "protection and respect for the welfare of animals as sentient beings" throughout the EU. An EU Council Directive in 2008 eventually added real teeth to the treaty, setting mandatory minimum standards for pig welfare, while some member states, including the Netherlands, went on to establish even higher standards on their own.

The new EU Directive specified a minimum area of unobstructed floor space for each pig, depending on the weight of the animals, and a minimum area of continuous solid floor space (not just slatted floors) for lying down. It required no tethering of sows, and it eliminated individual gestation crates by requiring group housing for pregnant sows. The directive, which came into force EU-wide at the start of 2013, also required that pigs have access to a clean, physically and thermally comfortable lying area big enough to allow all the animals to lie at the same time (pigs like to do things all at the same time), plus limits to noise levels and lighting above a minimum brightness for at least eight hours a day. Invasive procedures such as the castration of male pigs or tail docking could be carried out only by trained personnel or a veterinarian. To help the animals overcome boredom, the directive also specified that the pigs should have permanent access to "material to enable proper investigation and manipulation activities." In other words, toys.

These sweeping requirements increased housing and production costs for the European pig industry, a high-cost industry to begin with. One comparison found that in 2015 carcass-weight production costs in the EU averaged 19 percent higher compared to Canada, 38 percent higher than in the United States, and 58 percent higher than in Mato Grosso in Brazil. Yet on closer inspection these comparisons mostly reflected lower U.S., Canadian, and Brazilian feed costs, labor costs, and manure management costs, not housing costs. The higher building and capital costs associated with more spacious pig housing made a difference, but in countries like the Netherlands this category constitutes only a little more than one-tenth of total production costs.

Farm animal welfare rules in Europe are more stringent than in the United States partly because Europe is more densely populated, so the mistreatment of farm animals is harder to keep out of sight. Also, there is a greater cultural and political readiness in Europe to grant all animals independent moral status as sentient beings, with a number of European countries formally recognizing individual animal interests as matters of intrinsic constitutional concern. In addition, economic activity in Europe is more heavily regulated across the board.

When the new welfare rules for pigs were first promulgated in Holland, the task of implementation became a widely supported national project, one that was backed by groups ranging from the national farmers' organization to public schools and the Dutch chamber of commerce. Wageningen University & Research, widely recognized as the best agricultural university in the world, even sponsored a nationwide competition to design "toys for pigs," which recruited leading artists to submit entries. The winning design was made from hollow cylinders filled with different kinds of food. Schoolchildren learned and celebrated the "five freedoms" basic to animal welfare and they were encouraged to paint colorful wall murals showing happy pigs. To the present day, the side of one Wageningen research barn features the image of a cartoon pig enjoying its freedom in an open-cockpit airplane, smiling behind aviator's goggles.

Some in Holland would like to see even higher standards for farm animal welfare, including Annemarie Noordman. She is pleased that her family farm provides its animals with one quarter more space than the current law requires, but she has made it her mission to experiment with indoor systems that offer even greater comfort to the pigs. The extra-tall, triple-domed barn on the Noordman farm is where she puts her ideas into practice. She calls it Varkenshoff, or the "garden for pigs," spelled with an extra "f" so it will stand out in Google searches.

Annemarie is a thoroughly modern product of the Dutch countryside. She was raised on a farm but has also worked as a nurse. Her experimental barn attracts media attention and she welcomes veterinary students as visitors on a regular basis, but other pig farmers in the area are skeptical and tend to stay away. Inside the barn, from a second-floor visitor space, I could view the large sky-lit interior through a floor-to-ceiling glass wall (the glass wall allowed me to dispense with the usual biosecurity procedures such as washdowns, shoe changing, and coveralls). Immediately below and closest to me were three sows, each with more than a dozen nursing piglets, all born within the last three days. The sows weigh a quarter of a ton each but are not restrained by the "farrowing crates" widely used by the swine industry to protect piglets from being rolled on. This allows Annemarie's sows to periodically stand up, leave the straw in their nesting stalls, and walk to a "toilet" area with a slatted floor to relieve themselves of urine and dung. The tiny young piglets stay behind, warmed by a glowing heat lamp to keep them at a comfortable ninety degrees.

A bit farther away I saw weaned piglets in group pens and young, uncastrated boars, and also the gilts (females that have not yet had a litter). In still more distant pens, older pigs were eating their fill to be finished for the market. The inseminated sows going through gestation were separated and got a more restricted diet. Every stage in the life cycle of a pig could be seen from a single vantage point.

Annemarie's pigs are relaxed and visibly social. Pink skinned, they

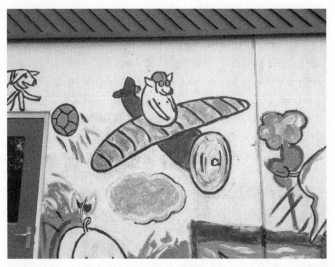

Mural of a happy pig enjoying his freedom, painted on a Dutch research barn, part of a national campaign to make housing for swine more humane.

lie in rows looking like careless beachgoers unaware they are getting a sunburn. They rest side by side, stir about together, and occasionally get excited together. Pigs like to synchronize their eating, and all the sows like to nurse at the same time. Watching this from the viewing area can be engrossing, since there is something new to see all the time. Visitors sometimes forgo their tour of the rest of the farm, telling Annemarie, "I'll stay here. Come back to get me at five."

The Varkenshoff demonstration barn exceeds Dutch welfare requirements by a wide margin, since it provides more extra space for the pigs and far more natural light. It also provides straw on the floor for the pigs to nest and root around in, which would be hard to enforce as an industry-wide requirement, because it would mean prohibitive labor costs. It takes Annemarie more than an hour every day to clean out straw for just twenty-five sows. In a less spacious facility more straw would inevitably fall between the floor slats along with the dung and urine, clogging up the waste slurry system, so extra conveyor belts would have to be installed below the slatted floors, costing still more money.

Annemarie's crate-free farrowing system could be scaled up to deliver welfare benefits for the sows, but this might put too many piglets at physical risk. Free farrowing is the rule in the organic pork sector, and the mortality rate for baby pigs can be as high as one in four, twice the rate in conventional operations. Organic standards that prohibit antibiotic use can also put the welfare of animals at risk if bacterial infections go untreated simply to preserve organic certification.

Annemarie has little use for the views of experts who are not farmers themselves. She trusts her own instincts with pigs because she spends so much time with them, talking to them, patting the ones that only eat when they get personal attention, and caring for the ones that get sick. She doesn't call a vet. "No, I can do what he does; I know more. He calls me," she says.

Pigs may not be as smart as primates and dolphins, but they come in well ahead of dogs and cats. As Annemarie confirms, "They can learn anything." But she stops short of treating them like pets. Her pigs are not given names, since they are for eating in the end, and Annemarie herself eats pork, poultry, or beef six days a week. She says her goal at Varkenshoff is to produce what she calls "high care" meat. When asked how it is possible to give individual care to so many different animals in a barn, she has another comeback: "Haven't you ever worked in a hospital?"

Some progressive pig farmers in the United States also exceed minimum animal welfare standards. Mark Legan raises pigs and grows corn and soybeans in Putnam County, Indiana, west of Indianapolis. Neither Mark nor his wife, Phyllis, grew up on a farm, which is unusual for commercial producers in the Midwest today. When Mark was sixteen, a neighbor with sixty sows hired him to work for two dollars an hour, which was two dollars more than his dad had been paying him to help with masonry work. Mark enjoyed the new responsibility and found the sows to be intelligent and responsive to careful management. He went on to study animal science at Purdue University, did summer internships on larger pig farms, took a job advising farmers as a county extension agent, then went back to the university to get a master's degree in agricultural economics.

Mark began pig farming for himself in the 1990s. At that time in Indiana, most sows were still gestated outside on dirt lots, where piglets born in the winter could be found dead from the cold in the morning. Mark decided to move his pigs indoors, and in 1998 he put up his first barn as part of a specialized "breeding to weaning" operation. Today the Legan farm has multiple barns that house more than two thousand pregnant and nursing sows, weaning about sixty thousand baby pigs a year. By modern standards this is not large; many pig farms in the United States now have more than ten thousand sows in a single location.

The Legan farm is very much a family operation. Mark's son-in-law Nick is now in charge of the sows, working along with eight full-time employees. Mark's daughter Beth manages finance and accounting, plus hedging and marketing. Beth made the local news when she was honored at the Obama White House in 2014 as one of America's fifteen "Champions of Change," setting an example for the next generation of farmers and ranchers. Phyllis Legan takes care of the hiring and ensures that all federal employment guidelines are met. Mark uses a consultant, but he provides the commercial vision for the operation himself, integrates the crop side with the animal side, and protects what he calls the core values. Every week he ships more than a thousand young weaned pigs to two other farms in Indiana, each with more than ten thousand pigs, to be finished for the market.

Two decades ago, when smaller pig farms were the rule, Putnam County had been home to at least one hundred separate pig operations, but now only three remain, with the Legan farm producing significantly more than the other two combined. Mark knows he is part of the global marketplace; a quarter of his pork will eventually be destined for export, most likely to Mexico, Canada, Japan, or China.

The Legan farm now enjoys a marketing advantage, since all of its pregnant sows are kept in open pens rather than in cramped gestation stalls. Mark has always kept sows in group pens—ten to a pen—a choice he originally made to save on capital costs. Keeping the animals this way requires more management, since the dominant sows often try to take too much of the feed and may sometimes bite the more submissive sows, but this cost is offset by the higher price big companies like Smithfield are now willing to pay for crate-free pork.

On welfare grounds, Mark is not a strong advocate for one specific sow housing system over another. He says the well-being of the animals will depend most of all on the attention and skill of the farmer, a view I also heard from Annemarie in the Netherlands. "As much as we want to make it a science," Mark says, "it still comes down to the people that care for the animals day in and day out, making sure their needs are being met."

Veterinarians have tried to study the welfare advantage of keeping sows in group pens rather than individual stalls, by measuring stress in the pigs through cortisol secretions. Some studies have shown no difference at all between group pens versus gestation crates, but in others the results have varied animal by animal, according to their relative status within the group. High-ranking sows, the so-called "boss sows," experience less stress in group pens, while low-ranking sows are less stressed in individual crates. Other studies have suggested the best way to relieve stress overall would be to switch to larger crates, big enough for the animals to turn around. In one study, young female pigs that were placed in larger turnaround stalls did turn an average of seventy-five times a day, suggesting this might offer the optimal combination to balance freedom with protection.

Smaller crates are criticized on welfare grounds even from some who are close to the industry. One swine veterinarian task force in 2005 found that it served "no direct animal health or welfare purpose" to keep a pregnant sow in a stall that prevents her from walking or turning. This report concluded, "Gestation stalls, particularly when used in conjunction with feed restriction, may adversely affect welfare by restricting behavior, including foraging, movement, and postural changes." These swine veterinarians depend on the pork industry for their own employment, so it took some professional courage to publish this critical judgment.

Mark is aware that even his ten-to-a-pen system will be criticized by some animal welfare advocates, but he says, "I'm not ashamed of the way we breed pigs. We are involved in the community. We're here on a state highway, and we don't want people to look at this farm and see a factory farm. We want them to look at it and see that this is the Legan family, and they're taking care of their animals." An advocate for transparency, Mark welcomes student tours from the local university.

When I asked Mark about waste disposal, he said he had been shifting away from the older "lagoon" systems for handling waste. Some of his lagoon waste is still hauled away in semitankers, to be applied as fertilizer on fields with low enough phosphorus levels, but he has mostly transitioned toward anaerobic manure treatment, a more efficient method that also helps contain odor. His fields are planted with cover crops in the winter, a measure that takes up any excess nitrogen and reduces downstream pollution when it rains, in addition to protecting the soil. Mark knows these issues well, having spent twelve years on the Indiana Water Pollution Control Board overseeing state regulations for wastewater and drinking water, including water used in animal operations such as his own. In 2016, Mark and Phyllis were jointly honored by the state's water and conservation districts for managing a River-Friendly Farm.

The Legan barns are essentially nurseries for producing thousands of baby pigs. Following artificial insemination in individual breeding stalls, the sows are pregnant for a surprisingly standard three months, three weeks, and three days. Once a pregnancy is confirmed, the animals are moved through interconnecting corridors into a separate gestation barn, ten to a pen. When nearly ready to give birth, they are then moved again to a farrowing barn, where they will be loosely restrained in metal frames (the farrowing crates *not* used by Annemarie) to prevent them from rolling on the nursing newborns. After the piglets are weaned and shipped off, the sows will be inseminated again. It's vaguely like a *Handmaid's Tale,* but with pigs.

Farm animal welfare standards are beginning to tighten in the United States, but for pigs they remain far less demanding than in Europe. Mark Legan's sows are not in crates, but they are still crowded together, and with no toys for enrichment. The ventilation fans make noise, the floors are inevitably unclean, and the rows of windows on the sides of the barn provide natural light that is uneven at best. Yet Legan's sows move about freely and maintain a sociable peace with each other most of the time. A visiting vet observed that Mark's animals did not flee to the far side of the pen when confronted by a stranger, an indication of humane treatment. Animal welfare regulations in the United States need to move more quickly toward the higher European standard, and we should cheer organizations like the Humane Society for making some progress toward that goal, but farmers like Mark Legan are showing that progressive improvements are possible even without tighter regulations.

Mark is not, however, a fan of the Humane Society. He may not use gestation crates on his farm, but he still sees that organization as an adversary. When asked what he thought it would take to satisfy HSUS, Mark comes back quickly with a simple answer: "Just don't raise pigs."

CHAPTER 8

The Brave New Future of Food

History's most famous prediction about the future of food was also the most mistaken. The English economist Thomas Robert Malthus predicted in 1798 that human population growth would soon outrun the earth's capacity to produce food, resulting in widespread famine. He was mostly right about the rapid growth in human numbers, but wildly wrong about food production and famine. The human population increased from one billion to almost eight billion over the next two centuries, yet food production more than kept pace. So much so, that Malthusian fears of famine are now being replaced by a growing global burden of chronic disease linked to overeating.

Some significant famines did occur in the twentieth century but they had little to do with Malthusian limits on food production, since most were caused by either policy mistakes or violent conflict. The biggest famine of all killed thirty million in China after 1959, during Mao Zedong's disastrous Great Leap Forward. This was a completely unnecessary tragedy caused by a misguided government program—the creation of rural people's communes—that reduced food production incentives. When Mao's unrealistic policies were relaxed, production revived and the famine ended.

At roughly this same time, green revolution breakthroughs in crop science were expanding food production potential throughout Asia, bringing an end to famine fears in countries like India. Industrial

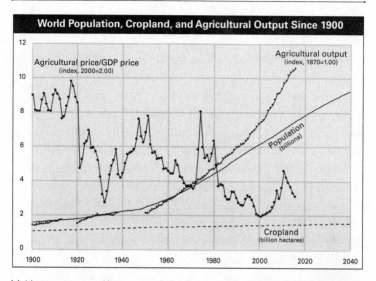

World Population, Cropland, and Agricultural Output Since 1900

Agricultural price/GDP price
(index, 2000=2.00)

Agricultural output
(index, 1870=1.00)

Population
(billions)

Cropland
(billion hectares)

Malthus was wrong. Human population increased fourfold over the past century, but agricultural output more than kept up. As a result, agricultural prices in real terms declined by roughly three-quarters. Cropland area barely increased at all.

development then took off in East and Southeast Asia in the decades that followed, bringing rapid income gains in these regions, an event described at the time as the "East Asia Miracle." Not only did this give more people the means to purchase food; industrialization also led to the rise of an urban middle class that demanded greater democracy, which greatly improved the accountability of governments responding to temporary food shortages.

Thanks to all these fortunate trends working together, hunger went into a broad retreat even though human numbers continued on a rapid rise. Poverty persisted in the countryside, and small famines continued to occur, but they usually took place in societies torn apart by violent conflict, where Malthusian limits were not the issue. Overall, a remarkably beneficial economic corner was being turned. As Steven Pinker has shown, in the second half of the twentieth century the share of the world's citizens living in extreme poverty fell from 60 percent down to just 10 percent, and the numbers killed by famine dropped to almost nothing. By the second decade of the twenty-first century, famine deaths relative to the number of people on earth had fallen essentially to zero.

Despite this good news on the famine front, significant numbers of poor people, particularly young children, have continued to suffer from chronic undernutrition, which compromises their physical strength, health, and cognitive development. Worst hit are the rural poor in destitute farming communities that still lack things like all-weather roads, electricity, irrigation, improved seeds, or fertilizers. Recall the previously mentioned example of rural Ethiopia. In these communities, children can be stunted or wasted due to protein and calorie deficits, and many also suffer from diseases linked to diets deficient in iron, zinc, iodine, or vitamin A.

Fortunately, chronic undernutrition of this kind is now also in retreat. The United Nations has estimated that the share of individuals in the developing world who suffer from chronic undernourishment fell from 36 percent in 1970 to 20 percent in 1990, and most recently to just 11 percent in 2018. Climate change, if not addressed,

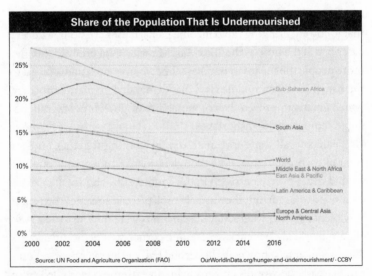

Changes in the undernourished share of the population, globally and by region. The undernourished share remains highest in sub-Saharan Africa and South Asia, but hunger prevalence has been in a long-term decline even there.

threatens to reverse some of this progress by making food more costly to grow, especially for poor farmers in tropical regions. A 2019 report from the Intergovernmental Panel on Climate Change (IPCC) explicitly warned of this danger, but continued scientific gains and farming investments have so far kept most of the world's food producers out ahead of this threat.

For Americans, poor and non-poor alike, having too much to eat is now a bigger health problem than having too little. There is still hunger in America, but this condition is in retreat thanks in part to successful food assistance programs such as the Supplemental Nutrition Assistance Program (SNAP) and the Women, Infants, and Children (WIC) program. On an average day in 2018, fewer than 1 percent of households in America experienced what the USDA calls "very low food security." Meanwhile, the body weight of an average American adult increased by more than thirty pounds between 1960 and 2018, making more than four out of ten American adults clinically obese.

Excessive food consumption is also on the rise in other countries, including some that were poor and hungry just a decade or two ago. In 2018 the World Health Organization reported that nearly half of the world's overweight children now live in Asia, and the number in Africa has increased by almost half since 2000. Of the world's six hundred million obese adults, two-thirds now live in the developing world. China, home to the world's largest famine just sixty years ago, is today home to the world's largest population of overweight people.

Eating too much food harms personal health, but producing all that food also harms environmental health, by polluting water supplies, destroying wildlife habitat, and speeding climate change. New technologies of precision agriculture have been reducing the damage for each bushel produced in wealthy regions like North America and Europe, but because the total quantity being produced keeps rising, the overall environmental damage can continue to grow even there. The harm is even more acute in developing countries where populations are still growing rapidly, and where diets are now being enriched by rapid income gains. In these countries dietary enrichment typically includes an increased consumption of animal products such as meat, milk, and eggs, which requires still larger crop production and expanded grazing to feed still more animals, compounding the environmental burden.

Eighty-three percent of the Earth's agricultural land is now being used to feed animals, even though they provide only 18 percent of total food calories. Modern livestock systems have reduced pasture requirements in rich countries, and the same has been happening in many developing countries, although not yet in sub-Saharan Africa. Total pasture area globally has actually declined for the past two decades according to the FAO, which is good news for habitat protection. Yet global demand for meat, dairy, and egg products is expected to increase by an additional 60 percent between now and 2050, and this will happen mostly in developing countries, intensifying environmental pressures whether the animals are on pastures or in feed lots. The consumption of red meat such as beef, lamb, and goat is projected to increase nearly 90 percent by 2050, a worrying trend because beef production emits twenty times more greenhouse gas compared to plant-based sources of edible protein such as beans, peas, or lentils. Globally, livestock production is responsible for 14 percent of total greenhouse gas emissions. Problems such as these linked to excessive food consumption could not be further from the starvation predicted by Malthus, but they are emblematic of our modern age, one of growing material excess rather than scarcity.

There is, of course, an elegant solution. Since consuming too much food is damaging our health, and since producing all that food (particularly from animals) is damaging our environment, we could address both problems simply by producing and eating less, especially less meat, and particularly less red meat. If we substituted plant-based protein for today's excessive red meat and dairy consumption, nutrition and health would improve and environmental pressures would be eased at the same time.

Powerful economic and cultural forces, until now, have blocked us from taking this plant-based protein path. Animal-based foods are both convenient and tasty, and in moderate quantities they can be good for nutrition, so those now eating such foods will resist being coerced into a reduction. In democratic societies, elected leaders know they will be punished at the polls if they resort to coercive measures. There are also equity concerns. Many in poor countries have been waiting for their chance to eat more meat, so they can live like the rich. Why should they curb their still modest appetites for meat to help solve a climate problem that was mostly caused by overconsumption elsewhere?

Meat consumption remains an important cultural aspiration. The original Chinese character for "family home" depicted a house with a pig inside. In European cultures, meat consumption has long been a signifier of social status and material success. In the sixteenth century, Henry IV of France said he wanted "no peasant in my realm so poor that he will not have a chicken in his pot every Sunday." In the Western Hemisphere, after the Europeans arrived bringing cattle, grazing these animals for food emerged as a still celebrated way of life for cowboys on the American plains and gauchos on the Argentine pampas. Cooking meat even hangs on—alas—as a signifier for masculinity. Men no longer need hunting, riding, or roping skills to put a steak on the grill, but doing so remains a valued ritual of manly prowess.

The real problem, once again, is excess. If meat consumption, especially red meat consumption, could simply be contained within standard dietary guidelines, significant benefits would result. A research team at Oxford in 2016 calculated that if global eating patterns were changed according to such a standard, red meat consumption would decline 56 percent and global mortality in 2050 would fall nearly 10 percent compared to a business-as-usual scenario. The environment would also benefit, as food-related greenhouse gas emissions overall would fall somewhere between 29 and 70 percent. The dietary shift imagined under this scenario would of course require major farming changes. Total fruit and vegetable consumption would increase by a quarter, so the production of these crops would have to increase as well. Total calorie consumption would decline by 15 percent overall, so food intake in rich countries would have to shrink as well as shift, but this would be good for health, with the greatest per capita health benefits captured in the countries cutting their consumption the most.

A parallel study the same year, from the World Resources Institute, focused more on the environmental benefits from a reduced consumption of animal-based foods. The WRI modeled the probable results if a hypothetical reduction in animal protein consumption had been initiated by high-consuming countries in 2009. This would not only move the diets of two billion people in a healthy direction; by 2050 it would spare an area of agricultural land roughly twice the size of India, land that could then be used to feed the added two billion people expected on earth by 2050. The WRI believed such changes were possible, noting that per capita beef consumption in the United States had already declined 27 percent since the 1970s (even though the benefit of this change was partly offset by increased poultry consumption). If the United States could simply continue reducing its beef consumption down to a world average level, health outcomes would improve and greenhouse gas emissions from American agriculture would decline by one-third.

What would happen if animal-based foods were avoided entirely? One study published in *Science* in 2018 tried to estimate the global environmental impact of eliminating animal product consumption. This study was based on data from forty thousand farms in more than one hundred countries, and it covered forty different food products that currently supply 90 percent of all consumption. It concluded that completely eliminating animal products from our diet would reduce the use of land for food (mostly pastureland) by more than three-quarters, with a 19 percent reduction in cropland specifically. The leader of this study, Joseph Poore at Oxford, concluded, "A vegan diet is probably the single biggest way to reduce your impact on planet Earth." Vegan diets do not work, at the moment, for pastoralist herdsmen on the drylands of Africa, where getting protein from crops is not an option.

Regional differences of this kind were considered more carefully in a 2019 study produced by the EAT-*Lancet* Commission, made up of thirty-seven world-leading scientists from sixteen countries, convened to develop targets for healthy diets and sustainable food production. This study estimated the health and environmental benefits that would come from shifting current eating patterns toward a prescribed "planetary health diet," one that would differ region by region depending on the cultural acceptance and availability of different food groups. The overall goal would be to remain within the boundaries set simultaneously by human health and environmental sustainability, including climate protection. For most societies this would require a shift toward plant-based diets supplemented with just modest amounts of fish, meat, and dairy foods. Globally, the consumption of healthy foods such as fruits, vegetables, legumes, and nuts would have to double, while global consumption of added sugars and red meats would have to be reduced by more than half.

The EAT-*Lancet* study delivered a particularly harsh message to the United States. To stay within planetary boundaries, Americans would have to eat 84 percent less red meat and six times more beans and lentils. The livestock industry erupted with scorn. The National Pork Producers Council called the report "irresponsible," saying it was "based on dubious science." The North American Meat Institute called it a "fad diet solution," out of step with genuine nutrition science. This was not a convincing charge since the cochair of the study was Dr. Walter Willett from Harvard's T. H. Chan School of Public Health, one of the world's leading nutrition scientists.

One interesting critique of the EAT-*Lancet* benchmark diet came from a team of economists, who pointed out that the diet was not yet affordable for about 1.6 billion of the world's poor. This was a good reminder that food scarcity, not excess, remains a leading problem for many. The EAT-*Lancet* message drew harsher fire from ordinary meat-eating Americans. Only one out of twenty Americans identifies as a vegetarian, and only 3 percent are completely vegan. Many on low-carb or paleo diets tweeted their objections to the study, using the hash tag #yes2meat. Diana Rodgers, the previously mentioned dietician and paleo cookbook author and spouse of Andrew Rodgers on Clark Farm, complained about the EAT-*Lancet* diet on her blog, asserting the real problems in America's diet come from refined oils and highly processed grains, not from meat.

Resistance to the EAT-*Lancet* message was also reinforced in 2019 by a mischievous statistical study from Dalhousie University, which concluded that the evidence of adverse health effects from red meat consumption was not particularly strong. The lead author summarized his message this way: "It's uncertain whether there are true health concerns related to moderate consumption of red or processed meats." The study was mischievous because it used an impossibly high standard of certainty, one that is normally reserved for clinical drug trials. Also, the lead author had earlier dismissed the health risks surrounding sugar by using the same technique, and had a history of accepting research support from private food industries. The bogus message nonetheless got wide play, making the task of moderating unhealthy red meat consumption that much more difficult.

Most American eaters clearly dislike personal deprivation. Efforts to reduce animal product consumption, if framed this way, are likely to fail. Better to present the problem as one of substitution. Consider the fashion industry, which reduced its use of animal fur by substituting low-cost, high-quality imitation fur products. The shoe industry reduced its use of animal hides by substituting microfibers that simulate leather in their durability, flexibility, breathability, and appearance. If modern science can imitate the fur and the hide of animals, perhaps it can also imitate the meat, the milk, and the eggs.

Success for such a project is just around the corner according to some enthusiasts. Richard Branson, the billionaire business magnate who created the Virgin Group, blogged in 2018 that "in thirty years or so, I believe we will look back and be shocked at what was the accepted way we killed animals en masse for food. I think that in the future, clean and plant-based meat will become the norm, and in thirty years it is unlikely animals will need to be killed for food anymore." In 2019 a think tank named RethinkX, which studies disruption, produced a report on imitation animal products that predicted an even quicker substitution, leading to a 70 percent drop in demand for cow-based products as early as 2030.

Predictions of such a large and rapid replacement of animal products in the diet will probably not fare any better than the original Malthus prediction, but even a modest substitution of imitation meat for the real thing would be a gain. If faux meats replace only half of our ground beef and half of our pork sausage, the benefits to the environment, the welfare of animals, and also to personal health would be considerable.

The simulated meats currently being developed and sold differ from yesterday's veggie burgers because they are being pitched not to vegetarians or vegans but to meat lovers. In fact, many vegetarians do not like them because they look and taste too much like the real thing. The imitation beef burgers currently on the market still suffer from a detectible taste and appearance gap if measured against real hamburgers, but the gap has been shrinking fast. Beyond Burgers (made of pea protein, canola oil, and coconut fat) became available in retail meat cases in 2016, and in that same year Impossible Burgers (originally made with wheat, soy, potato protein, coconut oil, and soy leghemoglobin) began appearing in restaurants. Cell-grown meat products have lagged behind, but in the end it may be easier for these to get over the final taste hurdle, since biologically they *are* real meat, just not from a slaughtered animal.

The market penetration of all these products in the United States is still less than 1 percent of total retail "meat" sales, but growing fast. In 2019 the investment firm UBS projected that the market for meat alternatives would increase from $4.6 billion to $85 billion by 2030. This would parallel an earlier growth trajectory seen for plant-based dairy products, including "milk" from almonds, coconut, rice, soy, and other nonanimal sources. These nondairy milk sales increased over a decade from 1 percent to 13 percent of America's fluid milk market. More than one-third of American households now buy at least some plant-based dairy products, and sales increased more than 60 percent over one five-year period, at a time when sales of authentic dairy milk were falling 15 percent.

These sales of faux milk mean fewer cows housed in confinement along with fewer emissions of climate-changing methane. A company named Perfect Day has developed a yeast-grown product that mimics many of the same proteins found in cow's milk, so not only does it taste like milk but it also works in an emulsion to give foods a softened texture. Get ready for cow-free mozzarella cheese, yogurt, and ice cream. Plant-based egg substitutes are also moving ahead. Just Egg, a San Francisco–based tech company, began selling mung-bean-based egg substitutes in grocery stores in September 2018, and by January 2019 the sales were up to the equivalent of one million real eggs a month. These plant-based eggs use 98 percent less water, 86 percent less land, and have a carbon footprint 93 percent smaller than real eggs from hens.

The scale-up challenge will nonetheless be huge. It's not enough just to have a substitute. Despite decades of competition from would-be substitutes like stevia, allulose, and monk fruit, real sugar still claims more than three-quarters of the global sweetener market. Real sugar even persists in the face of strong personal health reasons to substitute. What today's faux beef, faux pork, and faux poultry products will need to capture a significant market share is continued innovation. The plant-based substitutes will have to keep improving their taste and texture, and the cell-grown products will have to lower their production costs. This means still more costly R & D investment.

But the money just might be there. Over the past decade investors have put more than $16 billion into plant-based and cell-cultured meat companies, and more than four-fifths of that has come in just the last two years. The California-based Beyond Meat company attracted venture capital from thirty-four separate investors (including the Humane Society) before it went public in 2019, with an initial market capitalization of nearly $4 billion. Its chief rival, Impossible Foods, had raised $1.3 billion by 2020, and increased its retail footprint fiftyfold. Bill Gates was an investor in both companies, and cell-grown meats have been backed by celebrities like Leonardo DiCaprio and billionaires like Sergey Brin and Li Ka-shing. Richard Branson is an investor in Memphis Meats, a leading cell-based start-up.

Newer players keep coming to the table. Lightlife Foods rolled out its own plant-based burger early in 2019 and made plans to introduce plant-based bratwurst and Italian sausages as well. Lightlife is part of Maple Leaf Foods, a subsidiary of Canada's top packaged-meat provider, which has its own significant R & D capacity plus an existing distribution network and valuable client relationships. Like the Beyond Burger, Lightlife's product uses pea rather than soy or wheat protein. Impossible Foods went gluten-free in 2019 by introducing an Impossible Burger 2.0 without wheat protein. This new product was unveiled at the International Consumer Electronics Show in Las Vegas. Consumer electronics? The alt-meat industry grooms itself to please tech-oriented innovators, not nostalgia-driven traditionalists.

The Impossible Burger 2.0, which began appearing in supermarkets in the fall of 2019, was designed to be as versatile in the kitchen as regular ground beef. According to J. Michael Melton, the technical sales and culinary manager at Impossible Foods, "Veggie patties of the past were basically a reheatable puck. The dynamic nature of our product allows it to be used in any way that you can use conventional ground meat. You can use our bulk product to do crumbles, meatballs, meat loaf, lasagna. Ultimately, you take what we offer and utilize it in any way that you would use traditional ground beef." By 2020, Impossible Burgers were in more than three thousand grocery stores. "The more we do," says Melton, "the closer we get to ubiquity, which is always the goal for us. We want to convert the world." Impossible Foods says it wants to replace animals as a food production technology by 2035, a time frame more ambitious than Branson's.

Traditional meat companies in the United States have also been putting money into the faux-meat sector, to the dismay of livestock producers. Tyson Foods originally invested in both Beyond Meat and cell-based Memphis Meats. Then in 2019 Tyson sold its Beyond shares and announced a plan to launch its own alternative protein products, and to initiate the sale of plant-based nuggets in four thousand retail stores. "We have a deep understanding of how to develop new products, brands, and categories," said Tyson CEO Noel White. "Our distribution reach will allow us to move quickly into the marketplace."

Other deep-pockets food companies, including Cargill Meats, Conagra Brands, and the Swiss giant Nestlé have also become players. Cargill is an investor in Memphis Meats, headquartered in Berkeley, which raised $161 million in its latest investment round. In 2020, Trader Joe's released its own store-brand plant-based burger. Conagra bought the meatless-meat producer Gardein, and Nestlé launched an Awesome Burger and Awesome Grounds (a ground meat substitute) in the American market as well. The Awesome Burger has a better nutrition profile—more protein and fiber—than the Beyond or Impossible Burger. Nestlé will soon be selling Stouffer's Meatless Lasagna. In 2019 the MorningStar Farms company added a new "Cheezeburger" to its growing list of completely plant-based items, a line that also includes Chik'n nuggets and Tex-Mex burgers. Not using the words *cheese* or *chicken* allows MorningStar to avoid legal challenges from the livestock industry. The company expects to have a portfolio of totally vegan offerings by 2021, allowing its parent company Kellogg to claim it has eliminated the use of more than three hundred million egg whites a year.

Growing tissues of real meat in a lab from animal cells is a different approach. One early visionary here was Winston Churchill, who predicted as far back as 1931 that in half a century, "we shall escape the absurdity of growing a whole chicken in order to eat the breast or wing, by growing these parts separately under a suitable medium." Churchill exaggerated the timing but had the concept just right. Today's cell-based meat products begin with real animal muscle and fat cells, taken in a biopsy then cultured into tissue with a growth serum. Using such methods, the company Just Inc. has cultured chicken nuggets, and Israel's Aleph Farms claims to have a lab-grown steak that takes just three weeks from cell samples to finished product. New Age Meats in the United States has produced the first cultured pork sausage. Mosa Meat in the Netherlands is hoping to bring products to the market by 2021.

It may be easier for these cell-cultured products to deliver real meat tastes, because they will be real meat. Memphis Meats allowed Amanda Little, who was authoring a book, to taste a two-ounce piece of its cell-cultured duck breast meat, ultimately intended for the Chinese market. According to Little, the duck tasted as advertised: "meaty." Memphis Meats will have competition in China. In 2017, China signed a $300-million lab-grown meat deal with three Israeli companies—SuperMeat, Future Meat Technologies, and Meat the Future. Late in 2019, Impossible Foods rolled out its plant-based burger at a Shanghai trade fair attended by President Xi Jinping. Buddhists in China, who have been consuming meat alternatives for centuries, will have some new options.

The innovators leading this new race to provide imitation meats usually present environmental sustainability as their primary goal. The founder of Impossible Foods, a Stanford scientist named Patrick Brown, had concluded that the continued use of animals as a food technology was an unacceptable threat to climate, water, and wildlife, yet he also knew most people would not easily give up their taste for animal-derived foods. Being a biochemist, his solution was to identify with precision the molecular properties that give meat its distinctive taste and then re-create these same properties using molecules of plants. He set out to "invent a better way to transform plants into delicious, nutritious, safe and affordable meat, fish and dairy foods that consumers love."

Environmental benefits remain at the center of Brown's pitch. His company claims that the carbon footprint of an Impossible Burger is almost 90 percent smaller than that of a real beef burger, and at the same time 87 percent less dependent on water and 96 percent less dependent on land. The environmental savings from cell-grown meat are projected to be comparable: 90 percent less land and water and 90 percent fewer greenhouse gasses, compared to meat from slaughtered animals.

The Impossible Burger is designed to mimic ground beef in texture, flavor, chewiness, and sensory experience. It sears and caramelizes like the real thing, and it even has a simulated beef-like "blood," provided by an iron-containing molecule named heme. To produce enough heme without using animals, Impossible Foods introduced a gene from a soybean plant into yeast cells, which then manufacture the molecule as they multiply.

Impossible Burgers first showed up in select higher-end restaurants in New York and San Francisco in 2016, priced at about $14 each, and they got positive reviews. Joshua Katcher, a men's lifestyle writer who is also a vegan, said, "I had to sit there and tell myself 'This is not a burger.'" The targeted market was committed meat eaters, so the most important product rollout took place in Texas, where a skeptical meat-loving reviewer for *Texas Monthly* wrote that the product lived up to its name. When Impossible Burgers are served in restaurants, they arrive already garnished inside a toasted bun, which helps to mask some of the taste and texture differences compared to a real burger. Restaurant closings after COVID-19 did not slow sales growth, thanks to a recently expanded in-store retail presence, plus a new online option providing home delivery in just two days, and free shipping. Since 39 percent of all beef sales in the United States take the form of fresh ground beef, there is room for a significant marketplace substitution.

Fast-food restaurants are another scale-up pathway. Over one thousand Carl's Jr. restaurants began serving Beyond Burgers early in 2019, and later that year McDonald's tested a specially formulated "P.L.T." (plant, lettuce, and tomato) burger, provided by Beyond Meat on menus in Canada. Dunkin' Donuts began selling a Beyond Sausage Sandwich, served with egg and cheese, postering its walls with a new "Great Taste, Plant-Based" slogan. Burger King began selling "Impossible Whoppers," through its own partnership with Impossible Foods. On April Fools' Day 2019, Burger King sneaked in the imitation meat covertly at one of its St. Louis locations, hoping the switch would not be noticed by regular customers. When one burger lover was told about the switch, he blurted out an unprintable endorsement: "No f——ing way. This is a f——ing cow!"

Burger King's version of the Impossible Burger has the same amount of protein as its traditional Whopper, but 15 percent less fat and 90 percent less cholesterol. Both the Impossible Burger and the Beyond Burger are higher in sodium than a real burger, and nutrition scientists have criticized them for being far less healthy as a source of protein than beans, lentils, or sunflower seeds. Impossible's chief marketing officer, Fernando Machado, is trusting the clear environ-

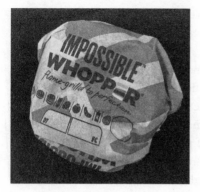

The Impossible Whopper no longer hides its identity. It is served in an attractive sea-foam-green-and-white wrapper and is dressed like a real Whopper with ketchup, mayonnaise, lettuce, tomato, onions, and pickles.

mental benefit to drive sales. "I have high expectations that it's going to be big business," he says, "not just a niche product." Impossible Foods has struggled to keep up with demand; it had to install a second production line at its Oakland, California, plant, and in 2020, the work force was expanded to 653 full-time employees.

Burger King's April Fools' stunt did not amuse Arby's, a rival chain that likes to brag "We have the meats." Arby's tried to counter with a tongue-in-cheek promotion of its own first-ever "meat-based carrot," which it called a marrot. The chief marketing officer at Arby's, Jim Taylor, claims he told his culinary innovation team it was time to reverse the paradigm of plant-based meats by offering meat-based plants. "Universally, people know we're supposed to eat vegetables every day. But ninety percent of Americans don't eat that recommended amount," said Taylor. "So, we said if others can make meat out of vegetables, why can't we make vegetables out of meat?"

Cell-cultured products are lagging because they have not yet reached a competitive price point. An individual cultured pork sausage from New Age Meats, as of 2018, would have cost more than two hundred dollars. The two-ounce cell-grown duck breast served to Amanda Little by Memphis Meats would also have been a several-hundred-dollar item. Just Inc., the San Francisco start-up making faux eggs, hopes to offer cell-grown chicken nuggets soon, but only in restaurants. Some visionaries want cell-grown animal products to go far beyond food. The founder of the Cellular Agriculture Society,

Kristopher Gasteratos, imagines that animal tissues will someday be grown as clothing for military environments, or possibly interplanetary travel.

Farmers who raise living animals want no part of faux meat, milk, or eggs. Livestock producers are fighting to stop sellers of plant-based or lab-based food from using the word *meat,* having seen what happened in dairy once sellers of almond and soy drinks were allowed to use the word *milk.* By 2019, beef producers and other farm industry groups had persuaded seven different state legislatures to prohibit use of the word *meat* for plant-based foods, and for cell-based foods as well. The National Cattleman's Beef Association calls it "fake meat."

Some livestock producers have even tried to convince environmentalists that raising living animals is a better way to fight climate change, so long as well managed grazing systems are used to sequester more carbon in the soil. Applegate Farms, a natural and organic meat company, launched a new line of pork sausages in 2019 from pigs raised on small farms using such "regenerative" agricultural practices. Applegate's president, John Ghingo, said his company was "making a big bet on regenerative agriculture as one of the paths to show the world that raising animals and eating meat doesn't have to be a problem."

True believers in one regenerative method called "holistic" grazing even say meat can be produced with *negative* greenhouse gas emissions. Holistic grazing seeks to imitate the feeding patterns of large ruminant animals in nature, on the grasslands of Africa. The key is to bunch the animals closely together and move them constantly from one place to the next, something done by wild animals to protect against predators. Allan Savory, who grew up in Zimbabwe, has promoted this method since the 1970s, originally as a way to combat overgrazing and desertification, but now he and his followers say it captures enough carbon in the soil to fight climate change.

This is slippery ground. Changes in the carbon content of pasture soils are a challenge to monitor, in multiple places, and of multiple depths, over time. This does not stop holistic grazing advocates from making startling claims. In 2019, a private life cycle analysis firm named Quantis presented findings from a study of cattle grazing practices on a farm in Georgia named White Oak Pastures, operated by rancher Will Harris. Quantis concluded that the grazing methods used were moving so much carbon into the soil that the system was greenhouse gas *negative,* and thus superior on climate protection grounds even to Beyond and Impossible Burgers.

I happened to attend a large climate-focused conference in Tennessee late in 2019 where Will Harris was on hand to speak up for this grazing system, wearing his signature Stetson hat. He threw in a complaint about the "greenwashing" he saw coming from the faux meat companies. "I could name names," said Harris. When shouts from the floor encouraged him to do so, he responded slyly in a Georgia drawl, "I'm not going to mention the Impossible Burger."

The improbable claim that grass-fed beef under holistic grazing can be better for climate protection than imitation beef is still being tested. The closest thing to a solid peer-reviewed defense of this claim, published in the journal *Agricultural Systems,* examines a Michigan State University experiment. This study conceded that the direct greenhouse gas emissions from holistic-grazed cattle were half again higher than from feedlot cattle, which was not a surprise given the longer time it takes for grazed cattle to reach a market weight. But once captured soil carbon was added to the calculation, the emissions became negative. The carbon capture rate calculated in this study was suspiciously high—nearly nine times as high as in a 2003 study of "management intensive grazing"—but the study became a debating point for defenders of "regenerative" real meat.

Faux meat has triggered an interesting range of reactions from food movement leaders, many of whom reject it for being inauthentic, corporate, industrial, and too heavily processed. "If you're combining a bunch of powders and turning it into something that looks like meat," says Mark Bittman, "I'm not sure you're doing anybody any good. I don't think it moves people in the direction of real food—which is the ultimate goal." Brian Niccol, CEO of Chipotle, says he won't serve plant-based meats "because of the processing." Whole Foods CEO John Mackey, although himself a vegan, has a similar re-

action: "If you look at the ingredients, they are super, highly processed foods." The livestock industry has decided to adopt this same
messaging. The Center for Consumer Freedom, which fronts for the
meat, restaurant, and alcohol industries, put a full-page ad in the
New York Times in October 2019, warning readers that "Fake meats
are ultra-processed imitations with dozens of ingredients including
methylcellulose, titanium dioxide, tertiary butylhydroquinone, disodium inosinate." Fake meat, they call it, but with "real chemicals."

Vandana Shiva, weighing in from India, dismissed plant-based faux
animal products as a "Fake Food Goldrush," led by profit-making
firms. Michael Pollan does not go that far but suggests caution:
"Foods that we've been eating for tens of thousands of years have
kind of proven themselves out, and we are talking about introducing
some novel foods and so we need to be careful." Later, after tasting a
plant-based meatball from Impossible Foods, Pollan remained uncon-
vinced. "By my standards, it's not food," he said. "Doesn't mean I'm
against it."

The surprise is that so many environmental groups have failed to
endorse faux meats. In 2017, the ETC Group and Friends of the Earth
called on Impossible Foods to remove their burger from the market,
pending further safety testing and stronger regulation from the FDA.
These organizations took issue with the genetically engineered yeast
that was producing the essential heme molecules. They accused Impossible Foods of "attempting to capitalize on animal welfare concerns
through 'molecular farming.'" Seth Itzkan, an environmental futurist
who advocates for regenerative land management instead, says fake
meat is not food. "It's software, intellectual property—14 patents."

Impossible Foods defended itself mostly with gauzy messaging.
In 2018 the company produced a ninety-second short film titled *The
Return,* showing an astronaut who has just come back to Earth. Our
planet is now a verdant paradise, with flowers, trees, birds, friendly
insects, turtles, people, and happy toddlers. Impossible's product is
never mentioned in the film, but it ends with an inspiring coda on
the screen: "We're on a Mission, and it's not to Mars." If the mission is successful, hog producer Mark Legan's facetious solution to

the animal welfare problem—"Just don't raise pigs"—may come true after all.

Faux meat products might eventually open the door to faux fish, delivering a second round of environmental benefits. Early in 2019, Whole Foods Market began selling a plant-based tuna from Good Catch Foods. The product is shelf stable, ready to eat, and claims to deliver the flavor and the flaky texture of chunk albacore tuna, but without the high mercury levels, PCBs, or dioxins found in some ocean-sourced fish. It has no unpleasant smell, allowing millennials to use the product in an open office space with no fear of food shaming from fellow workers. Connoisseurs of real tuna salad will find the aftertaste a drawback, but early in 2020, a real tuna company, Bumble Bee, announced a joint distribution venture with Good Catch, to promote "alternative ways for consumers to enjoy ocean-inspired foods."

Cell-cultured seafood products will be coming next. The California-based company Finless Foods has plans to launch cell-cultured bluefin tuna in high-end restaurants, and San Diego start-up BlueNalu wants to grow broad sheets of whole muscle tissue from mahi-mahi. A Singapore company named Shiok (which means "delicious" in Malay slang) is developing shrimp, crab, and lobster products by using stem cells taken from these crustaceans, fed with a nutrient mix. As of 2019, cell-based fish products were not yet available to taste, but Blue-Nalu was already producing seafood medallions and fillets at pilot scale. Viable commercial products may still be years away, but the science keeps getting better, so faux fish will also be a part of our future.

I f imitation meat and fish can help address problems with animal welfare and the environment, the next challenge will be upgrading America's dietary health. Even Nestlé's Awesome Burger won't be a healthy meal if consumed with fries and a sugary drink. Food science has been used in the past to develop irresistible items that are bad for health, so perhaps tomorrow's food scientists will devise craveable products that deliver positive nutrition benefits. Some of this is starting to happen, but only around the edges.

First, food companies will not take an interest in making more nutritious processed foods unless they are allowed to advertise a promised health benefit. When the FDA in 2004 finally allowed food manufacturers to claim that omega-3 fatty acids could reduce the risk of coronary heart disease, companies like Tropicana and Minute Maid did begin incorporating more omega-3 into their product offerings. Plant sterols, which lower LDL cholesterol and may fight cancer, are another "nutraceutical" additive highlighted now by food manufacturers. Probiotics and CLA (conjugated linoleic acid) are two more. Chemical compounds from the stevia plant are now delivering products that are sweet tasting but sugar-free. When Whole Foods listed its top ten food trends for 2019, it included new frozen desserts that are plant based, and shelf-stable probiotics added to products like granola, oatmeal, nut butters, soups, and nutrition bars.

Not all novel products promising better health sell. In 2016 scientists at Nestlé developed a "hollow" sugar that was more porous and dissolved faster in the mouth, so eaters could taste the same level of sweetness while consuming less. Nestlé then designed a Milkybar Wowsomes product around this technology, and launched in 2018, but discontinued the product amid low demand in 2020.

Big food companies alert to wellness concerns have been recruiting new leaders with experience in the nutrition space. In 2017, Kellogg's named as its CEO Steve Cahillane, the former president of Nature's Bounty, a company that sold vitamins and nutritional supplements. Nestlé appointed as its CEO Mark Schneider, who came from a health-care background. Indra Nooyi's twelve years of service as CEO at PepsiCo made the company more health-forward. In 2018, PepsiCo doubled-down on Nooyi's goal of moving away from sugary drinks when it spent $3.2 billion to purchase a sparkling water company named SodaStream. PepsiCo had already acquired the probiotics manufacturer KeVita and was selling a bottled water drink named LifeWTR.

When the tradition-bound Grocery Manufacturers Association then dragged its feet on wellness issues, it paid a price. Seven major food manufacturers quit the GMA in 2018 when the organization resisted a new FDA requirement to list added sugars on the nutrition facts panel, and when it opposed mandatory disclosure of GMO food ingredients. These defections cost the GMA half of its total revenue. Four of the breakaway companies—Danone North America, Mars, Nestlé USA, and Unilever USA—later joined to form their own association, the Sustainable Food Policy Alliance, committed to consumer transparency as well as sustainability. Publicly shamed, the GMA said it would change its name in 2020 to the Consumer Brands Association and stop lobbying on nutrition issues.

Some visible moves toward wellness have also emerged in food retail. In 2016, Aldi replaced the candy and chocolate products in its checkout area with packets of nuts, trail mix, dried fruits, and granola bars. In September 2018, the Raley's chain, with more than one hundred stores in Northern California and Nevada, announced it was removing all conventional candy and soda from its checkout lanes, offering instead seaweed snacks, rolled rice cakes, reusable grab-and-go packs of pitted and sliced black olives, and other healthy options. This was also the year Ahold Delhaize announced it would be extending the Guiding Stars nutrition-guidance shelf-tag system to all its American stores.

When food companies innovate, wellness is not always the central objective. Conagra, which makes Slim Jim jerky and Hunt's Ketchup, recently used advanced artificial intelligence to discover that younger eaters had a fascination with unicorns. Then it employed another AI-enabled development system to identify the looks and tastes consumers associated with unicorns, and the result was a pastel-colored Snack Pack pudding with cotton candy flavors, packaged with cartoon unicorns. An eight-page 2019 *Wall Street Journal* report titled "The Future of Food" described one innovation of this kind after another, but never once mentioned nutrition balance, dietary health, or obesity.

Finding healthy new products to put on supermarket shelves or add to restaurant menus may actually be the easy part. Persuading consumers to drop their current choices and select these items remains far more difficult. Greg Drescher, the vice president for strategic initiatives at the Culinary Institute of America (the other CIA), appreciates the new "plant-forward" menu offerings coming out in many national restaurant chains, but he says it won't be enough for these better-for-you items simply to taste good. The healthy new dishes will be competing with juicy, cheese-laden, fully craveable animal-based items, so if the restaurants want to move a significant share of customers plant forward they will have to meet a far more demanding standard, one he calls "deliciousness." "If we can't deliver this," says Drescher, "we've really got nothing." Darren Seifer, a leading food and beverage industry analyst, has gone further. Reporting on new survey results early in 2020, he said, "It could cure cancer, but if it doesn't taste great people won't adopt it."

Another innovative path to future wellness might be "personalized" foods, custom formulated to the unique clinical needs, gut biome, or genetics of individual eaters. Some restaurants are already trying to personalize, including Vita Mojo in the City of London, which offers touch screens that allow lunch customers to dial up exactly the combination of protein, vegetables, side dishes, and sauces they desire. Other restaurants are experimenting with "molecular cuisines" based on fractionated and recombined methods that offer food essences in enticing new forms, but not always to improve health. Personalized meals will also be fabricated in the years ahead by 3D food printers, machines programmed to deposit edible pastes, gels, powders, and liquid ingredients onto an appropriate cooking surface. The Chef 3D printer, from a company named BeeHex, uses a technology first developed for NASA's deep space missions. The BeeHex can print chocolates or entire pizzas (no health focus here quite yet) in a variety of food consistencies using a no-drip extrusion platform. After successful demonstrations at multiple events across the country, BeeHex entered a commercial partnership with Donatos, a pizza delivery restaurant chain headquartered in Columbus, Ohio.

Another company named Natural Machines makes the Foodini, which prints and cooks chicken nuggets in any shape that a child might select—like stars, or dinosaurs (or unicorns). Just insert ground chicken and bread crumbs. When parents input lower limits for fat or calorie content, the Foodini will adjust the size of the nugget coming out.

For tech-loving experimentalists, 3D food printing offers itself as a creative alternative to the home microwave. Digital countertop fabricators will print and then cook foods employing the user's favorite ingredients, creating flavors and textures that would be unobtainable with conventional kitchen devices. The machines will also talk to and learn from other fabricators. Visionaries are imagining "the evolution of a networked food culture intrinsically connected to our networked information society." By distributing, purchasing, sharing, and sampling new fabricator recipes these machines could make creative cooking as effortless and affordable as today's consumption of digital music.

Any such move toward digital food is likely to trigger a struggle for control between food companies and tech companies. Tech companies tend to be more nimble and innovative than habit-bound food companies, and whoever controls primary access to the consumer data could win the struggle. Amazon's acquisition of Whole Foods Market in 2017 suggests that Big Tech will have the edge.

We have seen that farms were already going digital, but this trend will push much further in the years ahead. Farmers will continue to optimize plant growth and reduce wasteful inputs through an increased deployment of drone-based sensor systems, improved precision guidance, artificial intelligence, and machine learning. Farm management decisions will be based on big data combined with farm-level and field-level real-time data, all gathered and analyzed using web-connected devices. With better information, each bushel of food production will require even less water, energy, or chemical use, and farming will move still farther down an ecomodernist path.

Reduced water use in almond production illustrates the opportunity. California produces more than four-fifths of all the almonds in the world, and every year each acre of almond trees uses three to four acre-feet of water (one acre of water a foot deep), which is not sustainable in water-stressed California. During one recent drought, producers of almonds in the Central Valley ran short of water from canals and had to dig more wells to pump groundwater. They pumped so much that in some places the ground began to subside, buckling roads and damaging bridge abutments. Farmers without wells were forced to cut water use sharply; they kept their valuable almond trees alive by leaving their normally productive vegetable fields dry and unplanted.

Almond growers have long used drip irrigation to reduce water waste, but the waste is now even better controlled thanks to improved real-time information. On one current operation in the Central Valley a farm manager divided his almond groves into smaller blocks, each separately irrigated by "smart" drip lines linked to soil moisture probes that send data back to a control location by radio signal. Soil moisture levels are monitored by location and also soil depth, and after the data is normalized it is relayed to a mobile app used by the farm manager. Instead of dripping water twenty-four hours a day, the lines operate block by block only when needed, delivering only as much as needed.

Variable rate irrigation (VRI) systems of this kind can be integrated into conventional systems simply by adding the appropriate controllers and software. A setup is costly, since it has to be custom tailored to each crop on each farm, but uptake will increase as equipment manufacturers develop better standards to facilitate setup, ease of use, and interchangeability.

VRI irrigation systems can also be paired with other smart farming tools, such as drones equipped with remote sensing platforms. Unlike remote sensing from manned aircraft or satellites, these small unmanned aerial vehicles (UAVs) can be tasked at any time to provide actionable same-day information on field and crop conditions. When flown at three hundred feet, drones generate valuable field-level data, but at lower altitudes they now can deliver images showing not just individual plants but individual plant leaves, the margins of those leaves, and even the small auricles that attach to plant stems. When near-infrared light is employed along with a red-edge light system,

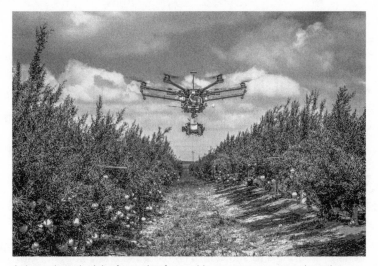

A drone does the job of scouting for trouble on a pomegranate plantation.

drone-based sensors are able to see more than the human eye. With drones to scout their fields, farmers can spot problems before they spread, then contain the damage with less extreme and less wasteful methods.

Drones also can map elevation variability within a field, which improves the precision of land leveling and the design of subsurface drainage tiles. Laser-based sensors on drones can measure gases such as ammonia or water vapor in a field, or collect canopy-level information on crop color, size, and shape. This data can be combined with ground-level measurements to create sophisticated within-field models of crop growth, allowing farmers to apply only the inputs required, only where they are required, and only at the moment they will do the most good.

Wasteful input use will also be reduced in the future through machine learning. One example is a machine developed by the Blue River company and named the See & Spray, an eight-row rig that can be pulled through a cotton field to identify very young weeds then spray herbicides onto them with laser-jet precision. Using a multi-camera array and powerful algorithms, the machine learns to locate, identify, and separately spray each individual weed. This is a vast improvement over today's practice of planting cotton varieties that can resist herbicides, then spraying a whole field indiscriminately. See & Spray rigs can keep a cotton field free of weeds with, on average, less than one-tenth the quantity of weed killer now being used on herbicide-tolerant crops.

The livestock sector is also going smart and digital. A machine vision company in Ireland named Cainthus has developed facial and hide-pattern recognition systems capable of identifying individual dairy cows, which allows food and water intake to be individually monitored, delivering individualized health benefits. If a cow deviates from its normal routine, an alert will be sent to the farm manager's smartphone. By the end of 2018, Cainthus cameras were installed in barns housing a total of fourteen thousand cows, both in North America and in Europe. Farmers have learned that the video cameras have to be placed out of reach of the curious cows' tongues. As Cainthus president David Hunt explained, "Any way you can think an animal with no hands could possibly cause problems with a camera—the cows did that." Thanks to a large investment by Cargill, Cainthus hopes to extend its facial recognition technology to hogs, poultry, and possibly even farmed fish.

Highly engineered "smart" technologies such as these are too expensive for undercapitalized smaller farms. Even for large almond growers, an investment in VRI drip irrigation may not pay off for up to seven years. An expensive See & Spray rig will pay off only if it gets steady use, making it a poor choice for cotton farms with limited acreage, except perhaps on a cooperative or rental basis. The operation of these new systems also requires a technical facility well beyond the grasp of most older farmers, and the repairs and maintenance can't be done using hand tools out in the barn. The data analysis can also be overwhelming.

Service providers are springing up to solve some of these problems. Site Specific Technology Software (SST) offers farmers desktop access to geographical information systems (GIS) and automated task processing. SST now manages and analyzes data for more than one hundred million acres in more than twenty different countries. Another provider is Climate Corp., owned by the (former) Monsanto Company, which sells its subscribers access to a Climate FieldView digital agricultural platform. As of 2016, FieldView services were in use on ninety-two million acres of U.S. cropland. Farmers with a Climate FieldView account receive a multilayered big data analysis of the information they provide from their own farm, plus access to companies selling soil sensors or drone companies supplying advanced aerial imagery. Beginning in 2019, farmers using Climate FieldView were also able to access high-resolution images of their own farm from Airbus satellites.

These smart farming systems further invalidate the charge that modern farming treats all landscapes the same. Wendell Berry, the farmer-poet from Kentucky, made this charge in 2015: "The great and characteristic problem of industrial agriculture is that it does not distinguish one place from another. In effect, it blinds its practitioners to where they are." This might have been true for industrial farming three or four decades ago, but farmers now have an unmatched ability to know exactly where they are in a field, and where everything else is, with sub-inch accuracy if necessary.

The capacity for precision agriculture (PA) to reduce excessive inputs is now well established. Drawing from a summary published by Cornell University in 2016, one New York State study found that the use of PA techniques had reduced environmental nitrogen losses by 39 percent. A 2013 study in Hungary found that the overall environmental burden from agriculture declined by a little less than one-third with the embrace of PA, partly depending on farm size and farming intensity. An earlier German study found that PA decreased herbicide use by more than half. A 1996 study of variable rate applications on corn and soybeans in the United States and Denmark found insecticide use decreased by roughly one-third, which helped prevent the emergence of insects resistant to the chemicals. For wheat, Jayson Lusk at Purdue University points out that precision agriculture has sharply reduced fertilizer use without any reduction in yield or grain quality.

PA practices still have plenty of room to grow on American farms.

In 2016 the Department of Agriculture published a study indicating that the practice of spatial yield mapping had tripled for most crops since 2000, but two-thirds of total planted acres have yet to begin using this method. GPS soil mapping and variable rate application were also on the rise, yet more than three-quarters of the nation's planted area had yet to benefit. The only PA technique that had spread to more than half of all planted acres for some crops was GPS auto-steering for tractors and harvesters.

The uptake of PA is easier on large farms. Fewer than one-fifth of America's farms smaller than 1,300 acres have been using variable rate technology, but 40 percent are using VRT on farms larger than 3,800 acres. This large farm bias may not be all bad from the standpoint of environmental protection. Recall that 81 percent of America's agricultural sales are made by just 7 percent of its farms—the larger farms with annual sales above half a million dollars—so it may be an environmental benefit that the farms producing most of our food are also the ones most likely to go digital.

Small farms in the developing world lack both the financial means and the scale of operations needed to adopt today's PA equipment, but they have different needs that are now taking them down a paral-lel path. On the small fields still worked by hand in Africa and Asia, farmers do not need a GPS system to know exactly where they are in a field, and they work with a hand hoe that can take out weeds almost as precisely as a See & Spray. In addition, reducing excessive water, chemical, or fuel use is not the first challenge for these farmers, because few farms are irrigated in Africa, most are currently using too little fertilizer rather than too much, and very few burn any diesel fuel. What these farmers are more likely to need is accurate informa-tion on the condition of their crops and soils, and this is something they can get now with highly affordable new tools.

Leaf color charts (LCC) and chlorophyll meters (SPAD) are cheap handheld tools that small farmers can use to judge the nitrogen status in their rice fields, to help in timing their fertilizer applications. In India, nitrogen management using LCC has helped farmers reduce chemical use by forty kilograms per hectare with no loss of yield. A handheld "GreenSeeker" nitrogen meter with an active light source works even better. For detecting fields contaminated with dangerous aflatoxins, farmers can now use compact goggles called AflaGoggles, with no advanced training required. Poor farmers in Africa can also benefit from countertop soil testing at a local NGO office or an agro-dealer shop. Battery-powered ion-sensitive electrode (ISE) devices test soil samples brought in, measuring not just pH but also nutrient deficits, enabling customized fertilizer recommendations.

To improve water management, small farmers can now join with their neighbors to hire laser-guided land-leveling services, which eliminate runoff and increase water use efficiency on rice fields by 65 percent. This has allowed rice and wheat farmers in India to gain an added $144 per hectare annually. Small farms also can profit from more precise drip irrigation through contracting or out-growing schemes. In India, Jain Irrigation provides over sixteen hundred farmers with drip equipment plus inputs and services, then it buys back the produce at a promised price. In Burkina Faso, farmers in ten different provinces have been purchasing their own simple drip irrigation kits, which allow them to grow vegetables all year long on small plots just twenty meters square.

Engineers are also developing affordable subsoil moisture sensors with traffic light displays that tell farmers at a glance whether moisture is adequate at three different depth levels in the soil. The data from these sensors can be georeferenced by a smartphone, then displayed on Google Earth to improve water management in irrigation systems that have multiple users. Using such systems, poor rice farmers in Asia will be able to enjoy water management options nearly as precise as those of rich California almond growers.

Farm robots and increased automation will also be part of the future. Powered machines have already replaced traditional hand labor almost everywhere in American farming. The one exception has been in harvesting easily bruised fresh fruits and vegetables, but now these tasks are also being automated, thanks to artificial intelligence, robotics, and machine learning. Some may see this as a loss for farm-workers, but the physically punishing and poorly compensated job of hand-picking fruits and vegetables is not something a progressive society should want to preserve. Manual labor in farming is not only repetitive and low-paying; it also tends to be physically punishing. Performing stoop labor with a bent back under the hot sun breaks people down. Historically, this kind of work was frequently done by slaves who had no choice in the matter, and today it often goes to socially marginalized immigrants. Much of the banana harvest in Malaysia is performed by Indonesians, and much of the coffee farming in Costa Rica is done by Nicaraguans. Likewise for the United States, where two-thirds of all hired workers in the crop sector originally came from Mexico. Even America's prison population will not do this kind of work. When the state of Georgia, facing a farm labor shortage, offered inmates a chance to do field work on farms for pay, very few signed up. Those who took the offer soon quit, having discovered the work was too hard.

Machines began replacing hand labor on America's farms more than a century ago. Horse-drawn reapers saved individuals from scything wheat by hand. Self-propelled harvesters eventually made it unnecessary to pick corn by hand. Cotton-picking machines replaced sharecropper labor in the South, and automatic milking machines eventually transformed the dairy sector. A great deal of fruit and vegetable farming has now been mechanized as well. Machines started harvesting tomatoes grown for canning as early as 1962, and Florida's sugar cane harvest has been mechanized since the 1990s. Machines today also harvest root crops like potatoes and carrots, most nuts, and many tree fruits grown for processing. Raisin grape harvesting is in the process of being mechanized, and Florida citrus fruits are also on the verge.

The more delicate fruits and vegetables grown for direct human consumption are the greatest challenge, so they are still largely picked by hand, but robots with improved sensors will eventually take over this job as well. California's Blue River company, developers of the See & Spray, also developed a LettuceBot, a robotic machine that thins young iceberg lettuce plants. Towed behind a tractor, a single LettuceBot can do the work of twenty human thinners. Video cameras and machine-learning visual recognition software allow the machine to select which plants will be killed with a concentrated squirt of fertilizer. This adds nutrients to the soil while giving the saved plants more space to grow.

Another California company, Vision Robotics in San Diego, has developed a lettuce-thinning robot of its own that is capable of replacing a crew of up to thirty individuals. Vision Robotics is also developing a smart pruner for wine grapes, with cameras that photograph and create computerized models of the vines, allowing the robotic pruner to figure out the orientation of the canes then select which to cut down with its precision guided arms. Similar algorithms developed by researchers at Washington State University allow robots to scan cherry trees branch by branch, identifying where the branches are best grasped and shaken to loosen the largest number of ripe cherries. The cherry trees themselves have been bred with upright rather than bushy branches (the branches are known as "upright fruiting offshoots" or UFOs), to make things easier for the robots.

Many salad greens are now both planted and harvested by machine, usually in uniform greenhouse environments. It is more difficult to mechanize the picking of ripe fruits and vegetables, even in greenhouses, but a Massachusetts start-up named Root AI has tested a robot named Virgo, equipped with a three-fingered gripper that squeezes just hard enough to pull cherry tomatoes off the vine. Virgo uses a built-in video-processing chip and AI software to identify which tomatoes are ripe.

Designing robots to work in open fields on delicate fruits and vegetables is more difficult still. Stavros Vougioukas is an engineer at the University of California, Davis, with a doctorate in robotics. He originally came to the United States from Greece on a Fulbright fellowship. Like so many of his countrymen, he had kept a few olive trees back home but otherwise had no exposure to farming. Stavros is committed to what robots can do on farms but also sees the many challenges.

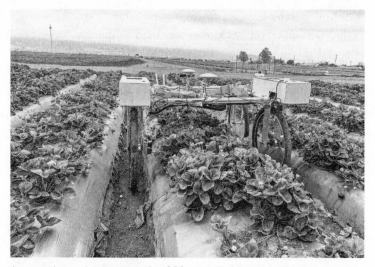

An experimental prototype of a GPS-controlled harvest-aid robot wheeling picked strawberries back from the field between raised beds.

At Davis, Stavros is known for developing the Fragile Crop Harvest-Aiding Mobile Robot (FRAIL-bot) to assist in strawberry picking. The first prototype looked a bit like a toy dump truck with four small bicycle wheels, plus an electric engine, multiple sensors, a GPS receiver, and a tilted holder for the trays of berries. In the field, this FRAIL-bot made its way back and forth between the long rows of plants, retrieving trays of picked strawberries, which saved the pickers from having to make repeated trips of their own. The FRAIL-bot does not do the picking, but it serves as a harvest aid. A later prototype with a wider frame straddles the strawberry beds.

Since the biggest labor demands are in harvesting, Stavros believes thinners like the LettuceBot are likely to have only limited value. The closest thing to a robotic harvester for lettuce uses a water-jet, but it works only for head lettuce and it isn't truly robotic since somebody has to drive it. When the John Deere company purchased the Blue River company for more than $300 million in 2017, the motive was not to get the LettuceBot. What Deere wanted instead were the technologies incorporated into the See & Spray weed-killing machine.

Picking crews can have skeptical reactions, even to a harvest aid. When Stavros shows his FRAIL-bot to pickers, he brings along a fluent Spanish speaker who opens with a basic reassurance: "This is a harvest aid. It is not going to pick. It's going to help you pick more trays because you won't have to walk as much." He recalls one suspicious picker replying with a clear warning: "If this machine is a picker, I'm going to crash it." Stavros acknowledges the anxiety. "If you ask the average picker how do you feel about robotic strawberry pickers, they will say 'I will hate the idea; I would lose my job.'"

Growers, however, feel increased pressures to automate the harvest because hiring pickers has become more difficult. Data from the USDA show that the number of unauthorized immigrants from Mexico living in the United States declined by almost one-fifth between 2007 and 2015. The reasons included reverse migration following the U.S. recession, increased risks associated with illegal border crossings, better employment opportunities in Mexico, much smaller families in rural Mexico, and education gains in Mexico as well. Growers seeking a solution to this labor shortage have repeatedly asked Congress for a streamlined temporary guest worker program, but this effort failed twice in 2018, and the Trump administration's immigration reform proposal in 2019 did not address the issue.

Paying higher wages might seem the obvious solution, but farm wages in California have already topped twenty dollars an hour and the shortages persist. In one 2019 survey, three-fifths of farmers in California reported they had not been able to hire all the employees they needed, at some point over the previous five years, even though 86 percent had increased wages in their efforts to do so. Some strawberry growers unable to find pickers in 2018 decided not to plant a crop at all the following year. Developing a robot capable of picking strawberries would solve these problems.

Some robots can already pick apples, but only from trees pruned flat into a "fruit wall" where each separate apple can be visible to the machine's cameras, a solution that does not work for strawberries growing on the ground. A Japanese company developed a system that moves boxes of strawberry plants within reach of a robot that identifies the ripe berries, then snips them by the stem, but this system only works in a greenhouse.

R & D investments in robotic solutions for harvesting specialty fruits and vegetables are often insufficient because each crop has a different geometry and poses a different problem to solve. Also, the market for any one crop—peaches, for example—may be too small to ensure a financial payoff. Because adequate corporate investments were not being made in strawberry picking, America's growers finally organized to take matters into their own hands, joining to invest in a Tampa company named Harvest CROO Robotics. In relatively short order, this company developed a robotic strawberry picker that it hopes can be in commercial use by 2022.

This Harvest CROO robot first positions itself over the plant, then grabs and gathers the plant leaves to expose the berries. Next it employs machine vision to evaluate the berries, identifying which are ripe. Finally, a rotor of revolving spokes with rubber claws picks and cleans the ripe fruit. The machine requires eight seconds to pick each plant and less than two seconds to move to the next plant. It can work in the dark if necessary, and without any lunch breaks. A single harvester replaces roughly thirty pickers and covers eight acres in a day. Each separate strawberry plant has its own GPS coordinates and a distinct geometry, so the harvester can learn to recognize them individually.

One University of Florida engineer advising Harvest CROO has speculated that in the next ten to twenty years half of all specialty

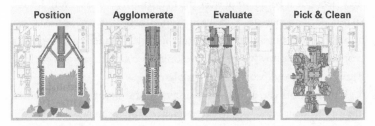

In a total of eight seconds, the Harvest CROO robot performs four separate functions over each strawberry plant, then moves on.

crops in the United States will be harvested by machines of this kind. If so, what will happen to the hired pickers? Following the depression of the 1930s, the mechanization of cotton picking in the South pushed millions of African American sharecroppers off the land and up north to work in factories, a labor shift known as the Great Migration. Fortunately, factory jobs were abundant at the time. The families that pick strawberries in California today, mostly foreign-born and often without documents, could find such adjustments more difficult if a new Harvest CROO takes over.

Ray Rodriguez was raised as a farmworker in California's Central Valley and learned about the hardships of field work at an early age. He has vivid memories of what it was like to pick cotton: "You had a bag called a choke-sack that went over the head and shoulder, 50 pounds for the kids, 100 pounds for the women, 150-pound sacks for the men. My dad would compete with the other men to see how much they could pick in a day, 300, 400, or 500 pounds. And I said I'm never doing this again. It's nothing you want to expose people to unless you have to."

Rodriguez broke away from a life in the fields by going to Fresno City College, and then earned a Ph.D. in genetics at UC Santa Cruz. He went on to an accomplished career in molecular biology but always kept one eye on farm labor issues in the Central Valley. When it became clear that automation was on its way, Ray knew how many families in the Valley would be left with no options, so he branched out and began to envision and promote the education and training programs that would be needed to help transition the next generation into higher-skill occupations in the local economy. He hoped to spare them the disruptions of a great migration that might not end so well.

Rodriguez says he would have no regrets if hand labor in the fields disappeared entirely. He quotes Cesar Chavez, the charismatic union organizer from the 1960s and 1970s, who always said he supported farmworkers, but not the farm work itself, because it was simply too tough. Ray sees it as "almost inhumane" to expect Mexican women and children to pick strawberries on their knees in the sun all day long; they know they need the job but nearly all hate doing it. They would welcome automation if they knew it would be accompanied by better work choices for their children.

Robotic harvesters would be fine with Rodriguez if he knew the school-age children of today's farmworkers were getting the training and education needed to find better jobs, including jobs in the local farm economy. He is not talking about low-skilled jobs like washing and packing vegetables, since these are scarcely better than field work. Packinghouses for leafy greens in Salinas, California, are kept at 35 degrees, so the workers must wear multiple layers of clothing and earmuffs. What's more, the packinghouse jobs will themselves be automated before long. What Rodriguez has in mind are the well-paying skilled jobs that will open up in agriculture for young men and women who have some training in fields like mechanical engineering, biology, fabrication, drones, and computers. Ray says today's farmworkers have little or no exposure to these occupations, so they will need help moving their children onto this ladder of advancement. Rodriguez wants this to become a primary mission for local community leaders, private companies, universities, and schools, all generously supported by taxpayers. The preparation must start in grades K–12. "We have to plan for this," says Rodriguez. "We need to get underrepresented people interested early."

The food future I have described should not surprise anyone. The digital revolution has already swept through medicine, manufacturing, finance, and entertainment, so we should expect it to take over food and farming as well. A return to the analog past would be unacceptable in any one of these other sectors, so we should not wish for it in food and farming either. Reverence for the past is fine, as long as we don't attempt a return.

There are many reasons to be hopeful about this future. Agricultural science will continue to boost farm productivity, so the price of farm commodities traded on the world market will almost certainly continue their long-term decline, a progressive outcome for the poor.

Because of parallel gains in worker productivity, individual purchasing power will also continue to rise, another reason the food choices available to poor as well as rich consumers will expand. As choice expands, eating practices will become increasingly diverse. Some consumers will opt for improved nutrition and health, even while others yield to the lure of taste gratification and convenience. Foodies will be able to find plenty of slow-paced artisanal authenticity, while others will continue to devour super-sized helpings of sugary or salt-laden foods. New food choices and new eating fads, both good and bad, will emerge all the time. It will bring improved health for some, and persistent dietary imbalance for the rest.

Since most basic appetites will be satisfied, eating decisions will more often be based on matters going beyond the food. Concerns over climate change and farm animal welfare will push us toward less-polluting faux meat products that require no living animals. On the larger farms that grow most of America's food, digital technologies will allow field operations to become better informed and more precise, enabling growers to produce more food while using less land and labor, less water, less energy, and fewer chemicals. Chemical use will decline, not through a switch to organic, but by an embrace of digital, smart, and precise. Small farms will survive in considerable numbers in America, but increasingly as a lifestyle choice sustained by nonfarming income. For hired farmworkers, laborious tasks like picking strawberries will more often be done by robotic machines, putting at risk those workers not prepared to find other breadwinning options.

This future will hardly be a utopia. Too many Americans will continue their unhealthy eating, unless health consciousness grows or industry resistance to policy reform can somehow be weakened. Academics like me will continue to endorse interventions to nudge consumers away from bad food choices, and some of this advice will eventually be taken, but probably too little and too late for a dramatic turnaround. Most Americans will continue to resist being told by their government what they should or should not eat, but their freedom will come at a price. If the nation's bad eating habits are not corrected, more Americans will find themselves living with chronic illness, then using up resources to treat the adverse medical consequences. Those born into disadvantage, with less education, less insurance, and less money to spend, will be those treated last, and least.

Straight Talk to Commercial Farmers

❧

Commercial farmers have so far gotten off easy in this book. Criticism has been leveled at food companies and the organizations that represent them; at supermarkets and restaurant chains; at advocacy organizations fixated on local food and organic food; and also at those who push for agroecology or food sovereignty over green revolution farming. So now it's the turn of commercial farmers, and especially the organizations trying to represent their interests. These organizations are understandably tired of being blamed by food movement activists for making eaters obese, polluting the environment, and torturing animals. I sympathize, but they have been missing out on one easy way to soften the criticism. The critics would be less harsh if commercial farm organizations were seen, at least occasionally, advocating for reforms to promote dietary health.

Patronizing attitudes from city people can worsen the problem. Massachusetts, where I live, is not a farm state. For the past half century our best-known export has been presidential candidates. First came the three Kennedy brothers, then in quick succession Michael Dukakis, Paul Tsongas, John Kerry, and Mitt Romney. Four more actually tried in 2020: Senator Elizabeth Warren, Congressman Seth Moulton, and two former governors, William Weld and Deval Patrick. When these Bay State politicians travel out to campaign in the nation's heartland they usually come off as tone-deaf on agriculture.

Michael Dukakis, who grew up in Boston as a son of Greek immigrants, had an impressive front-yard tomato garden at his home in Brookline, but was conspicuously out of touch with the agricultural Midwest. At one farm policy forum in Iowa during his presidential run in 1988, he offered his view that corn and soybean farmers would do well to switch to fruits and vegetables, perhaps growing crops like Belgian endive. "When the laughter died down," the *New York Times* reported, "the Republicans realized that they now had a ready-made issue in farm states, to show that Mr. Dukakis was one of those Cambridge elitists who not only ate that stuff but knew little about the needs of farmers in the Midwest." Following this early misstep, Dukakis added some midwesterners to his advisory team (full disclosure: I was one of those), but his reputation in farm country never recovered.

Four years later I was advising Paul Tsongas, who encountered a similar Iowa farm policy debate challenge, but handled it with greater aplomb. One of his midwestern opponents drew a big laugh by saying, "The Senator from Massachusetts knows so little about farming, he thinks a combine is a kind of martini." Tsongas managed to get a bigger laugh with his deadpan response: "What's a martini?"

John Kerry faced his own challenge a dozen years after that, when he held a campaign rally in Missouri on a cattle and soybean farm. His spouse, Teresa Heinz Kerry, tried to help by suggesting that farmers in Missouri should use organic production methods. A hog farmer in the audience, who claimed to be a loyal Democrat, jumped up and interrupted: "Mrs. Kerry, you've got to understand that hog farmers just freak out when they hear people telling them to go organic." Ms. Kerry seemed genuinely surprised, underscoring her cultural disconnect.

Commercial farmers who live in the middle of the country have little patience with East Coast know-it-alls, but they need to pull back on that attitude in their own self-interest. The nonfarmers who are now taking a much keener interest in how their food is grown are not just the final customers in the marketplace; they also shape the public policies that will govern food and agriculture. Overly defensive farmers like the one who interrupted Ms. Kerry should therefore sit back down, listen, and reconsider how they look to the rest of us.

A good start will be to stop bragging. During the 2018 Farm Bill debate, Representative Mike Conaway from Texas, then the chair of the House Agriculture Committee, claimed that "Americans enjoy the safest, most abundant and affordable food supply of any developed nation in the world." This kind of talk antagonizes critics because it ignores the obvious unsolved problems with chemical pollution from farms, excessive confinement of farm animals, and the growing public health crisis linked to dietary excess. For farm leaders, a better strategy will be to listen to the critics, be ready with the facts, and then highlight the values both sides can share.

At a "Food for Tomorrow" conference organized by the *New York Times* in 2014, two leading urban critics of industrial farming, Mark Bittman and Michael Pollan, backed off a bit when a midwestern pork producer who was brave enough to attend spoke up. She jokingly introduced herself as part of "the Big Ag you were taught to hate," then shared some positive information about modern livestock production not found in the pages of the *New York Times*. Her bravery was admired. By the end of the conference, Bittman's tone had changed from an initial declaration of "war" on industrial farming to an assertion that "we all want the same thing."

Agricultural leaders seeking to communicate across the cultural divide also should work harder to show that "industrial" farms are still family farms. The Illinois Farm Bureau does this with its "Adopt-a-Legislator" program, encouraging downstate farmers to identify legislators from Chicago and then invite them, along with some of their big-city constituents, to engage in reciprocal home visits. Welcoming outsiders onto a modern commercial farm breaks down stereotypes and builds valuable personal relationships at both ends. Even America's biggest farms tend to be family run, and urban legislators will take a softer view once they have seen the family values at work firsthand. American agriculture looks much less industrial after you have had a mug of coffee at the kitchen table, met the kids, and patted the farm dog.

But this will be the easy part. The bigger challenge for farmers, and for the organizations speaking for them, is to start showing adequate concern for dietary health. Farm organizations constantly champion food abundance but say little or nothing about dietary balance. Their critics won't care about the mug of coffee or the dog if they sense a persistent indifference toward healthy eating. Until commercial farm organizations exhibit greater concern for the nation's dietary crisis, they will fail to win over the critics.

The blind support farm organizations routinely give to food manufacturing companies is one big part of this problem. When it comes to nutrition, the companies have given our entire food system a bad name. They take perfectly healthful commodities produced on our farms and transform them into packaged goods harmful to personal health, then market them aggressively to our children. If farm organizations can't bring themselves to criticize these practices, activist critics will naturally see them as allied with the enemy.

The misbehaving food companies eagerly welcome support from farm organizations since it provides political cover, making them feel less isolated. Consider what took place at a public forum during the annual Farm Bureau convention in Nashville in 2018. The Farm Bureau, the nation's biggest lobby group speaking for commercial agriculture, had invited the head of the Grocery Manufacturers Association to lead the forum. Having consistently downplayed consumer wellness concerns, the GMA at that very moment was driving away some of its own most valued members, but the Farm Bureau apparently didn't care. The GMA president told her audience of farmers, "Your harvest becomes our product." She then made a second claim: "We work together to tell the story of American agriculture . . . [We] are the link between you and the consumers in the cities."

The farmers in the audience should have been thinking, Wait, I don't want *my* story told by the companies that turn my wholesome harvest into Frosted Flakes and Doritos! Farm organizations need to see that their own reputation suffers when they accept an embrace from the food companies; they should be building political ties instead to advocates for dietary health and improved nutrition.

Opportunities to do this keep coming their way, but the farm groups always seem to take a pass.

Consider First Lady Michelle Obama's highly regarded "Let's Move!" initiative, a campaign launched in 2010 to reduce childhood obesity. All of the organizations that speak for commercial farmers, including the Farm Bureau and the Farm Foundation, should have jumped at the chance to support this goal, but when I suggested such a move at a Farm Foundation meeting at the time, there was nothing but stony silence. Rather than support Michelle Obama's fight against obesity (which even the food companies were pretending to do), the farm organizations opted to sulk over the First Lady's earlier decision to plant an *organic* vegetable garden on the White House lawn, an act that they thought denigrated commercial farming.

Farm organizations missed an even bigger opportunity when they offered no support in Congress in 2010 for the Healthy, Hunger-Free Kids Act, a measure that improved school lunch menus. Rather than voicing support, the Montana Farm Bureau expressed alarm about "federal bureaucrats taking over the most important role of parents—feeding our children." Multiple commodity groups fought against the new menu standards, not on principle but for transparently self-serving reasons. The potato lobby blocked an effort to place limits on "starchy vegetables" like French fries, while the dairy lobby pushed to allow higher-fat chocolate milk.

On the importance of healthy eating, America's commercial farming establishment projects surprising indifference. Sonny Perdue, who became secretary of agriculture in 2017, grew up on a dairy farm in Georgia and worked for a while as a consultant to the dairy industry. He not only defended high-fat chocolate milk for the school lunch program; he laughed away the health implications by making jovial references to his own conspicuous girth. Speaking to a room full of grade-schoolers in Leesburg, Virginia, Perdue said, "I wouldn't be as big as I am today without chocolate milk." Michelle Obama expressed disbelief later at a public health forum, asking her audience, "Think about why someone is OK with your kids eating crap."

Agricultural groups missed yet another chance to champion

healthy eating during the 2018 Farm Bill debate in Congress. A bipartisan group led by two former secretaries of agriculture, Democrat Dan Glickman and Republican Ann Veneman, was proposing that sugary beverages be removed from the SNAP program, better known as food stamps. The American Heart Association favored this proposal while the soda industry was opposed. The farm lobby could have sided with the Heart Association, but instead it went with the soda companies, and with its own sugar lobby, by refusing to support even a pilot study to determine the health gains a restriction on sugary beverages might deliver.

If you want to see genuine discomfort, try criticizing "junk food" before an audience of commercial farmers. At the 2015 Farm Bureau convention, the featured speaker was Jay Leno, the celebrity comedian and former host of *The Tonight Show*. Leno got big laughs at first, but when he launched into an extended bit about America's poor eating habits the convention hall fell silent. One attendee later explained on Twitter, "Listening to Jay Leno crack junk-food jokes in front of an audience of commodity farmers is kinda awkward." The comfort level farm organizations show toward junk food is even more awkward.

The sources of farm organization behavior are easy to identify. The companies that manufacture junk food are all buyers of farm products, so farmers see them as valued customers. Most of these companies are also headquartered in the nation's agricultural heartland, making them cultural neighbors. General Mills is headquartered in Minneapolis, Kellogg's in Michigan, Frito-Lay in Texas, and Kraft-Heinz in Illinois. Add to this the bond formed by facing a common adversary. Food companies and commercial farmers are both under attack from the same food movement critics, so the enemy of an enemy can easily look like a promising friend.

Another factor is political partisanship. Commercial farmers and food companies strongly identify with the Republican Party. They both tend to dislike the higher taxes, trade barriers, and tighter government regulations, including environmental regulations, traditionally favored by Democrats. But this partisan attachment is now blinding farmers to the advantage they would gain if they could break ranks and side with Democrats at least on dietary health issues.

Deep partisanship seems to make this impossible. Food companies over the past two decades have given more than two-thirds of their political contributions to Republicans, and commercial farmers are more Republican still. Eighty percent of farmers voted for Donald Trump in the 2016 presidential election, and Trump carried all but two midwestern states, capturing 90 percent of the vote in some agricultural counties. Once in office, Trump took the Republican Party away from its farm-friendly tradition of supporting free trade agreements, but this did not stop farmers from continuing to support Trump and the Republicans, despite the damage their export sales in China and elsewhere has sustained. According to a *Wall Street Journal* poll in January 2020, 83 percent of farmers and ranchers still approved of the president's job performance. This comes partly from a reflexive mistrust of Democrats, so joining Democrats to champion dietary health policies will be an uncomfortable move.

When commercial farmers formed their current partisan preferences decades ago, ignoring dietary health carried little or no penalty, because the nation did not yet face an acute obesity crisis. Commercial farmers did little or nothing to bring on this crisis, as was argued earlier, but some of the blame will continue to be laid at their feet until they learn to speak up for better diets, and to distance themselves at least a bit from food companies. If commercial farmers were to begin to champion healthy eating, important food policy goals would become easier to reach. The food companies would feel more pressure to change if denied the political cover they currently get from farmers.

The preceding pages have described multiple policy moves available to bring progressive food system change, many already taken by countries in Europe to ward off dietary excess and imbalance. Introducing a front-of-package nutrition guidance system similar to the traffic light system used in the United Kingdom is one place to start. Similar government-endorsed systems are also in place in Belgium, Croatia, the Czech Republic, Denmark, Finland, France, Iceland, Israel, Lithuania, the Netherlands, Norway, Poland, Slovenia, and Sweden. Some of these systems consist of just a simple endorsement logo (such as a check mark, a heart symbol, a green keyhole, or a green squiggle) signposting for shoppers the "healthier choice" foods. Beginning in 2016, some Latin American countries even began requiring warning labels on packaged foods high in sugar, salt, calories, or fat. Guidance of this kind can be criticized for being imperfect and incomplete, but it beats the U.S. system of just numbers and fine print on the side of the box.

Front-of-package nutrition labeling systems remain mostly voluntary in Europe, since EU regulations do not allow different mandatory schemes country-by-country, but most food companies have participated just the same. In the Netherlands, more than one hundred retail and food service companies (in fact, four-fifths of the food service market) now participate in the Choices Programme. Less than a year after the launch of the Nutri-Score system in France in 2017, more than seventy manufacturers and retailers were committed to the label. In Britain two-thirds of the market for prepackaged foods and drinks was covered by that nation's front-of-package scheme by 2016.

The government of the United States has yet to create a front-of-package labeling system, voluntary or otherwise, and it does not yet endorse either the Facts Up Front system designed by private grocery manufacturers or the alternative Guiding Stars front-of-shelf system. With adult obesity rates now roughly twice as high as in Europe, it is well past time for the American government to take a cue from Europe and endorse either front-of-package or front-of-shelf labels, or both, to improve nutrition guidance.

The United States also remains a policy laggard in the struggle against excess consumption of sugary beverages. In 2018 the U.S. deputy secretary for health and human services actually blocked the World Health Organization from endorsing taxes on sugary drinks.

Two years earlier the United States did not object when the WHO endorsed such taxes, but the new Trump administration said no to taxes. The WHO is forced to listen because America provides a significant share of the organization's budget. Instead of persisting in this fight against sugary beverage taxes, America should follow the lead of Catalonia, Chile, France, Hungary, Malaysia, Mexico, Norway, Panama, Peru, the Philippines, Portugal, South Africa, and the United Kingdom, and adopt taxes of its own.

Another unfortunate instance of American exceptionalism in food policy is the nation's failure to promote sensible restraints on food advertising to children. This problem goes back to a troublesome 1976 Supreme Court ruling that classified corporate advertising as commercial speech, protected by the First Amendment so long as it was not deceptive or untruthful. The Federal Trade Commission tried to get past this ruling two years later when it proposed restrictions on television advertising to children, but private industry objected and persuaded Congress in 1980 to pass a law explicitly prohibiting any FTC action of this kind.

Three decades later, after childhood obesity had become a national epidemic, the Obama administration revived the issue by attempting to develop guidelines for food ads to kids. The guidelines were only intended to be voluntary, but private industry still rejected the move. The top lobbyist for the Grocery Manufacturers Association branded Obama's proposed guidelines a "dramatic overreach," and in 2011 Congress passed a measure killing the effort once again.

In contrast to America's experience, a number of countries in Europe have successfully regulated food advertising to children. Ireland prohibits the advertising of foods high in fats, sugars, and salt during children's TV and radio programming, and maintains overall limits for other times of the day. The United Kingdom has a similar rule for viewers under sixteen. Norway prohibits marketing to children under eighteen years of age along with ads on children's programs. Sweden prohibits any TV or broadcast advertising to children below the age of twelve. Hungary prohibits all advertising in schools directed at children under eighteen. In schools in Poland, advertising foods that do not meet nutrition standards is prohibited. Chile now bans the advertising of unhealthy foods to children.

In France, all TV advertising for processed foods and drinks that contain added fats, sweeteners, or salt must be accompanied by messages such as "For your health, avoid eating too many foods that are high in fat, sugar, or salt." In 2011, Spain declared that schools and kindergartens should be completely free of advertising. Denmark limits advertising to children all foods that exceed guideline limits for salt, sugar, or fat content.

Because most Americans are proud of their exceptionalism, it is not easy for politicians to be seen following the lead of other countries, even when they know it might be a good idea. During a CNN debate early in the 2015 presidential primary campaign, Hillary Clinton expressed frustration over the tendency of her opponent Bernie Sanders to praise so many European policies he considered superior to our own. Clinton finally raised her voice in exasperation, "We are not Denmark!" True enough, but in the area of public health and nutrition, this is nothing to be proud of. European governments have seen the benefit of nudging food companies and food consumers toward more healthy diets and America should follow.

My hope is to see America's farmers join with public health advocates to promote policy pathways such as these to encourage better eating. Farmers won't have to change the way they farm to do this. In fact, the dramatic progress farmers have already made adopting modern precision agriculture methods would be easier for nonfarmers to appreciate if joined with a more progressive position on dietary health. By endorsing better policies at the table, farmers might finally get some of the credit they deserve for having improved their own performance on the farm.

Acknowledgments

This book is built on a career's worth of collaboration. I have gathered insights over the years not just from other scholars but also from government officials, representatives from international organizations, advocacy leaders, food company veterans, retailers, restaurant chain specialists, and many individual farmers in the United States and abroad. I have been drawn to these practitioners for their engagement and the difference they try to make, so I thank them here for the wisdom they have shared.

I have also learned from my students over the years, both at Wellesley College and at Harvard University. I take energy from their enthusiasm and get my own thoughts straight trying to answer the hard questions they ask. Some of the content in this book will be familiar to my Kennedy School students, since it was road-tested in classroom lectures. I put students to an interesting test, since many arrive committed to a vision of food and farming different from my own. They have been told that our food should be grown on small, local, diverse, organic farms. When they learn how many economists, agronomists, and nutritionists do not share this view, they are at first surprised, but then intrigued. They hold off reaching a conclusion until they have reviewed the evidence for themselves. I ask nothing more from the readers of this book.

My earliest teachings about farming came from my father, Don Paarlberg, who grew up on a small family farm in Indiana where he labored through the depths of the Great Depression. Working on the farm delayed my dad's university education, but he eventually went on for a Ph.D. in agricultural economics, became a professor, and then a prominent government official. Listening to my dad when he talked about farm policy with his colleagues and relatives taught lessons not found in academic journals or government reports. Sharing work routines on the Paarlberg farm with my brother and cousins during summer visits also gave me lifelong respect for the diverse skills needed to make a living in commercial agriculture, along with a lifelong itch to learn more.

My international interests deepened after a trip to visit my older brother, Don Jr., while he was serving in a rural village in Nepal as a Peace Corps volunteer. I had seen some rural poverty growing up in Indiana, but nothing like the destitution that was (and still is) pervasive in so much of the South Asian countryside. Improving farming and farm policy to reduce rural poverty and hunger, in Africa as well as South Asia, became a touchstone of my own research career. I want to thank and honor my brother for introducing me to this still urgent challenge.

A research career built around global food and farming means costly travel to out-of-the-way destinations, not possible for me without generous support from a long list of foundations, international organizations, think tanks, and government agencies. I am grateful as well for the numerous paid leaves from teaching I was given over the years by my longtime academic employer, Wellesley College. Time is as important as money.

To enliven this book with human voices, I approached engaged specialists to request personal meetings. Many of the informants I contacted were strangers to me, but nobody turned me down. I am indebted to all these individuals for the time, and the trust, they were willing to share. Talking to these experts was the most rewarding part of writing this book. Those I spoke with included John Nidlinger, a corn and soybean farmer in Indiana; Julie Greene, a former grocery marketing specialist with a supermarket chain who is now providing nutrition guidance to shoppers; William C. Hale, a consultant to the restaurant industry; Andrew Rodgers, an organic farmer who manages a successful community supported agriculture (CSA) farm; Pamela Ronald, a senior rice scientist who defends genetic engineering; Bruce Webster, a poultry scientist who consults on animal welfare with meat companies; Delia Grace, a veterinarian who works with farm animals in Africa; Mark

Legan, a breed-to-wean hog farmer in Indiana; Annemarie Noordman, a hog farmer from the Netherlands; Karel de Greef, a livestock scientist from the Netherlands; Jennifer Fearing, a successful lobbyist promoting farm animal welfare; Stavros Vougioukas, an engineer who designs agricultural robots; and Raymond Rodriguez, a former field hand from California's Central Valley who became a scientist and now studies what robots might mean for farmworkers. These individuals, along with many others, were uniformly generous with their time and patient when answering my questions.

Academic researchers attempting to write for a wider audience require coaching. I found an agent, Carolyn Savarese, who was familiar with this challenge and gave me the guidance I needed. Carolyn then helped me find a superb editor at Knopf, Jonathan Segal, who was willing to work with someone trying a book like this for the first time. Jonathan was blunt when he had to be, but kept me going with his commitment and respect. I soon learned that his deletions and penciled suggestions in the margin were guided by a clear editorial vision, one I valued for its consistency. I also wish to thank Jonathan's quick and superbly well-organized assistant, Erin Sellers, who was always available to help on matters both large and small.

Halfway through my writing process I shared drafts of individual chapters with Ronald Herring and Jack Kyte, friends with much deeper expertise than I in key areas. I then shared an early draft of the complete manuscript with Nora Ng, a professional writer, editor, and personal friend with a keen and sensitive eye for both style and content. Nora helped me avoid several missteps. For the missteps and errors that remain I take responsibility.

Along the way, others provided help of various kinds, including Raoul Adamchak, Yiannis Ampatzidis, Jeffrey Blumberg, Carolyn Chelius, Angela Chnapko, William C. Clark, Michael Fisher, Keith Fuglie, Ray Goldberg, Merilee Grindle, Missy Holbrooke, Robert Hoste, Mike Jacobson, Calestous Juma, Garry Levin, David Lindauer, Jayson Lusk, Susan MacMillan, Katie Marshall, Jim McBride, John McDermott, Renata Micha, Jim Mintert, Dariush Mozaffarian, Hoey Paarlberg, Michael Paarlberg, Philip Paarlberg, Rajul Pandya-Lorch, John Park, Carl Pray, Forest L. Reinhardt, Anne Stone, Timothy Taylor, and Don Villarejo.

Writing this book soaked up a great deal of personal time. Marianne Perlak, my spouse and longtime partner in all things, adjusted with little complaint to my slighting of other responsibilities. Marianne knew how important this project was to me and gave me both the space and the reassurance I needed to complete the task. She read drafts, helped in selecting illustrations, and took my author photo. As a former designer and art director at a major university press, she knows the book world well. She is also a skilled cook who knows a great deal about food. I could never have completed this work without her by my side, so I dedicate the book to her, with my everlasting thanks and love.

Notes

Introduction

5 "tortured billions of animals": Mark Bittman, "Fixing Our Food Problem," *New York Times,* January 1, 2013, A19.

5 "before it's too late": Bibi Van der Zee, "Why Factory Farming Is Not Just Cruel—but Also a Threat to All Life on the Planet," *Guardian,* October 4, 2017.

5 has not set foot in a supermarket: Kim Severson, "Alice Waters on Sex, Drugs and Sustainable Agriculture," *New York Times,* August 23, 2017, D1.

7 "costs are too high": Michael Pollan, "The Food Movement Rising," *New York Review of Books,* June 10, 2010.

8 "I got a free ride for a long time": Michael Pollan, interview, Food Revolution Network, April 24, 2013, https://www.youtube.com/watch?v=iGg7BxI6S2M.

9 80 percent lower than in 1972: Jorge Fernandez-Cornejo et al., "Pesticide Use Peaked in 1981, Then Trended Downward, Driven by Technological Innovations and Other Factors," *Amber Waves,* June 2, 2014.

10 produce more with fewer resources: John Asafu-Adjaye et al., *An Ecomodernist Manifesto,* April 2015, ecomodernism.org.

10 a term from fast-food culture: Severson, "Alice Waters on Sex, Drugs," *New York Times,* August 23, 2017, D1.

10 late-winter vegetables: Phoebe Maltz Bovy, "Food Snobs Like Mark Bittman Aren't Even Hiding Their Elitism Anymore," *New Republic,* March 25, 2015.

11 organic as of 2018: "U.S. Organic Sales Break Through $50 Billion

Mark in 2018," press release, Organic Trade Association, May 17, 2019, https://ota.com/news/press-releases/20699.

11 less than 1 percent of all farm sales: USDA, 2017 Census of Agriculture, vol. 1, AC-17-A-51, April 2019. Calculated from Table 2, p. 10.

11 "lessened their ardor amazingly": Barbara L. Packer, *The Transcendentalists* (Athens, GA: University of Georgia Press, 2007), 148–49.

12 folded after seven months: Carlos Baker, *Emerson Among the Eccentrics: A Group Portrait* (New York: Viking Press, 1996), 221.

13 less than 1 percent of total national farm sales: Calculated from USDA, "Cash Receipts by Commodity State Ranking," 2017, https://data.ers.usda.gov/reports.aspx?ID=17844.

Chapter 1: TESTING THE CASE AGAINST INDUSTRIAL FARMING

17 flour and cereal product consumption: Rosanna Mentzer Morrison et al., "Guess Who's Turning 100? Tracking a Century of American Eating," *Amber Waves*, March 1, 2010.

18 failed to qualify because of disabilities: Susan Levine, *School Lunch Politics: The Surprising History of America's Favorite Welfare Program* (Princeton, NJ: Princeton University Press, 2008), 56.

18 an astonishing 42 percent: Craig Hales et al., "Prevalence of Obesity and Severe Obesity Among Adults: United States 2017–2018," NCHS Data Brief No. 360, Centers for Disease Control and Prevention, February 2020.

18 now die from eating processed meats: Dariush Mozaffarian, "Want to Fix Health Care? First, Focus on Food," *Tufts Now,* September 15, 2017.

18 too fat to enlist in the military: Roxana Hegeman, "Report: Nearly 1 in 3 Young Adults Too Fat for Military," *Military Times,* July 15, 2015.

18 half as high as in the United States: A. Marques et al., "Prevalence of Adult Overweight and Obesity in 20 European Countries, 2014," *European Journal of Public Health* 28, no. 2 (April 1, 2018): 295–300.

19 traced poor eating not to farms: Anthony Winson, *The Industrial Diet: The Degradation of Food and the Struggle for Healthy Eating* (Vancouver: UBC Press, 2013).

19 a trait associated with nutrition: Mark Schatzker, *The Dorito Effect: The Surprising New Truth About Food and Flavor* (New York: Simon & Schuster, 2015).

19 38 percent drop for riboflavin: D. R. Davis et al., "Changes in USDA Food Composition Data for 43 Garden Crops, 1950 to 1999," *Journal of the American College of Nutrition* 23, no. 6 (2004): 669–82.

20 a new variety of amaranth: Jane Black, "Our Future Tastes Fresh," *Wall Street Journal,* October 6–7, 2018, D5.

20 consumption in the United States . . . increased: USDA, Food Availability (Per Capita) Data System, https://data.ers.usda.gov/data-products /food-availability-per-capita-data-system/.

20 "it's because we're eating more": Quoted in Ray A. Goldberg, *Food Citizenship: Food System Advocates in an Era of Distrust* (New York: Oxford University Press, 2018), 3.

20 ninety more calories: Tiffany Hsu, "Bigger, Saltier, Heavier: Fast Food Since 1986 in 3 Simple Charts," *New York Times,* March 4, 2019.

21 started within the normal range: Anahad O'Connor, "Cutting 300 Calories a Day Shows Health Benefits," *New York Times,* July 16, 2019.

21 far too many carbohydrates: "The Truth About Fats: The Good, the Bad, and the In-Between," Harvard Health Publishing (website), August 13, 2018, https://www.health.harvard.edu/staying-healthy /the-truth-about-fats-bad-and-good.

21 still more calories were then consumed: Gary Taubes, *Good Calories, Bad Calories: Fats, Carbs, and the Controversial Science of Diet and Health* (New York: Knopf, 2007), 437.

22 consume too much salt: USDA and HHS, *Dietary Guidelines for Americans 2015–2020,* December 2015, https://health.gov/dietaryguidelines /2015/guidelines.

22 "cheapest calories in the supermarket": Nilagia McCoy, "Michael Pollan on Improving Food Policy and Its Coverage in the Media" (lecture, Shorenstein Center on Media, Politics, and Public Policy, Harvard Kennedy School, October 31, 2017).

23 none of this enters: National Oilseed Processors Association, "Top 10 Destinations for U.S. Soy Exports 2018," https://www.Nopa.Org /Resources/datafacts/Top-10-Destinations-U-S-Soybean-Exports-2016 -2018/.

23 "this has happened so quickly": David Karp, "Most of America's Fruit Is Now Imported: Is That a Bad Thing?" *New York Times,* March 14, 2018.

23 were all being propped up: Julian M. Alston et al., "Farm Subsidies and Obesity in the United States: National Evidence and International Comparisons," *Food Policy* 33, no. 6 (2008): 470–79.

24 64 percent higher: Mark J. Perry, *Carpe Diem,* American Enterprise Institute, February 14, 2013, https://www.aei.org/carpe-diem/protectionist -sugar-policy-cost-americans-3-billion-in-2012/.

24 phone call from Alfonso Fanjul: Independent Counsel Kenneth Starr's
    report to the House on President Clinton, Narrative Pt. III, Septem-
    ber 11, 1998.

25 not push them down: Robert Paarlberg, *Fixing Farm Trade: Policy Op-
    tions for the United States* (Cambridge, MA: Ballinger Publishing Com-
    pany, 1988), 81.

25 hardly a plague of cheap corn: Tristan Hanon, "The New Normal: A
    Policy Analysis of the U.S. Renewable Fuel Standard," *SS-AAEA Journal
    of Agricultural Economics*, no. 22 (2014), https://econpapers.repec.org/
    article/agsssaaea/232730.htm.

26 more than 90 percent of all commercial value: Economic Research
    Service (USDA), Food Dollar Series, 2017, https://data.ers.usda.gov
    /reports.aspx?ID=17885.

27 adjusted for quality and seasonality: Fred Kuchler and Hayden Stew-
    art, "Price Trends are Similar for Fruits, Vegetables, and Snack Foods,"
    Economic Research Service Report No. ERR-55, March 2008.

27 snacks that were less nutritious: Laura Lloyd, "Myth-buster: USDA
    Tackles Whether Fruits, Vegetables Are More Expensive Than Other
    Snacks," *Food Business News,* December 20, 2012.

28 two dollars per person per meal: Hayden Stewart et al., "The Cost of
    Satisfying Fruit and Vegetable Recommendations in Dietary Guide-
    lines," Economic Research Service (USDA), Economic Brief No. 27,
    February 2016.

28 raised food prices for consumers: Vincent H. Smith et al., "Agricultural
    Policy in Disarray: Reforming the Farm Bill—an Overview," Report,
    American Enterprise Institute, October 13, 2017.

28 "on an unprecedented scale": Union of Concerned Scientists, "Indus-
    trial Agriculture: The Outdated, Unsustainable System That Domi-
    nates U.S. Food Production," https://www.ucsusa.org/our-work
    /food-agriculture/our-failing-food-system/industrial-agriculture
    #.W46at34nZmA.

29 one-tenth the output of today: Bruce L. Gardner, *American Agriculture
    in the Twentieth Century: How It Flourished and What It Cost* (Cambridge,
    MA: Harvard University Press, 2002), Figure 1.2, p. 5.

29 "depredations on the landscape": Stanley W. Trimble, "Perspectives
    on the History of Soil Erosion Control in the Eastern United States,"
    Agricultural History 59, no. 2 (1985): 162–80.

29 over the next five decades: Gardner, *American Agriculture in the Twentieth
    Century,* Figure 1.1, p. 4.

33 with sub-inch accuracy: Jamie Condliffe, "A New Technique Makes GPS Accurate to an Inch," *Gizmodo*, February 11, 2016.

35 total acreage planted to corn *declined*: Jesse H. Ausubel, "The Return of Nature: How Technology Liberates the Environment," *Breakthrough Journal* (Summer 2015), https://thebreakthrough.org/journal/issue-5/the-return-of-nature.

35 compared to intensive tillage: USDA, 2017 Census, Table 47, p. 58.

35 livestock breeds and crops: Organisation for Economic Co-operation and Development, *Environmental Performance of Agriculture in OECD Countries Since 1990*, Paris, 2008, http://www.oecd.org/greengrowth/sustainable-agriculture/44254899.pdf.

36 production continued to increase: Ausubel, "Return of Nature."

36 fallen by more than 80 percent: Jorge Fernandez-Cornejo et al., "Pesticide Use in U.S. Agriculture: 21 Selected Crops, 1960-2008," *Amber Waves*, June 2, 2014.

36 rice, soybeans, and sugar beets: Field to Market, "Environmental and Socioeconomic Indicators for Measuring Outcomes of On-Farm Agricultural Production in the United States," December 2016, Table 1.6, https://www.ncga.com/uploads/useruploads/key_messages_for_ftm_2012_indicators_report-final.pdf.

36 far from being stabilized: Char Miller, "Farmers Are Drawing Groundwater from the Giant Ogallala Aquifer Faster Than Nature Replaces It," *Conversation*, August 7, 2018.

37 "into the Mississippi River system": Doyle Rice, "Near-Record 'Dead Zone' Predicted in the Gulf of Mexico This Summer," *USA Today*, June 10, 2019.

37 fewer storms that year: John Seewer, "Voluntary Efforts Aren't Enough to Stop Lake Erie Pollution, Study Shows," online post, WOSU Public Media, April 23, 2018.

37 suspected to come from livestock farms: Nicole Rasul, "Factory Farms Are Polluting Lake Erie: Will the Lake's New Legal Rights Help?," *Civil Eats*, April 9, 2019.

37 from a C− to a D+: "Report: In 2018, the Chesapeake Bay 'Suffered a Massive Assault,'" *Virginia Mercury*, January 7, 2019, https://www.cbf.org/news-media/newsroom/2019/cbf-in-the-news/report-in-2018-the-chesapeake-bay-suffered-a-massive-assult.html.

38 sixfold and fourteenfold, respectively: Karl Blankenship, "Path to a Clean Chesapeake Poses Problems for Key Bay States," *Bay Journal*, September 30, 2019.

38 a tripling of the nation's population: Don Paarlberg and Philip Paarl-
    berg, *The Agricultural Revolution of the 20th Century* (Ames, IA: Iowa
    State University Press, 2000).

38 farm size more than doubled: Carolyn Dimitri et al., "The 20th Cen-
    tury Transformation of U.S. Agriculture and Farm Policy," Economic
    Research Service (USDA), Economic Information Bulletin Number 3,
    June 2005.

38 classified as a farmer: Maggie Koerth-Baker, "Big Farms Are Getting
    Bigger and Most Small Farms Aren't Really Farms at All," *Five Thirty-
    Eight,* November 17, 2016.

39 just 7 percent of all farms: USDA, 2017 Census, Vol. 1, AC-17-A-51.
    Calculated from Table 2, p. 9.

39 "no reason to be there": Ted Genoways, *This Blessed Earth: A Year in the
    Life of an American Family Farm* (New York: Norton, 2017).

40 "few months before he died": Quoted in Albert H. Sanford, *The Story
    of Agriculture in the United States* (New York: D.C. Heath, 2016), 364.

40 had indoor plumbing: Gardner, *American Agriculture in the Twentieth
    Century,* 76.

40 just one-third the nonfarm level: Gardner, *American Agriculture in the
    Twentieth Century,* Figure 3.12, p. 78.

40 three fewer years of schooling: Gardner, Table 4.6, p. 116.

40 every year from farm accidents: Gardner, 124.

41 land they did not own: Gardner, 95.

41 95 percent of farm producers: USDA, 2017 Census, Table 63, p. 81.

41 "death on women and oxen": *Prairie Farmer* (Chicago), July 1847, 222.

41 less likely to come back: Gardner, *American Agriculture in the Twentieth
    Century.*

41 to double after the 1950s: Dimitri et al., "20th Century Transformation
    of U.S. Agriculture."

41 about one by 2000: Dimitri et al.

42 had fallen to just six minutes: Paarlberg and Paarlberg, *Agricultural
    Revolution of the 20th Century.*

43 "not of great consequence": Glenn Johnson and Joel Smith, "Social
    Cost of Agricultural Adjustment," in *Problems and Policies of American
    Agriculture* (Ames, IA: Iowa State University Press, 1959), 267.

43 not the primary occupation: "Farm Structure: Classifying Diverse
    Farms," Economic Research Service (USDA), https://www.ers.usda
    .gov/topics/farm-economy/farm-structure-and-organization/farm
    -structure.

43 14 percent of all U.S. households: Vincent H. Smith et al., "Agricultural

Policy in Disarray: Reforming the Farm Bill—an Overview," Report, American Enterprise Institute, October 2017, p. 16, https://www.aei .org/research-products/book/agricultural-policy-in-disarray/.

43 an impressive $912,000: "Income and Wealth in Context," Economic Research Service (USDA), April 26, 2019, https://www.ers.usda.gov /topics/farm-economy/farm-household-well-being/income-and -wealth-in-context/#wealth.

44 still family owned: USDA, 2017 Census, vol. 1, AC-17-A-51.

Chapter 2: FOOD SWAMP NATION

45 two hundred calories: Laura Lloyd, "Myth-Buster: USDA Tackles Whether Fruits, Vegetables Are More Expensive Than Other Snacks," *Food Business News,* December 20, 2012.

45 3 percent annual rate: Jessi Devenyns, "Impulse Snack Purchases Decline as Shopping Goes Online," *Food Dive,* January 4, 2019.

48 paying the retailers: Gary Rivlin, "Rigged: Supermarket Shelves for Sale," Center for Science and the Public Interest, September 2016, p. 34, https://cspinet.org/sites/default/files/attachment/CSPI_Rigged_4 _small.pdf.

49 in the District of Columbia: Jonathan Ringen, "Why This Is the Golden Age of Grocery Shopping," *Washingtonian,* March 25, 2018.

49 "best ice-cream custard": Ringen, "Golden Age of Grocery Shopping," 85.

50 controlled for food swamps: Kristen Cooksey-Stowers et al., "Food Swamps Project Obesity Rates Better Than Food Deserts in the United States," *International Journal of Environmental Research and Public Health* 14, no. 11 (November 2017): 1366.

50 grocery store access and healthful diets: Janne Boone-Heinonen et al., "Fast Food Restaurants and Food Stores," *Archives of Internal Medicine* 171, no. 13 (July 11, 2011): 1162–70.

50 closer proximity to supermarkets: Parke Wilde et al., "Population Density, Poverty, and Food Retail Access in the United States: An Empirical Approach," *International Food and Agribusiness Management Review* 17, special issue (2014): 171–86.

51 versus low-income households: Hunt Allcott et al., "Food Deserts and the Causes of Nutritional Inequality," *The Quarterly Journal of Economics* 134, no. 4 (November 2019): 1793–1844.

51 to reset their taste buds: Michael Moss, "The Extraordinary Science of Addictive Junk Food," *New York Times Magazine,* February 20, 2013.

52 triggering still more calorie consumption: David Ludwig, "Examining the Health Effects of Fructose, *JAMA* 310, no. 1 (July 3, 2013): 33–34.

52 reward circuit in our brains: A. Y. Onaolapo and O. J. Onaolapo, "Food Additives, Food, and the Concept of 'Food Addiction': Is Stimulation of the Brain Reward Circuit by Food Sufficient to Trigger Addiction?," *Pathophysiology* 25, no. 4 (December 2018): 263–76.

52 sends intense reward sensations: David Kessler, *The End of Overeating: Taking Control of the Insatiable American Appetite* (New York: Rodale Books, 2010).

52 "great public health crises": David Kessler, interviewed by Ira Flatow, "How Tasty Foods Change the Brain," *Science Friday,* National Public Radio, July 10, 2009.

52 brain scans that reveal more: Robert L. Shewfelt, *In Defense of Processed Food: It's Not Nearly as Bad as You Think* (Switzerland: Copernicus Books, 2017).

53 sugary drinks, and unhealthy snack brands: Erica Sweeney, "Unhealthy Food Brands Spend More on TV Ads Targeting Black, Hispanic Youth, Study Finds," *Food Dive,* January 16, 2019.

53 gained it all back: Alison Fildes et al., "Probability of an Obese Person Attaining Normal Body Weight: Cohort Study Using Electronic Health Records," *American Journal of Public Health* 105, no. 9 (September 2015):e54—e59.

53 they avoided some foods: Coast Packing Company, "Consumers Read Food Labels, But Don't Always Understand or Trust Them, New Coast Packing/Ipsos Survey Reveals," press release, June 29, 2016, https://www.prnewswire.com/news-releases/consumers-read-food-labels-but-dont-always-understand-or-trust-them-new-coast-packingipsos-survey-reveals-300291564.html.

54 "select a healthier alternative": Hank Cardello, *Stuffed: An Insider's Look at Who's (Really) Making America Fat and How the Food Industry Can Fix It* (New York: Harper Collins, 2009), 10–11.

54 So you're sort of trapped: Moss, "Extraordinary Science."

55 " 'guys in white coats are worried about obesity' ": Moss.

55 80,000 in the previous year: Jessi Devenyns, "Onward and Upward: Clean Label Trend Shows No Signs of Slowing," *Food Dive,* January 14, 2019.

55 brought back the synthetic original: Patti Zarling, "Kraft Heinz Gives Legacy Brands a Healthy Makeover to Stay Relevant," *Food Dive,* August 14, 2008.

56 "I'll give you indulgent products": Indra Nooyi, interview, *New York Times,* March 24, 2019, 4.

56 "enable them to live healthier lives": Access to Nutrition Foundation, "Leading U.S. Food and Beverage Companies Fall Short on Efforts to Help Consumers Eat Healthy and Combat High Rates of Obesity and Diet-Related Diseases," Boston Common Asset Management website, November 15, 2018, http://news.bostoncommonasset.com/access-to-nutrition-us-spotlight.

57 increased purchases of plain water: M. A. Colchero et al., "Beverage Purchases from Stores in Mexico under the Excise Tax on Sugar Sweetened Beverages: Observational Study," *The BMJ,* January 6, 2016.

57 just 47 liters by 2018: John Henley, "Sweet Spot: Norwegians Cut Sugar Intake to Lowest Level in 445 Years," *The Guardian,* November 20, 2019, https://www.theguardian.com/world/2019/nov/20/norwegians-cut-sugar-intake-to-lowest-level-in-44-years.

57 reducing direct medical costs: Y. C. Wang et al., "A Penny-per-Ounce Tax on Sugar-Sweetened Beverages Would Cut Health Costs of Diabetes," *Health Affairs* 31, no. 1 (2012): 199–207.

57 Coke Zero Sugar also increased: Jack Winkler and Tam Fray, "UK Sugar Tax: Historic Sales Shift to Sugar Free," *Beverage Daily,* May 21, 2019.

58 nobody in Congress was talking: Robert Paarlberg, *The United States of Excess: Gluttony and the Dark Side of American Exceptionalism* (New York: Oxford University Press, 2015).

58 especially Bloomberg Philanthropies: Robert Paarlberg et al., "Viewpoint: Can U.S. Local Soda Taxes Continue to Spread?," *Food Policy* 71 (August 2017): 1–7.

58 purchases in neighboring towns: Associated Press, "Soda Sales in Philly Dropped After Tax on Soft Drinks, Study Says," May 14, 2019.

59 just thirty-seven for Democrats: "State Legislative Elections, 2018," Ballotpedia, https://ballotpedia.org/State_legislative_elections,_2018.

59 just under half by 2017: Food Marketing Institute, "U.S. Grocery Shopper Trends 2017," July 18, 2017, https://www.fmi.org/docs/default-source/webinars/trends-2017-webinar-7-18-2017.pdf.

59 15 percent annual rate: Jessica Dumont, "Report: Online Grocery Sales Grew 15% This Year," *Grocery Dive,* September 13, 2019.

59 online at least once a month: Jeffrey M. Jones and Sean Kashanchi, "Online Grocery Shopping Still Rare in U.S.," Gallup website, August 20, 2019, https://news.gallup.com/poll/264857/online-grocery-shopping-rare.aspx.

60 online for candies and snacks: Heather Haddon, "E-Commerce Re-shapes Grocery Stores," *Wall Street Journal,* October 3, 2018, R2.

60 discounts from food and beverage companies: Rivlin, "Rigged."

61 faster comprehension for shoppers: Food Standards Agency (UK), Department of Health, "Guide to Creating a Front of Pack (FoP) Nutrition Label for Pre-Packaged Items Sold Through Retail Outlets," November 2016.

62 at-a-glance color-code: Erica van Herpen and H. C. Trip, "Front-of-Pack Nutrition Labels: Their Effect on Attention and Choices When Consumers Have Varying Goals and Time Constraints," *Appetite,* August 2011, 148–60.

62 "willing to do at the time": David L. Katz, "Nutrition GPS for All," posted July 22, 2016, davidkatzmd.com.

62 "brutal honesty about the food supply": David L. Katz, "The Rise and Fall of NuVal Nutritional Guidance," Yahoo! Finance, November 17, 2017.

62 NuVal algorithm "fatally flawed": Katz, "Rise and Fall of NuVal."

63 quietly discontinued in 2017: "NCL Welcomes Nationwide Removal of Misleading Nutritional Scoring System from Grocery Shelves," National Consumers League, *NCL Communications,* November 9, 2017.

63 available in 2,500 retail locations: Jeff Wells, "Ahold Delhaize Will Add Guiding Stars Rating System to More Banners," *Food Dive,* April 4, 2018.

64 only about a quarter of meats: Frequently Asked Questions, Guiding Stars website, accessed January 12, 2020, https://guidingstars.com/what-is-guiding-stars/frequently-asked-questions.

64 "sizeable population effects": There was a decline of 8 percent in the share of zero-star products purchased. Erin Hobin et al., "Consumers' Response to an On-Shelf Nutrition Labeling System in Supermarkets; Evidence to Inform Policy and Practice," *Millbank Quarterly* 95, no. 3 (2017): 494–534, 523.

65 FDA and USDA have not joined: "U.S. Surgeon General Touts Guiding Stars at Weight Conference," *Progressive Grocer,* July 27, 2009.

65 more than four times a week: Michelle Saksena et al., "America's Eating Habits: Food Away from Home," Economic Information Bulletin No. (EIB-196), USDA, September 2018.

65 identical to annual grocery sales: "Restaurant Industry Facts at a Glance," National Restaurant Association website, https://restaurant.org/research/restaurant-statistics/restaurant-industry-facts-at-a-glance.

65 more saturated fats and sodium: Saksena et al., "America's Eating Habits."

65 by 2012 that had doubled: Saksena et al.

66 total restaurant use: Hale Group, "Strategic Overview: Foodservice Market and Industry Dynamics," November 15, 2017.

66 silicone used in Silly Putty: Holly Van Hare, "McDonald's French Fries Contain a Chemical That Could Cure Baldness," *Chicago Tribune*, February 7, 2018.

66 twice the recommended daily level: Anthony Winson, *The Industrial Diet: The Degradation of Food and the Struggle for Healthy Eating* (Vancouver: UBC Press, 2013).

67 total for a single meal: Amy H. Auchincloss et al., "Nutritional Value of Meals at Full-Service Restaurant Chains," *Journal of Nutrition Education and Behavior* 46, no. 1 (2014): 75–81.

67 more calories, fat, and sodium: H. W. Wu and R. Sturm, "What's on the Menu? A Review of the Energy and Nutrition Content of US Chain Restaurant Menus," *Public Health Nutrition* 16, no. 1 (2013): 87–96.

67 children's entrées that are less healthy: Brian E. Saelens et al., "Nutrition Environment Measures Study in Restaurants," *American Journal of Preventive Medicine* 32, no. 4 (2007), 273–81.

67 "That's the role we play": "Applebee's Is Betting on Stress Eaters, and It's Paying Off," CNN Wire, November 4, 2018.

67 set a fourteen-year record: "Applebee's Is Betting on Stress Eaters."

67 15 percent of total sales: Auchincloss et al., "Nutritional Value of Meals."

68 future of the food service industry: Hale Group, "Foodservice 2025: Digitalized, Democratized & Disrupted," 2018, http://www.hale group.com/wp-content/uploads/2018/01/Foodservice-2025-White -paper.pdf.

70 increased by more than 80 percent: Johannah M. Frelier et al., "Trends in Calories and Nutrients in Beverages in U.S. Chain Restaurants, 2012–2017," *American Journal of Preventive Medicine* 57, no. 2 (August 2019): 231–40.

70 food fads and fashions: William Hale, "Strategic Overview: Food-service Market and Industry Dynamics," Lecture, Harvard Kennedy School, November 19, 2015.

71 more calories than the average dessert: Tiffany Hsu, "Bigger, Saltier, Heavier: Fast Food Since 1986 in 3 Simple Charts," *New York Times*, March 3, 2019.

72 Dunkin' Donuts, and Jack in the Box: Charlie Heller, "Panera and Chipotle's Antibiotic Free Meat Tops Industry Report Card," *Food & Wine*, September 27, 2017.

72 use of medically important antibiotics: "McDonald's Moves to Protect Public Health by Reducing Antibiotics Use in Beef," NRDC (Natural Resources Defense Council), *Expert Blog,* December 11, 2018.

72 fell short of healthy eating guidelines: Sarah Rainey, "Celebrity Chefs—Are They Making Us Ill?" *The Telegraph,* April 24, 2013.

73 separate menu labeling requirements: Center for Science and the Public Interest, "Calorie Counts on Chain Restaurant Menus Become Mandatory on Monday, Result of 15-Year-Long Campaign," May 2, 2018, https://cspinet.org/news/calorie-counts-chain-restaurant-menus -become-mandatory-monday-result-15-year-long-campaign.

73 had not noticed menu calorie counts: New York University, "Fast-Food Calorie Labeling Unlikely to Encourage Healthy Eating, Finds NYU Study," news release, October 20, 2016, https://www.nyu.edu/about /news-publications/news/2016/october/fast-food-calorie-labeling -unlikely-to-encourage-healthy-eating-.html.

74 "no significant change" in reported calories: Thaisa M. Cantu-Jungles et al., "A Meta-Analysis to Determine the Impact of Restaurant Labeling on Calories and Nutrients (Ordered or Consumed) in U.S. Adults," *Nutrients* 9, no. 10 (2017): 1088.

74 bring some benefit nationwide: "New Cochrane Review Evidence Suggests That Nutritional Labeling on Menus in Restaurants and Cafes May Reduce Our Calorie Intake," Wiley, press release, February 27, 2018, https://newsroom.wiley.com/press-release/cochrane-library/new -cochrane-review-evidence-suggests-nutritional-labelling-menus-res.

74 might order more: Carrie Dennett, "Will Calorie Counts on Menu Items Do More Harm Than Good?" *Washington Post,* April 18, 2018.

74 local menu labeling law: Barbara Bruemmer et al., "Energy, Saturated Fat, and Sodium Were Lower in Entrées at Chain Restaurants at 18 Months Compared with 6 Months Following the Implementation of Mandatory Menu Labeling Regulation in King County, Washington," *Journal of the Academy of Nutrition and Dietetics* 112, no. 8 (2012): 1169–76.

74 "nuts and legumes": Scott Gottlieb, "Reducing the Burden of Chronic Disease," remarks, National Food Policy Conference, March 29, 2018, https://www.fda.gov/news-events/speeches-fda-officials/reducing -burden-chronic-disease-03292018.

75 reduced consumption of trans fats: Dong D. Wang et al., "Trends in Dietary Quality Among Adults in the United States: 1999–2010," *JAMA Internal Medicine* 174, no. 10 (September 1, 2014): 1587–95.

75 had no trans fat: Walter C. Willett, quoted in Ray A. Goldberg, *Food Cit-*

izenship: Food System Advocates in an Era of Distrust (New York: Oxford University Press, 2018), 55.

75   remaining sanctioned uses of PHOs: Ryan McCrimmon, "FDA to Kill Trans Fat Once and for All," Politico, October 18, 2018.

75   has continued to widen: Wang et al., "Trends in Dietary Quality."

Chapter 3: THE LIMITS OF LOCAL FOOD

78   continued to become more global: Economic Research Service (USDA), "U.S. Agricultural Trade, Overview," https://www.ers.usda.gov/topics/international-markets-us-trade/us-agricultural-trade/.

78   less than 1 percent: USDA, 2017 Census of Agriculture, Vol. 1, AC-17-A-51, April 2019. Calculated from Table 2, p. 10.

78   still less than 1 percent: USDA, 2017 Census. Calculated from Table 2, p. 10.

79   total U.S. food and beverage spending: "Sales of Local Foods Reaches $12 Billion," Packaged Facts, press release, January 28, 2015; Lauren Manning, "Buy 'Local'? The Term Is Murky for Shoppers, Survey Says," *Food Dive*, May 6, 2019.

79   "a gift of the Earth": Larry West, "What Is a Locavore?," ThoughtCo., April 5, 2018.

79   "your great-grandmother wouldn't recognize": Michael Pollan, *In Defense of Food: An Eater's Manifesto* (New York: Penguin, 2008).

79   "beginning in about 1880": Michael Pollan, "You Are What You Cook," *Talk of the Nation*, National Public Radio, May 3, 2013.

81   not year-round residents: Daniel Baker et al., "Who Shops at the Market?," *Journal of Extension* 7, no. 6, 2009, https://joe.org/joe/2009december/a2.php.

81   a graduate or professional degree: Daniel Lass et al., *Community Supported Agriculture Entering the 21st Century: Results from the 2001 National Survey,* 2003, http://www.cias.wisc.edu/wp-content/uploads/2008/07/csa_survey_01.pdf.

81   will also, most likely, be white: Julie Guthman, "Bringing Good Food to Others: Investigating the Subjects of Alternative Food Practice," *Cultural Geographies* 15, no. 4 (2008): 431–47.

82   reliance on experience and intuition: Dwight Garner, "In Wendell Berry's Essays, a Little Earnestness Goes a Long Ways," *New York Times*, May 20, 2019.

82   "re-establishment of the local community": Quoted in Kupfer, "Wendell Berry," *Earth Island Journal*, Winter 2015, https://www.earthisland.org/journal/index.php/magazine/entry/wendell_berry/.

84 role animal products can play: Diana Rodgers, with Andrew Rodgers, *The Homegrown Paleo Cookbook* (Las Vegas: Victory Belt Publishing, 2015).

87 "picked un-ripened": Carrie A. Furman and Faidra Papavasiliou, "Scale and Affect in the Local Food Movement," *Food, Culture & Society* 21, no. 2 (February 2018), 8.

87 still involved with CSA: Marcia Ruth Ostrom, "Community Supported Agriculture as an Agent of Change: Is It Working?," in *Remaking the North American Food System: Strategies and Sustainability,* ed. C. Clare Hinrichs and Thomas A. Lyson (Lincoln, NE: University of Nebraska Press, 2007).

87 net income becomes negative: Warren Lizio and Daniel A. Lass, "CSA 2001: An Evolving Platform for Ecological and Economical Agricultural Marketing and Production," Department of Resource Economics, University of Massachusetts, Amherst. Unpublished manuscript, 2005.

87 a quarter fewer weekly boxes: Greg Trotter, "Fewer Consumers Opting for That Weekly Box of Veggies, so Local Farmers Are Struggling to Survive," *Chicago Tribune,* October 20, 2018.

87 "small part of the food system": Cheryl Brown and Stacy Miller, "The Impacts of Local Markets: A Review of Research on Farmers Markets and Community Supported Agriculture (CSA)," *American Journal of Agricultural Economics* 90, no. 5 (2008): 1296–1302.

88 may be impossible to market later: Robert L. Shewfelt, *In Defense of Processed Food: It's Not Nearly as Bad as You Think* (Switzerland: Copernicus Books, 2017).

90 "unidirectional tendency in human history": Gretel H. Pelto and Pertti J. Pelto, "Diet and Delocalization: Dietary Changes Since 1750," *Journal of Interdisciplinary History* 14, no. 2 (1983): 510.

91 hired to do this kind of work: Devra First, "Why Is It So Hard to Find Local Asparagus, Anyway?" *Boston Globe,* 2017.

91 imported share had increased: Statista Research Department, April 11, 2016, https://www.statista.com/statistics/193817/fruit-imports-as-a-share-of-total-us-domestic-fruit-consumption/.

91 triple that for fresh vegetables: "US Imports of Vegetables Make Up Increasing Share of Domestic Consumption," *Fresh Plaza,* North American Edition, April 18, 2017.

92 sold in America's supermarkets doubled: Phil Kaufman et al., "Understanding the Dynamics of Produce Markets," Economic Research

Service (USDA), 2000, https://www.ers.usda.gov/publications/pub
-details/?pubid=42295.

92 broccoli availability increased: Jeanine Bentley, "U.S. Trends in Food
    Availability and a Dietary Assessment of Loss-Adjusted Food Avail-
    ability, 1970-2014," Economic Information Bulletin No. 166, Economic
    Research Service (USDA), January 2017.

92 a full-time job by itself: Valerie A. Ramey, "Time Spent in Home Pro-
    duction in the Twentieth-Century in the United States: New Estimates
    from Old Data," Journal of Economic History 69, no. 1 (March 2009):
    1–47.

92 "threat of disease and decay": Dylan Gordon, "The Coming Conver-
    gence of Natural and Industrial Food," Idea Couture, 2017, https://idea
    couture.com/app/uploads/2017/05/ic-food-misc-food-series.pdf.

93 an albino variety of wheat: Gina Pace, "Wonder Bread to Offer Whole
    Wheat," CBS News, January 22, 2006, https://www.cbsnews.com
    /news/wonder-bread-to-offer-whole-wheat/.

93 ending the threat of rickets: Michael F. Holick, "Sunlight and Vitamin
    D for Bone Health and Prevention of Autoimmune Diseases, Cancers,
    and Cardiovascular Disease," American Journal of Clinical Nutrition 80,
    no. 6 (December 2004): 1678S—88S.

94 to prevent neural tube defects: Centers for Disease Control and Preven-
    tion, "Achievements in Public Health, 1900–1999: Safer and Healthier
    Foods," Morbidity and Mortality Weekly Report 48, no. 40 (October 15,
    1999).

94 calcium, magnesium, and iron: Connie M. Weaver et al., "Processed
    Foods: Contributions to Nutrition," American Journal of Clinical Nutri-
    tion 99, no. 6 (June 2014): 1525–42.

94 magnesium, calcium, or dietary fiber: Weaver et al., "Processed Foods."

94 heart-healthy fats along with protein: Jennifer LaRue Huget, "Pro-
    cessed Foods . . . Can Be Good for You?" Washington Post, Septem-
    ber 27, 2011.

95 it had been satisfied: Kevin D. Hall et al., "Ultra-Processed Diets Cause
    Excess Calorie Intake and Weight Gain: An Inpatient Randomized
    Controlled Trial of Ad Libitum Food Intake," Cell Metabolism 30 (July 2,
    2019): 67–77.

95 classified as ultraprocessed: "America's Packaged Supply Is Ultra-
    Processed," Northwestern University, news release, July 24, 2019.

96 formulated foods with added ingredients: Shewfelt, In Defense of Pro-
    cessed Food.

96 make the labels "cleaner": Anne Marie Chaker, "Packaged Foods' New Selling Point: Fewer Ingredients," *Wall Street Journal,* 2016.

97 no sanitation training to workers: Judy A. Harrison et al., "Survey of Food Safety Practices on Small to Medium-Sized Farms and in Farmers Markets," *Journal of Food Protection* 76, no.11 (2013): 1989–93.

97 diarrhea, cramping, abdominal pain: C. E. Park and G. W. Sanders, "Occurrence of Thermotolerant Campylobacters in Fresh Vegetables Sold at Farmers' Outdoor Markets and Supermarkets," *Canadian Journal of Microbiology* 38, no. 4 April 1992): 313–16.

97 likely to test positive for salmonella: Joshua Scheinberg et al., "A Microbiological Comparison of Poultry Products Obtained from Farmers' Markets and Supermarkets in Pennsylvania," *Journal of Food Safety* 33 (2013): 259–64.

97 shop at a farmers market: Oklahoma Farm Report, June 15, 2016, http://www.oklahomafarmreport.com/wire/news/2016/06/00105 _OSUFoodDemandSurvey06152016_103320.php#.Xh8tZKeZOu4.

98 after eating at a Chipotle: Siddharth Cavale and Uday Sampath Kumar, "Chipotle Slumps 9 Percent after Ohio Outlet Linked to Food Poisoning Complaints," *Business News,* 2018.

98 "quality control guidelines": Nicole Torres, "Why Sourcing Local Food Is so Hard for Restaurants," *Harvard Business Review,* June 15, 2016, https://hbr.org/2016/06/why-sourcing-local-food-is-so-hard-for-restaurants.

99 "if regulations are properly instituted": Pew Charitable Trusts, "Putting Meat on the Table: Industrial Farm Animal Production in America: A Report of the Pew Commission on Industrial Farm Animal Production," 2008, 15.

99 reduced by over 90 percent: P. R. Davies, "Intensive Swine Production and Pork Safety," *Foodborne Pathogens and Disease* 8, no. 2 (2011): 189–201.

99 "eliminated about 15 diseases": Greg Cima, "Protecting Pigs, Cultivating Consumers: Consumer Perceptions, Swine Welfare, and Effective Practices Among American Association of Swine Veterinarians' Priorities," *JAVMA News,* April 18, 2010, https://www.avma.org/javma -news/2010-05-01/protecting-pigs-cultivating-consumers.

99 ready-to-eat meat: North American Meat Institute, "U.S. Achieves Public Health Goals for E. coli O157:H7 Cases for Second Straight Year," June 7, 2011, https://www.meatinstitute.org/ht/display/Article Details/i/69765/pid/206; North American Meat Institute, "Myth: Meat Is Less Safe Today Than It Was in the Past," *Meat Myth Crushers,*

https://www.meatmythcrushers.com/myths/myth-meat-is-less-safe
-today.php accessed January 15, 2020.

100 two hundred people hospitalized: Aneri Pattani, "Backyard Chickens Carry a Hidden Risk: Salmonella," *New York Times,* 2017.

100 load size and mode of travel: Pierre Desrochers and Hiroko Shimizu, *The Locavore's Dilemma: In Praise of the 10,000-Mile Diet* (New York: Public Affairs, 2012).

100 4,200 miles from Nairobi: Desrochers and Shimizu, *Locavore's Dilemma,* 100.

100 transport from producer to retailer: Pierre Desrochers and Hiroko Shimizu, "Eating Local Hurts the Planet," Salon, June 16, 2012.

100 imported tomatoes grown outdoors: Desrochers and Shimizu, *Locavore's Dilemma,* 96.

101 Total fertilizer and chemical use: Steve Sexton, "The Inefficiency of Local Food," *Freakonomics Blog,* November 14, 2011.

101 forage land area by half: Daimon C. Meeh et al., "Feeding a Population with Smaller Scale and Alternate System Production: An Examination of Farm Requirements with a Multi-Species Pasture System to Feed 10 Million People," *Renewable Agriculture and Food Systems* 29, no. 2 (2014): 176–85.

101 but also with other shoppers: Lisa McNeill and Olivia Hale, "Who Shops at Local Farmers' Markets? Committed Loyals, Experiencers, and Produce-Oriented Consumers," *Australasian Marketing Journal* 24, no. 2 (May 2016): 135–40.

101 "citizens, neighbors, parents and cooks": Michael Pollan, "Vote for the Dinner Party," *New York Times Magazine,* October 10, 2012.

102 staring at a glowing screen: Craig J. Thompson and Gokcen Coskuner-Balli, "Countervailing Market Responses to Corporate Co-optation and the Ideological Recruitment of Consumption Communities," *Journal of Consumer Research* 34 (August 2007): 135–52.

102 food as a community: Amory Starr, "Local Food: A Social Movement?" *Cultural Studies-Critical Methodologies* 10, no. 6 (2010): 479–90.

102 "Honey Nut Cheerios, and a loaf of bread": Krishna Thakker, "Hey Alexa, What's the Future of Voice Ordering for Groceries?" *Grocery Dive,* January 29, 2019.

102 don't expect a tip: Bradley Berman, "Burrito Delivered by Bot, as Long as Students Don't Trap It," *New York Times,* November 7, 2019.

102 appear to have peaked nationally: Luke Runyon, "Are Farmers Market Sales Peaking? That Might be Good for Farmers," *The Salt,* National Public Radio, 2015.

102 70 percent compared to peak sales: Todd M. Schmit et al., "Assessing the Barriers to Increasing Customer Participation and Farm Sales at Farmers Markets: Implications for Marketing Strategy," Charles H. Dyson School of Applied Economics and Management, Cornell University, August 2019, http://www.nyfarmersmarket.com/wp-content/uploads/Cornell-Dyson-eb1905.pdf.

102 drop in attendance in 2017: Jodi Helmer, "Why Are So Many Farmers Markets Failing? Because the Market Is Saturated," *The Salt*, National Public Radio, 2019.

103 came in frozen from India: Laura Reiley, "At Tampa Bay Farm-to-Table Restaurants, You're Being Fed Fiction," *Tampa Bay Times*, April 13, 2016.

103 produces only 1 percent: Stephanie Leydon, "Rhode Island Bets the Farm That Cheap Land Will Help Local Agriculture Thrive," *The Salt*, National Public Radio, 2018.

103 just 167 five years earlier: Corie Brown, "Feds Won't Make Good Food Happen: So Cities, Armed with Food Policy Councils, Will Do It Themselves," commentary, The New Food Economy, December 12, 2017.

104 subsidies were provided by public agencies: Jayne Pyle, "Farmers Markets in the United States: Functional Anachronisms?," *Geographical Review* 61, no. 2 (1971): 167–97.

105 two blocks from the White House: Michael Pollan, "Big Food Strikes Back: Why Did the Obamas Fail to Take on Corporate Agriculture?" *New York Times Magazine*, October 5, 2016.

105 forty thousand local and regional: "USDA Seeks Applications for Grants to Help Agricultural Producers Increase the Value of Their Products," USDA press release no. 0088.16, April 8, 2016.

105 "We are vigilantes": Kim Severson, "Alice Waters on Sex, Drugs and Sustainable Agriculture," *New York Times*, August 22, 2017.

106 "completely inefficient, economically": Quoted in Elizabeth Royte, "Urban Farming Is Booming, But What Does It Really Yield?" Ensia, April 27, 2015.

106 thirty times as high: William Larson, "New Estimates of Value of Land of the United States," Bureau of Economic Analysis, April 3, 2015.

107 a city of eighty thousand: Royte, "Urban Farming Is Booming."

107 "Foundation funding is critical": Funders' Network for Smart Growth and Livable Communities, "Investing in Healthy, Sustainable Places Through Urban Agriculture," Translation Paper 5, 2011, http://www

.fundersnetwork.org/files/learn/Investing_in_Urban_Agriculture
_Final_110713.pdf.

107 Among the foundations chipping in: Funders' Network, "Investing in Healthy, Sustainable Places."

108 $400,000 state grant: Sherri Welch, "$400,000 State Grant to Help RecoveryPark Through First-Phase Financing," *Crain's Detroit Business,* 2016.

108 GreenThumb continues: Winnie Hu, "From Around the World, Homegrown in New York," *New York Times,* 2017.

108 if they rent to gardeners: Conor Friedersdorf, "How Urban Farming Is Making San Francisco's Housing Crisis Worse," *Atlantic,* 2014.

108 the state of Missouri: National Council of State Legislatures, "Urban Agriculture State Legislation," updated 2014, https://www.ncsl.org /research/agriculture-and-rural-development/urban-agriculture-state -legislation.aspx.

109 A survey in 2013: Lydia Oberholtzer et al., "Urban Agriculture in the United States: Baseline Findings of a Nationwide Survey," National Center for Appropriate Technology, November 2016, https://www .planning.org/knowledgebase/resource/9136139/.

109 Brooklyn Grange: Royte, "Urban Farming Is Booming."

109 who agree to work without pay: Will Boisvert, "A Locavore's Dilemma: On the Fantasy of Urban Farming," *New York Observer,* January 15, 2013.

110 had to close early in 2017: Adele Peters, "The Future of Urban Farming Might Actually Be Suburban Farming," *Fast Company,* March 2, 2017, https://www.fastcompany.com/3068368/the-future-of-urban-farming -might-actually-be-suburban-farming.

110 vertical farm in downtown Vancouver: Jen St. Denis and Darryl Greer, "City of Vancouver Still Paying for Failed Urban Farm," *Business Vancouver,* May 15, 2015.

111 roll it out "everywhere": "Urban Farming Flourishes in New York," Phys.org, April 30, 2017, https://phys.org/news/2017-04-urban -farming-flourishes-york.html.

111 actually been bought in stores: Noam Cohen, "M.I.T. Shuts Down 'Food Computer' Project," October 25, 2019.

111 One study by city planners: Wylie Goodman and Jennifer Minner, "Will the Urban Agricultural Revolution Be Vertical and Soilless? A Case Study of Controlled Environment Agriculture in New York City," *Land Use Policy* 83 (April 2019): 160–73.

111 The "Plantagon": "Sweden: Construction of Plantagon Vertical Green-house Planned for 2017," HortiDaily, June 17, 2016, https://www.horti daily.com/article/6026957/sweden-construction-of-plantagon-vertical -greenhouse-planned-for-2017/.

Chapter 4: THE PANIC FOR ORGANIC

112 fewer than 2 percent of commodities: USDA, 2017 Census of Agricul-ture, calculated from Table 41, p. 55.

112 Processed and packaged foods: Organic Trade Association, "U.S. Or-ganic Sales Break Through $50 Billion Mark in 2018," press release, 2019, https://ota.com/news/press-releases/20699.

113 "insufficiently tested or are completely misguided": Louise O. Fresco, *Hamburgers in Paradise: The Stories Behind the Food We Eat* (Princeton, NJ: Princeton University Press, 2016), 241.

115 little more than a social fetish: Michael Specter, *Denialism: How Irratio-nal Thinking Hinders Scientific Progress, Harms the Planet, and Threatens Our Lives,* 2009.

115 2 percent of layer hens: Economic Research Service (USDA), "Over-view," organic production, September 22, 2016.

115 organic produce was 54 percent higher: Jaewon Kang, "Grocers Pick Produce for Healthy Growth," *Wall Street Journal,* December 27, 2019, B2.

115 organic salad mix cost 60 percent: Andrea Carlson, "Investigating Retail Price Premiums for Organic Foods," USDA, *Amber Waves,* May 24, 2016, https://www.ers.usda.gov/amber-waves/2016/may/investigating -retail-price-premiums-for-organic-foods/.

116 an adequate diet and malnutrition: Vaclav Smil, "Nitrogen and Food Production: Proteins for Human Diets," *Ambio* 31, no. 2 (2002): 126–31.

117 earlier lost continent named Lemuria: Rudolf Steiner, *Cosmic Memory: Prehistory of Earth and Man* (1959), Rudolf Steiner Archive.

117 lacked "biodynamic" force: William Bechtel and Robert C. Richardson. "Vitalism," in E. Craig, ed., *Routledge Encyclopedia of Philosophy* (Lon-don: Routledge, 1998).

117 forces from Mars, Jupiter, and Saturn: Rudolf Steiner, "The Agricultural Course," Lecture 1, Koberwitz, June 7, 1924, Rudolf Steiner Archive.

118 "so it is also with the hoofs": Rudolf Steiner, "The Agricultural Course," Lecture 4, Koberwitz, June 12, 1924, Rudolf Steiner Archive.

118 were also treated biodynamically: Eric Kurlander, "Hitler's Supernatu-ral Sciences: Astrology, Anthroposophy, and World Ice Theory in the Third Reich," in Monica Black and Eric Kurlander, eds., *Revisiting the*

"Nazi Occult": Histories, Realities, Legacies (Suffolk, UK: Boydell and Brewer, 2015).

118 in German concentration camps: Peter Staudenmaier, *Between Occultism and Nazism: Anthroposophy and the Politics of Race in the Fascist Era* (Leiden: Brill, 2014).

119 foremost advocate for organic farming: P. Conford, *The Origins of the Organic Movement* (Glasgow, UK: Floris Books, 2001).

119 but not "artificial" fertilizers: Albert Howard, *An Agricultural Testament* (New York: Oxford University Press, 1943).

119 correcting specific soil nutrient limitations: Conford, *Origins of the Organic Movement*.

120 "to protect themselves against disease": Howard, *Agricultural Testament*.

120 one-tenth the size of corn today: Brad Plumer, "Here's What 9,000 Years of Breeding Has Done to Corn, Peaches, and Other Crops," *Vox*, May 12, 2016.

120 just like in nature: Albert Howard, *The Soil and Health* (New York: Schocken Books, 1972).

120 in diseases of all kinds: Howard, *Agricultural Testament*.

121 "after forty centuries of management": Howard.

121 population continued to increase: Krishan Saini, "The Growth of the Indian Economy: 1860–1960," *Review of Income and Wealth* 15, no. 3 (September 1969): 247–63.

121 imperialist India Defence League: P. Conford, "Organic Society: Agriculture and Radical Politics in the Career of Gerard Wallop, Ninth Earl of Portsmouth (1898–1984)," *Agricultural History Review* 53, no. 1 (2005): 78–96.

121 book called *Famine in England*: Conford, "Organic Society."

121 "widespread critical praise and discussion": Erin Gill, *Lady Eve Balfour and the British Organic Food and Farming Movement* (Ph.D. thesis, Department of History and Welsh History, Aberystwyth University, November 2010), 28.

121 organic versus chemical-based farming: Conford, "Organic Society."

122 Albert Howard never joined: Gill, *Lady Eve Balfour*.

122 "may be said to be proved": Lord Northbourne, *Look to the Land* (London: Dent, 1940), 173.

122 Howard to be his associate editor: J. I. Rodale, "An Introduction to Organic Farming," *Organic Farming and Gardening*, May 1942.

123 artificially softened water could cause cancer: Maria McGrath, "The Bizarre Life (and Death) of 'Mr. Organic,'" *New Republic*, August 8, 2014.

123 better for diphtheria than a vaccine: Kimiko de Freytas-Tamura, "Vaccine Skepticism Takes Root at Progressive Schools," *New York Times,* June 15, 2019, A18.

123 inorganic nitrogen use on American farms: Bruce L. Gardner, *American Agriculture in the Twentieth Century* (Cambridge, MA: Harvard University Press, 2002).

123 nitrogen fertilizer dressings: Keith W. Jaggard et al., "Possible Changes to Arable Crop Yields by 2050," *Philosophical Transactions of the Royal Society B* 27 (September 2010), https://royalsocietypublishing.org/doi/full/10.1098/rstb.2010.0153#.

124 by 1980 to ninety-one bushels: Economic Research Service (USDA), Feed Grains Database, Custom Query, January 2020, https://data.ers.usda.gov/FEED-GRAINS-custom-query.aspx#ResultsPanel.

124 less than five million by 1990: Gardner, *American Agriculture.*

125 "Chlorinated hydrocarbons like everyone else": "Rachel Carson 1907–1964," *A Science Odyssey: People and Discoveries,* Public Broadcasting System, WGBH, 1998, https://www.pbs.org/wgbh/aso/databank/entries/btcars.html.

125 "hazard from their misuse is greatly reduced": Rachel Carson, *Silent Spring* (New York: First Mariner Books Edition, 2002), 184.

125 "I think chemicals do have a place": Eliza Griswold, "How 'Silent Spring' Ignited the Environmental Movement," *New York Times Magazine,* September 21, 2012.

125 He also faulted Carson: Suzanne Peters, *The Land in Trust: A Social History of the Organic Farming Movement* (Ph.D. thesis in Sociology, McGill University, Montreal, August 1, 1979).

126 "the organic point of view": Robert Rodale, "Rachel Carson Makes a Television Conquest," *Organic Gardening and Farming,* June 1963, 36.

126 branded him "an eccentric": Samuel Fromartz, *Organic, Inc.: Natural Foods and How They Grew* (New York: Harcourt, 2006), 21.

126 not to acknowledge these contacts: John Paull, "The Rachel Carson Letters and the Making of *Silent Spring,*" *Sage,* July 2, 2013.

126 one-fifth lower per acre: Andrew R. Kniss et al., "Commercial Crop Yields Reveal Strengths and Weaknesses for Organic Agriculture in the United States," *PLOS ONE,* August 23, 2016.

126 lower forty-eight states: Steven Savage, "The Lower Productivity of Organic Farming: A New Analysis and Its Implications," *Forbes,* October 9, 2015.

126 pesticide use in the United States: Gardner, *American Agriculture.*

127 review of allowable residue levels: Centers for Disease Control and Pre-

vention, "Achievements in Public Health, 1900–1999: Safer and Healthier Foods," *Morbidity and Mortality Weekly Report* 48, no. 40 (October 15, 1999).

127 even as total crop production: Fernandez-Cornejo et al., "Pesticide Use in U.S. Agriculture: 21 Selected Crops, 1960–2008," Economic Research Service (USDA), Economic Information Bulletin 124, May 2014, https://www.ers.usda.gov/webdocs/publications/43854/46734_eib124.pdf.

127 80 percent below that peak: Jorge Fernandez-Cornejo et al., "Pesticide Use Peaked in 1981, Then Trended Downward, Driven by Technological Innovations and Other Factors," *Amber Waves,* June 2, 2014.

128 transported to multiple locations: Environmental Protection Agency, "Colony Collapse Disorder," updated April 26, 2018, https://www.epa.gov/pollinator-protection/colony-collapse-disorder.

128 more benign conclusion: Michael L. Goodis, "Dear Registrant" letter, Office of Chemical Safety and Pollution Prevention (EPA), August 7, 2019.

128 reduced to $69 million: Tina Bellon, "In Roundup Case, U.S. Judge Cuts $2 Billion Verdict Against Bayer to $86 Million," *Reuters,* July 25, 2019.

129 reaching more than three thousand: Warren Belasco, *Appetite for Change: How the Counterculture Took on the Food Industry* (Ithaca, NY: Cornell University Press, 2007).

129 attempting to grow their own food: Eleanor Agnew, *Back from the Land: How Young Americans Went to Nature in the 1970s, and Why They Came Back* (Chicago: Ivan R. Dee, 2005).

129 increase 40 percent: Brian K. Obach, *Organic Struggle: The Movement for Sustainable Agriculture in the United States* (Cambridge, MA: MIT Press, 2015).

129 "anything chemical, synthetic, or plastic": Warren Belasco, *Appetite for Change.*

129 "renounced energy-guzzling appliances": Agnew, *Back from the Land.*

129 not all were impressed: Jonathan Kauffman, *Hippie Food: How Back-to-the-Landers, Longhairs, and Revolutionaries Changed the Way We Eat* (New York: William Morrow, 2018).

129 stale, dry brown bread: Alice Waters, *Coming to My Senses* (New York: Clarkson Potter, 2017), 269.

129 consumer cooperatives, or health food stores: John Ikerd, "Organic Agriculture Faces the Specialization of Production Systems; Specialized Systems and the Economical Stakes," University of Missouri, paper presented at international conference titled Organic Agriculture

Faces the Specialization of Production Systems, Lyon, France, December 6–9, 1999.

130 one out of five organic growers in the United States: Obach, *Organic Struggle.*

130 including fewer chemical inputs: Donella H. Meadows and Dennis L. Meadows, *Limits to Growth* (New York: Universe Books, 1972).

130 consumers as well as farmers: USDA Study Team on Organic Farming, "Report and Recommendations on Organic Farming," July 1980, https://pubs.nal.usda.gov/report-and-recommendations-organic-farming-usda-1980.

130 "back to the stone age": Quoted in Obach, *Organic Struggle,* 50.

130 emissions would rise by 21 percent: Laurence G. Smith et al., "The Greenhouse Gas Impacts of Converting Food Production in England and Wales to Organic Methods," *Nature Communications* 10 (October 22, 2019), https://www.nature.com/articles/s41467-019-12622-7#auth-4.

131 "most potent cancer-causing agent": David Shaw, "Alar Panic Shows Power of Media to Trigger Fear," *Los Angeles Times,* September 12, 1994.

131 reducing fresh fruit consumption: John Tierney, "The Big City; The Apple and the Sins of Journalists," *New York Times,* August 18, 2000.

132 "appear to be insignificant": Carl K. Winter and Sarah F. Davis, "Organic Foods," *Journal of Food Science* 71, no. 9 (November/December 2006): R117–24.

132 slightly higher breast cancer risks: "Is Eating More Organic Food Tied to Lower Cancer Risk?," Medscape Education Clinical Briefs, November 21, 2018.

132 highest pesticide residue levels: Environmental Working Group, "EWG's 2019 Shopper's Guide to Pesticides in Produce," 2019, https://www.ewg.org/foodnews/dirty-dozen.php.

132 0.01 percent of the reference dose: Michael P. Holsapple et al., "Don't Believe Everything You Hear About Pesticides on Fruits and Vegetables," *Conversation,* April 12, 2017.

133 nutrient content or health benefit: Crystal Smith-Spangler et al., "Are Organic Foods Safer or Healthier Than Conventional Alternatives? A Systematic Review," *Annals of Internal Medicine* 157, no. 4 (September 2012): 348–66.

133 a single baked sweet potato: Joseph Rosen, *Claims of Organic Food's Nutritional Superiority: A Critical Review,* American Council on Science and Health, July 2008.

133 "panic for organic": Obach, *Organic Struggle.*

133 "process of making it workable": Quoted in Obach, *Organic Struggle,* 66.

134 animal welfare advocates: Obach, 71.

134 processing of certified organic foods: Obach, 103.

134 existing organic and natural food stores: Ikerd, "Organic Agriculture Faces the Specialization."

134 consistent grade and uniformly packaged: Ikerd.

134 "same industrial-size farming": John Cloud, "Eating Better than Organic," *Time,* March 2, 2007.

134 organic sales originate from California: Chuck Abbott, "Big Gains in Number of US Organic Farms, Value of Organic Sales," Food and Environment Reporting Network, September 20, 2017.

135 H. J. Heinz, and Kellogg: Michael Sligh and Carolyn Christman, *Who Owns Organic?,* Rural Advancement Foundation International, 2003.

135 Walmart, Costco, and Kroger: Cathy Siegner, "Why Are Organic Food Prices Dropping?" *Food Dive,* January 25, 2019.

135 from small farmers to consumers: USDA, "Organic Farming: Results from the 2014 Organic Survey," September 2015.

136 "Why the hell am I paying": Peter Whoriskey, "More Than a Million Hens, Filling Barns at Three Per Square Foot. And Yes, They're USDA Organic," *Washington Post,* July 13, 2017.

136 5.7 percent of all food sold: USDA, 2017 Census of Agriculture, Table 41, 55; "U.S. Organic Sales Break Through $50 Billion Mark in 2018," Organic Trade Association, press release, May 17, 2019, https://ota .com/news/press-releases/20699.

136 "other potential scofflaws": "Restaurants Frequently Misrepresent What's Organic," Cornucopia Institute, news release, January 14, 2019.

138 taken to a landfill: Rodale Institute, "Beyond Black Plastic," updated on May 31, 2019, https://rodaleinstitute.org/science/articles/beyond -black-plastic.

138 contain petroleum-based materials: Lisa Elaine Held, "Organic Farming Has a Plastic Problem: One Solution Is Controversial," *The Salt,* National Public Radio, 2019.

Chapter 5: SHOULD PEASANTS STAY POOR?

139 chronically undernourished: World Hunger Education Service, "Africa Hunger and Poverty Facts," accessed January 17, 2020, https://www .worldhunger.org/africa-hunger-poverty-facts-2018/.

141 stunted from malnutrition: Izabela Leao and Tenzin Lhaden, "Promoting Better Nutrition in Bhutan," *World Bank Blog,* May 4, 2018.

141 "embracing the complexity of nature": Olivier de Schutter, "Why We

Need an Agroecological Revolution," *Rural 21: The International Journal for Rural Development* 52 (June 2018), 6.

141 "wild areas and natural habitat": Quoted in Cathriona Russell, *Autonomy and Food Biotechnology in Theological Ethics* (Bern, Switzerland: Peter Lang, 2009), 14.

142 feed its fast-growing population: William Paddock and Paul Paddock, *Famine 1975! America's Decision: Who Will Survive?* (Boston: Little Brown and Co., 1967).

142 "battle to feed all of humanity is over": Paul R. Ehrlich, *The Population Bomb* (New York: Ballantine Books, 1968).

142 two a day leaving the docks: Lester R. Brown, *Breaking New Ground: A Personal History* (New York: W. W. Norton & Company, 2013).

143 ending the fear of famine: Robert Paarlberg, *Food Trade and Foreign Policy: India, the Soviet Union, and the United States* (Ithaca, NY: Cornell University Press, 1985).

143 doubled between 1971 and 1976: Robert Paarlberg, *Countrysides at Risk: The Political Geography of Sustainable Agriculture* (Washington, D.C.: Overseas Development Council, 1994).

144 made possible by the new seeds: Per Pinstrup-Andersen and Mauricio Jaramillo, *The Impact of Technological Change in Rice Production on Food Consumption and Nutrition* (Baltimore: Johns Hopkins University Press, 1991).

144 planted with these modern varieties: Prabhu L. Pingali, "Green Revolution: Impacts, Limits, and the Path Ahead," *PNAS*, July 31, 2012.

144 for wheat nearly 90 percent: Douglas Gollin, Michael Morris, and Derek Byerlee, "Technology Adoption in Intensive Post-Green Revolution Systems," *American Journal of Agricultural Economics* 87, no. 5 (December 2005): 1310–16.

144 both small and large farms had adopted: Vernon W. Ruttan, "Controversy About Agricultural Technology: Lessons from the Green Revolution," *International Journal of Biotechnology* 6, no. 1 (2004): 43–54.

145 green revolution seeds and methods: Peter B. R. Hazell, "The Asian Green Revolution," International Food Policy Research Institute, Discussion Paper 00911, November 2009, http://ebrary.ifpri.org/cdm/ref/collection/p15738coll2/id/29462.

145 James Lovelock and Patrick Moore endorsed: CIMMYT (International Maize and Wheat Improvement Center), *CIMMYT in 1992: Poverty, the Environment, and Population Growth, the Way Forward* (Mexico City: CIMMYT, 1993).

145 would have been malnourished: Robert E. Evenson and Douglas

Gollin, "Assessing the Impact of the Green Revolution, 1960 to 2000," *Science,* May 2003.

145 farming methods remain least improved: Bill Gates and Melinda Gates, "We Were Making Headway on Global Poverty. What's About to Change?" *New York Times,* September 22, 2018.

146 "vast numbers of peasant farmers": John Vidal, "Norman Borlaug: Humanitarian Hero of Menace to Society?" *Guardian,* April 1, 2014.

146 "death of peasants by the million": Alexander Cockburn, "Al Gore's Peace Prize," *Counterpunch,* October 13, 2007.

147 encouraged too much pumping: Paul Faeth, "Building the Case for Sustainable Agriculture: Policy Lessons from India, Chile, and the Philippines," *Environment,* January / February 1994.

147 Indonesia knew better than to stop: Food and Agriculture Organization of the United Nations, "Integrated Pest Management in Rice in Indonesia: Status After Three Crop Seasons" (Jakarta, Indonesia: FAO, May 1988).

148 "an exogenous, and high input one": Vandana Shiva, *The Violence of the Green Revolution: Third World Agriculture, Ecology, and Politics* (London: Zed Books, 1991), 29.

148 "narrow genetic base and monocultures": Shiva, *Violence of the Green Revolution,* 44–45.

148 "food supplies of millions precariously perched": Shiva, 81.

149 compared to traditional varieties: Food and Agriculture Organization of the United Nations, *Unlocking the Water Potential of Agriculture* (Rome: FAO, 2003).

149 for each pound of grain produced: Norman Borlaug, "The Green Revolution, Peace, and Humanity," Nobel Peace Prize Lecture, December 11, 1970.

149 "whatever people want to hear": Quoted in Michael Specter, "Seeds of Doubt: An Activist's Controversial Crusade Against Genetically Modified Crops," *New Yorker,* August 18, 2014.

149 "remarkable increase" since the 1960s: Marcelo A. Aizen et al., "Global Agricultural Productivity Is Threatened by Increasing Pollinator Dependence Without a Parallel Increase in Crop Diversification," *Global Change Biology* 25, no. 11 (July 10, 2019), 7.

149 variety of wheat or rice: Mark W. Rosegrant and Peter B. R. Hazell, *Transforming the Rural Asian Economy: The Unfinished Revolution* (New York: Oxford University Press, 2000).

149 polyculture of traditional varieties: Thomas R. DeGregori, "Green Myth vs. the Green Revolution," *Butterflies & Wheels* (blog), February 5, 2004.

149 "early years of the Green Revolution": Melinda Smale and Tim McBride, "Understanding Global Trends in the Use of Wheat Diversity and International Flows of Wheat Genetic Resources," abstract, CIMMYT 1995/96 World Wheat Facts and Trends, January 1996.

150 177 percent higher: Food and Agriculture Organization of the United Nations, FAOSTAT database, Fertilizers Archive, accessed May 30, 2017.

150 increased on a tonnage basis: Food and Agriculture Organization, FAOSTAT.

150 dollar value of agricultural exports: Alain de Janvry, *The Agrarian Question and Reformism in Latin America* (Baltimore: Johns Hopkins University Press, 1981).

150 3 percent controlled 79 percent: Merilee Grindle, *State and Countryside: Development Policy and Agrarian Politics in Latin America* (Baltimore: Johns Hopkins University Press, 1986).

150 lost between 1961 and 1990: Angus Wright, *The Death of Ramon Gonzalez: The Modern Agricultural Dilemma* (Austin, TX: University of Texas Press, 1990).

151 shading and cooling the soil: Francisco J. Rosado-May, "The Intercultural Origin of Agroecology: Contributions from Mexico," in V. Ernesto Mendez et al., eds., *Agroecology: A Transdisciplinary, Participatory and Action-oriented Approach* (New York: CRC Press, 2015), 123–34.

151 habitat for fish: Alfred H. Siemens, "Wetland Agriculture in Pre-Hispanic Mesoamerica," *Geographical Review* 73, no. 2 (April, 1983): 166–81.

152 "each plant in the chinampa": Miguel A. Altieri, "Applying Agroecology to Enhance the Productivity of Peasant Farming Systems in Latin America," *Environment, Development, and Sustainability* 1 (1999), 202.

153 270 person-days per hectare: Altieri, "Applying Agroecology," 202.

153 "maintain the productivity of the system": Organization of American States, *Source Book of Alternative Technologies for Freshwater Augmentation in Latin America and the Caribbean,* Unit of Sustainable Development and Environment, General Secretariat, Washington, D.C., 1997.

153 Globally Important Agricultural Heritage System: Dan Collyns, "The Three Wonders of the Ancient World Solving Modern Water Problems," *Guardian,* August 19, 2015.

154 resorts in Cancún and Tulum: Gabriel Popkin, "Mayans Have Farmed the Same Way for Millennia: Climate Change Means They Can't," *The Salt,* National Public Radio, February 3, 2017.

154 an ancient, proven practice: Popkin, "Mayans Have Farmed the Same Way."

154 "conservation model for the future": Anabel Ford, "Legacy of the Ancient Maya: The Maya Forest Garden," *Popular Archaeology*, December 15, 2010.

155 projects using green manures: Altieri, "Applying Agroecology."

155 might have delivered: Altieri.

155 nitrogenous fertilizers increased 139 percent: Food and Agricultural Organization, FAOSTAT.

155 another 43 percent: World Bank, Data Catalog, "Fertilizer Consumption (Kilograms per Hectare of Arable Land)," https://datacatalog .worldbank.org/fertilizer-consumption-kilograms-hectare-arable-land.

156 almost half between 1990 and 1994: Food and Agriculture Organization, FAOSTAT.

156 spread of agroecology methods: Peter Rosset et al., "The Campesino-to-Campesino Agroecology Movement of ANAP in Cuba," *Journal of Peasant Studies* 38, no. 1(2011).

156 "closes local production and consumption cycles": Miguel A. Altieri and Fernando R. Funes-Monzote, "The Paradox of Cuban Agriculture," *Monthly Review*, January 2012.

156 "more production from less": Food and Agriculture Organization of the United Nations, "Agroecology in Cuba: For the Farmer Seeing Is Believing," *52 Profiles on Agroecology*, 2012.

156 "an example on a global level": Food and Agriculture Organization of the United Nations, "Final Report: Regional Meeting on Agroecology in Latin America and the Caribbean." Brasilia, June 24–26, 2015 (Rome: FAO, 2016), 11.

157 more than one-third lower: Food and Agriculture Organization of the United Nations, FAOSTAT, "Cuba: Average Value of Food Production (Constant 1$ per Person), Three Year Moving Average," accessed September 2019.

157 widespread rationing of chicken: Associated Press, "Cuba Rations Staple Foods and Soap in Face of Economic Crisis," *New York Times*, May 11, 2019.

157 research on genetically engineered crops: Altieri and Funes-Monzote, "Paradox of Cuban Agriculture."

157 imports grew by more than half: Food and Agriculture Organization, "Cuba: Average Value of Food Production."

157 more than four-fifths of the items: Altieri and Funes-Monzote, "Paradox of Cuban Agriculture."

158 organic farming and agroecology: NGO Forum, "Profit for Few or Food for All," World Food Summit, Rome, November 17, 1996.

158 did nothing to dissuade them: Tony Hill, "Three Generations of UN-Civil Society Relations: A Quick Sketch," paper presented at the Global Policy Forum, April 2004.

158 only region not to have experienced: NGO/CSO Forum, "'Profit for Few or Food Food for All' Revisited Five Years Later," NGO/CSO Forum for Food Sovereignty, Rome, June 10, 2002.

158 endorse organic farming and agroecology: International Assessment of Agricultural Knowledge, Science and Technology for Development (IAASTD), *Agriculture at the Crossroads: Synthesis Report,* Executive Summary, 2009.

159 guarantee the human right to food: Olivier de Schutter, "Agroecology and the Right to Food," Report to the United Nations Human Rights Council, March 8, 2011.

159 "agro-ecological production methods": United Nations Conference on Trade and Development (UNCTAD), *Wake Up Before It Is Too Late: Make Agriculture Truly Sustainable Now for Food Security and Changing Climate* (Geneva, Switzerland: UNCTAD, 2013), 341.

159 transition process in twenty countries: Food and Agricultural Organization of the United Nations, "Scaling Up Agroecology to Achieve the Sustainable Development Goals (SDGs)," Second International Symposium on Agroecology, Rome, April 3–5, 2018.

159 "discussions about the future of agriculture": Hector Valenzuela, "Agroecology: A Global Paradigm to Challenge Mainstream Industrial Agriculture," *Horticulturae,* March 16, 2016.

160 "drought, pest and disease resilience": Gordon Conway, "Global Food Crisis: Towards a 'Doubly Green' World," *Guardian,* 2011.

160 side benefit from productivity gains: Jacqueline Loos et al., "Putting Meaning Back into 'Sustainable Agricultural Intensification,'" *Frontiers in Ecology and the Environment,* 2014.

160 nearly one-tenth of agricultural land: Jules Pretty et al., "Global Assessment of Agricultural System Redesign for Sustainable Intensification," *Nature Sustainability,* 2018.

161 resulting growth in industrial output: "Multinationals: The Retreat of the Global Economy," *Economist,* January 28, 2017.

162 had increased almost fiftyfold: "How the Indian Economy Changed in 1991–2011," *Economic Times,* September 15, 2011.

162 into the streets of Brussels: Gérard Choplin, "The Founding of La Via Campesina in Relation to Agricultural Globalisation," *La Via Campesina's Open Book: Celebrating 20 Years of Struggle and Hope,* March 2013.

162 to protest agricultural reforms: Douglas Imig and Sidney Tarrow, *Con-*

tentious Europeans (Lanham, MD: Rowman and Littlefield Publishers, 2001).

162 thirty-six different countries represented: Choplin, "Founding of La Via Campesina."

162 farmer-activist from Spain: Transnational Institute, video presentation, "Paul Nicholson: Food Sovereignty, a Critical Dialogue," February 21, 2014, https://www.tni.org/en/article/paul-nicholson-food-sovereignty-a-critical-dialogue.

162 named Rafael Algeria: Marc Edelman, "Transnational Peasant and Farmer Movements and Networks," in M. Kaldor et al., eds., *Global Civil Society* (Oxford: Oxford University Press, 2003).

162 Friends of the Earth International: Saturnino Borras, Jr., "Reply: Solidarity. Re-examining the 'Agrarian Movement-NGO' Solidarity Relations Discourse," *Dialectical Anthropology* 32 (2008), 208.

162 Action Network based in Germany: Borras, "Reply: Solidarity," *Dialectical Anthropology* 32 (2008): 203–9.

163 engaged in a symbolic planting: Annette Aurelie Desmaris, "The Power of Peasants: Reflections on the Meanings of La Via Campesina," *Journal of Rural Studies* 24 (2008): 138–49.

163 block the import of farm products: Edelman, "Transnational Peasant and Farmer Movements."

164 "and economic classes and generations": La Via Campesina, "Declaration of Nyeleni," February 27, 2007, http://www.cadtm.org/spip.php?page=imprimer&id_article=2464.

164 commodities to be bought and sold: Peter Rosset, "Re-thinking Agrarian Reform, Land and Territory in La Via Campesina," *Journal of Peasant Studies* 40, no. 4 (2013): 731, 753.

164 "problems facing the rural world": Maria Elena Martinez-Torres and Peter M. Rosset, "La Via Campesina: The Evolution of a Transnational Movement," *Global Policy Forum* 30, no. 1 (February 8, 2010): 149–76.

164 purchase seeds, chemicals, or farm equipment: Geoffrey Livingston et al., *Sub-Saharan Africa: The State of Smallholders in Agriculture,* International Fund for Agricultural Development, Rome, January 2011.

165 4 percent of total global investment: Lee Mwiti, "10 Trends on Foreign Investment in Africa," World Economic Forum, July 9, 2015; Don Gunasekera et al., "Effects of Foreign Direct Investment in African Agriculture," *China Agricultural Economic Review* 7, no. 2 (2015): 167–84.

165 eleven out of the bottom twenty: World Bank, "Rankings & Ease of Doing Business Score," 2019, https://www.doingbusiness.org/en/rankings.

165 surplus out to the market: Livingston et al., *Sub-Saharan Africa*.

165 less than $1.25 a day: Livingston et al.

165 nearly 60 percent of its food: Mestawet Gebru et al., "Food Systems for Healthier Diets in Ethiopia," International Food Policy Research Institute, April 2018, https://a4nh.cgiar.org/files/2018/04/DP1050 _Formatted.pdf.

166 agroecology and activist organizing skills: Christina Schiavoni, "The Venezuelan Food Sovereignty Experiment," *Solutions Journal* 5, no. 6 (November 2014): 46–53.

166 eggs, milk, and fruit: Ana Vanessa Herrero and Nicholas Casey, "In Venezuela That Empty Feeling," *New York Times,* September 3, 2017, 6.

166 searching through piles of garbage: Meridith Kohut and Isayen Herrera, *New York Times,* December 18, 2017, F9.

167 consistent with their vision of self-reliance: Christina Schiavoni and William Camacaro, "Special Report: Hunger in Venezuela? A Look Beyond the Spin," Food First, September 11, 2016; Christina Schiavoni, "The Contested Terrain of Food Sovereignty Construction: Toward a Historical, Relational and Interactive Approach," *Journal of Peasant Studies* 44, no. 1 (2017): 1–32.

167 integrate the physical and the personal: Internal Report on the Day of Dialogue on Knowledge for Food Sovereignty, the Hague, the Netherlands, January 25, 2014, https://www.tni.org/files/download/day_of _dialogue_on_knowledge_for_food_sovereignty-1.pdf.

167 Plan People to People: U.S. Food Sovereignty Alliance, "Food Sovereignty Prize 2019: Venezuela Awarded (Plan Pueblo a Pueblo)," *Orinoco Tribune,* August 29, 2019.

167 "if so, on what terms": "Food Sovereignty: A Critical Dialogue," International Institute of Social Studies (ISS). The Hague, The Netherlands, 24 January, 2014, https://www.iss.nl/sites/corporate/files/90 _Schiavoni.pdf.

167 "resisted, refracted, or reversed": Schiavoni, "Contested Terrain of Food Sovereignty."

Chapter 6: REJECTING BIOTECH FOOD

168 ripping genetically engineered crops: Will Storr, "Mark Lynas: Truth, Treachery, and GM Food," *Guardian,* March 9, 2013.

170 "most successful campaign": Mark Lynas, "Lecture to Oxford Farming Conference," January 3, 2013, Mark Lynas: Environmental News and Comment, http://www.marklynas.org/2013/01/lecture-to-oxford -farming-conference-3-january-2013.

173 should be regulated like GMOs: Erik Stokstad, "European Court Ruling Raises Hurdles for CRISPR Crops," *Science*, July 25, 2018.

173 same benign conclusion: Laura DeFrancesco, "How Safe Does Transgenic Food Need to Be?," *Nature Biotechnology* 31 (2013): 794–802; Allesandro Nicolia et al., "An Overview of the Last 10 Years of GE Crop Safety Research," *Critical Reviews in Biotechnology* 34 (2013): 77–88; Roberg Paarlberg, *Starved for Science: How Biotechnology Is Being Kept Out of Africa* (Cambridge, MA: Harvard University Press, 2008).

173 "conventional plant breeding technologies": European Commission, "A Decade of EU-Funded GMO Research (2001–2010)," Report 24473, Directorate General for Research, 2010.

173 "foods derived from GE crops": National Academies of Sciences, Engineering, Medicine, "Distinction Between Genetic Engineering and Conventional Plant Breeding Becoming Less Clear, Says New Report on GE Crops," News, May 17, 2016.

174 "however inconvenient that might be": Mark Lynas, "Confession of an Anti-GMO Activist," *Wall Street Journal*, June 23, 2018, C2.

175 ships bringing GMO soybeans: Thomas Bernauer and Erika Meins, "Technological Revolution Meets Policy and the Market," *European Journal of Political Research* 42, no. 5 (2003): 643–83.

175 starch from American corn: Les Levidow and Jos Bijman, "Farm Inputs Under Pressure from European Food Industry," *Food Policy* 27, no 1 (2002): 31–45.

175 recombinant therapeutic proteins: Paarlberg, *Starved for Science*.

176 journal retracted the paper: Barbara Casassus, "Study Linking Genetically Modified Corn to Rat Tumors Is Retracted," *Nature*, November 29, 2013.

177 "are bound to happen": William Hallman et al., *Public Perceptions of Genetically Modified Foods: A National Study of American Knowledge and Opinion*, Rutgers Food Policy Institute, 2003.

177 bit of sweet corn: Ronald Herring and Robert Paarlberg. "The Political Economy of Biotechnology," *Annual Review of Resource Economics* 8 (2016): 397–416.

177 planting materials ordered destroyed: Rosemary Mirondo, "Shock as Government Bans GMO Trials," *Citizen*, November 23, 2018.

177 staunchly opposed to GMOs: Joseph Opoku Gakpo, "Ghana's Scientists, Farmers, Reject Claim That GMO Crops Aren't Needed," Cornell Alliance for Science, March 20, 2019.

177 technically remained in place: Verenardo Meeme, "Kenya's Bt Cotton Approval Opens Door to Other GMO Crops," Cornell Alliance for Sci-

ence, December 20, 2019, https://allianceforscience.cornell.edu/blog/2019/12/kenyas-bt-cotton-approval-opens-door-to-other-gmo-crops/.

179 "dangerous to their health": "Zambia Refuses GM 'Poison,'" BBC News, World Edition, September 3, 2002.

179 "Keep Zambia GMO Free": Paarlberg, *Starved for Science,* 142.

179 "food the Americans are forcing": Brighton Phiri, "US Comes Under Attack Over GMOs," *Post* (Zambia), August 13, 2002.

179 Danish foreign assistance agency: Women for Change: WFC Networking. Zambia: Women for Change (WFC) 2007, https://www.wfc.org/zm/networks.html.

179 "they don't explain": Quoted in Mark Lynas, *Seeds of Science: Why We Got It So Wrong on GMOs* (London: Bloomsbury Sigma, 2018), 154.

180 before it could be taken away: IRIN News, "Zambia: WFP Delivers Non-GM Food Aid," January 30, 2003.

180 retrovirus similar to HIV: *Daily Telegraph* (UK), "Will Their Protests Leave Her Hungry?," November 23, 2002.

180 confirmed his negative view of GMOs: Government of Zambia, "Report of the Factfinding Mission by Zambian Scientists on Genetically Modified Foods, 10 September—2 October," Lusaka, Zambia, 2002, 1–56.

180 "possible ailments including cancers": Third World Network, "Don't Pressure Hungry Peoples to Accept GM Food Aid," September 2, 2002, https://www.twn.my/title/geletter.htm.

181 "NO to genetically modified foods": Genetic Food Alert UK, "UK Government Minister Condemns 'Wicked' USAID GM Food Policy," November 27, 2002, http://www.connectotel.com/gmfood/gf271102.txt.

181 genetic composition of the human body: "Interview with Fred Kalibwani of PELUM," *In Motion Magazine,* December 6, 2002.

181 "if it was true": Andrew Natsios, "Hunger, Famine, and the Promise of Biotechnology," in Jon Entine, ed., *Let Them Eat Precaution* (Washington, D.C.: American Enterprise Institute, 2006).

181 "question everyone is asking": Eric Hand, "Africa in the Middle of the U.S.-EU Biotech Trade War," *St. Louis Post-Dispatch,* December 12, 2006.

182 "developmental challenges our country faces": "Jairam Differs with PM, Says No NGO Forced Bt Brinjal Ban," *Hindustan Times,* February 26, 2012, https://www.hindustantimes.com/india/jairam-differs-with-pm-says-no-ngo-forced-bt-brinjal-ban/story-OIU7DRELEfbS1yBXEQP7dI.html.

182 research funding from Monsanto: Pamela C. Ronald and Raoul W. Adamchak, *Tomorrow's Table: Organic Farming, Genetics, and the Future of Food*, 2nd ed. (New York: Oxford University Press, 2018).

183 Mark Lynas and his friends: "GM Crops: A Bitter Harvest?" BBC News, June 14, 2002.

184 hardly a neutral referee: Genetic Literacy Project. "U.S. Right to Know (USRTK): Organic Industry Funded Anti-Bio Group Attacks Researchers," July 18, 2019.

184 no academic work had been compromised: Eric Lipton, "Food Industry Enlisted Academics in G.M.O. Lobbying War, Emails Show," *New York Times*, September 5, 2015.

184 had spoken out publicly: Tara Dugan, "Major Brands Reverse Course on Genetically Modified Food Labels," *San Francisco Chronicle*, 2016.

185 "mating and/or natural recombination": European Union, Directive (EU) 2015/412, 2015.

186 became CRISPR-Cas9: Eric S. Lander, "The Heroes of CRISPR," *Cell*, January 14, 2016.

186 toolkit for less than fifty dollars: Ian Haydon, "CRISPR Revolution: How Scientists Are Turning Gene-Editing Hype into Food and Medical Breakthroughs," Genetic Literacy Project, August 10, 2017.

186 better able to resist disease: Leena Arora and Alka Narula, "Gene Editing and Crop Improvement Using CRISPR-Cas9 System," *Frontiers in Plant Science* 8 (November 8, 2017: 1932.

186 APHIS replied it would not: Haydon, "CRISPR Revolution."

186 "CRISPRy fried vegetables": D. Zhang et al., "Targeted Gene Manipulation in Plants Using the CRISPR/Cas Technology," *Journal of Genetics and Genomics* 43, no. 5 (May 20, 2016): 251–62.

186 wheat, maize, and potato: Deepa Jaganathan et al., "CRISPR for Crop Improvement: An Update Review," *Frontiers in Plant Science*, July 17, 2018.

187 culling of millions of birds: Cathy Siegner, "Gene-Edited Chicken Cells May Stop the Spread of Bird Flu," *Food Dive*, June 19, 2019.

187 "biotechnology from undue regulation": "White House Calls for Light Regulation of Low-Risk Gene-Edited Crops and Livestock," *Hagstrom Report*, June 11, 2019.

187 shelf life than other soybean oils: Candice Choi, "Gene-Edited Food Quietly Arrives in Restaurant Cooking Oil," *Washington Post*, March 12, 2019.

188 long history of safe use: Court of Justice of the European Union, "Organisms Obtained by Mutagenesis Are GMOS and Are, in Principle,

Subject to the Obligations Laid Down by the GMO Directive," Press
Release No. 111/18, July 25, 2018.

188   "death blow for plant biotech": Erik Stokstad, "European Court Ruling
Raises Hurdles for Crispr Crops," *Science,* July 25, 2018.

188   "revision of the Directive": Gerardo Fortuna, "Commission in Search
of 'Robust Response' to Gene Editing Challenge," *Euractiv,* June 6, 2019.

189   "devastating effects of climate change": Sarantis Michalopoulos,
"Industry Shocked by EU Court Decision to Put Gene Editing Technique Under Gm Law," *Euractiv,* July 26, 2018.

189   compared to GMO crops: Tim Searchinger, "World Resources Report: Creating a Sustainable Food Future: Synthesis Report," World
Resources Institute, December 2018, 24.

189   as hard to commercialize as GMOs: Jason Daley, "Europe Applies Strict
Regulations to CRISPR Crops," Smithsonian.com, July 27, 2018.

189   "how stupid the European system is": Daley, "Europe Applies Strict
Regulations."

189   "contaminating" organic and GMO-free food: Organics International,
"Position Paper: Compatibility of Breeding Techniques in Organic Systems," International Federation of Organic Agriculture Movements
(IFOAM), 2017, https://www.ifoam.bio/sites/default/files/position
_paper_v01_web_0.pdf.

189   Belgium, Sweden and Finland: Daley, "Europe Applies Strict Regulations."

190   "most likely to display unintended effects": National Research Council,
*Safety of Genetically Engineered Foods: Approaches to Assessing Unintended
Health Effects* (Washington, D.C.: National Academies Press, 2004), 64.

190   an alarm for such groups: Nala Carlos, "Crispr Food Will Be Available
Within 5 Years, Says Geneticist," *Tech Times,* April 22, 2019.

191   reduces cardiovascular and cancer risks: Kathleen L. Hefferon and Ronald J. Herring, "The End of the GMO? Gene Editing, Gene Drives, and
New Frontiers in Plant Technology," *Review of Agrarian Studies* 7, no.
1 (January–June 2017): 1–32.

191   similar to new veterinary drugs: Carolyn Y. Johnson, "Gene-Edited
Farm Animals Are Coming: Will We Eat Them?," *Washington Post,*
December 17, 2018.

191   federal labeling and disclosure requirements": Johnson, "Gene-Edited
Farm Animals."

191   created with gene-editing tools: Cathy Siegner, "Gene-Edited Chicken
Cells May Stop the Spread of Bird Flu," *Food Dive,* June 19, 2019.

191   "my cows are not drugs": Helena Bottemiller Evich, "FDA to Issue

Guidance on Gene-Edited Plants and Animals in 2019," *Politico Pro,* October 30, 2018.

192 baby girls with immunity to HIV: Meera Senthilingam, "Chinese Scientist Was Told Not to Create World's First Gene-Edited Babies," CNN Health, January 7, 2019, https://www.cnn.com/2019/01/07/health/robin-lovell-badge-gene-edited-babies-intl/index.html.

192 all the mosquitoes were gone: Kyros Kyrou et al., "A CRISPR–Cas9 Gene Drive Targeting Doublesex Causes Complete Population Suppression in Caged Anopheles Gambiae Mosquitoes," *Nature Biotechnology* 36 (2018): 1062–66.

192 disease vector control: Virginie Courtier-Orgogozo et al., "Agricultural Pest Control with Crispr-Based Gene Drive: Time for Public Debate," *EMBO Reports: Science and Society,* May 16, 2017.

192 "significant parts of Africa": Nicholas Wade, "Giving Malaria a Deadline," *New York Times,* September 24, 2018.

193 spread rapidly across international borders: Valentino M. Gantz and Omar S. Akbari, "Gene Editing Technologies and Applications for Insects," *Current Opinion in Insect Science* 28 (August 2018): 66–72.

193 "laboratory to test risky technologies": Rob Stein, "Scientists Release Controversial Genetically Modified Mosquitoes in High-Security Lab," *Morning Edition,* National Public Radio, February 20, 2019.

193 without passing on the alteration: University of California, San Diego, "New CRISPR-Based Technology Developed to Control Pests with Precision-Guided Genetics," press release, January 8, 2019.

Chapter 7: THE FATE OF FARM ANIMALS

195 "better off euthanized": Bailey F. Norwood and Jayson L. Lusk, *Compassion by the Pound: The Economics of Farm Animal Welfare* (New York: Oxford University Press, 2011), 225, 229.

195 veal from tightly confined calves: "California Proposition 12, Farm Animal Confinement Initiative," 2018, Ballotpedia, https://ballotpedia.org/California_Proposition_12,_Farm_Animal_Confinement_Initiative_(2018).

195 "capitulation to the egg industry": Californians Against Cruelty, Cages, and Fraud, "The REAL Story of Prop 12," 2018, https://stoptherotten egginitiative.org.

196 moment it leaves the fairgrounds: "4-H Livestock Market Animal Auction, General Rules," San Juan County Fairground, Washington State, https://s3.wp.wsu.edu/uploads/sites/2054/2014/04/New-Livestock-Market-Auction-Requirements.pdf.

197 small amount of transparent mineral oil: Fallon/Carter County 4-H, "Showmanship Guide, Large Animal," December 2012.

197 "but you get over it": Tove Danovich, "For 4-H Kids, Saying Goodbye to an Animal Can Be the Hardest Lesson," *The Salt,* National Public Radio, August 30, 2017.

197 sun and the outdoors: "How to Raise and Show Pigs," July 2011, http://counties.agrilife.org/lasalle/files/2011/07/How_Raise_Show_Pigs_7.pdf.

197 no opening at all: "Housing Decisions for the Growing Pig," *National Hog Farmer,* July 26, 2019.

198 just three million by 1960: Emily R. Kirby, "The Demographics of the U.S. Equine Population," in Deborah J. Salem and Andrew N. Rowan, eds., *State of the Animals IV: 2007* (Washington, D.C.: Humane Society Press, 2007), http://www.humanesociety.org/sites/default/files/archive/assets/pdfs/hsp/soaiv_07_ch10.pdf.

198 to produce chicken meat: Don Paarlberg and Philip Paarlberg, *The Agricultural Revolution of the 20th Century* (Ames, IA: Iowa State University Press, 2000).

199 more than one hundred billion: "History of Commercial Egg Production," American Egg Board website, 2019, https://www.aeb.org/farmers-and-marketers/history-of-egg-production; USDA, Economics, Statistics and Market Information System, 2017.

199 more than one million hens: American Egg Board, accessed 12/2/2015, www.aeb.org/farmers-and-marketers/industry-overview.

199 almost nine billion: National Chicken Industry, Broiler Chicken Industry Facts, accessed January 18, 2020, https://www.nationalchickencouncil.org/about-the-industry/statistics/broiler-chicken-industry-key-facts/.

199 required for indoor waste removal: Chris Mayda, "Pig Pens, Hog Houses, and Manure Pits: A Century of Change in Hog Production," *Material Culture,* 2004.

200 disappeared from the marketplace: Mayda, "Pig Pens, Hog Houses."

200 five thousand animals each: "U.S. Hog Industry, Then and Now," *Farm Journal AgWeb,* December 22, 2016, https://www.agweb.com/blog/straight-from-dc-agricultural-perspectives/the-us-hog-industry-then-and-now.

200 no pasturing at all: Larry Muller, "Pasture-Based Systems for Dairy Cows in the United States," PennState Extension website, updated May 9, 2016, https://extension.psu.edu/pasture-based-systems-for-dairy-cows-in-the-united-states.

200 increasing by more than half: Brian W. Gould, "Consolidation and Concentration in the U.S. Dairy Industry," *Choices* 25, no. 2 (2010): 1–15.

201 finished entirely on grass: Allen R. Williams, "Financial Analysis Shows Grass-Fed Beef Is Good for Producers," *Organic Producer,* July / August 2014.

201 beef production per animal since 1950: James McGrann, "The United States Beef Cattle Industry," Texas A&M University, August 9, 2010, http://agrilife.org/coastalbend/files/2012/06/The-United-States -Beef-Cattle-Industry-8-9-2010.pdf.

201 89 percent fewer animals: Judith L. Capper et al., "The Environmental Impact of Dairy Production: 1944 Compared with 2007," *Journal of Animal Science* 87 (2009): 2160–67.

201 have fallen by almost half: Erik O'Donoghue et al., "Changing Farming Practices Accompany Major Shifts in Farm Structure," *Amber Waves,* 2011.

201 declined more than one-third: "U.S. Broiler Performance," National Chicken Council website, accessed January 17, 2020, https://www .nationalchickencouncil.org/about-the-industry/statistics/u-s-broiler -performance/.

201 generating 18 percent less manure: Judith L. Capper, "The Environmental Impact of Beef Production in the United States: 1977 Compared with 2007," *Journal of Animal Science* 89, no. 12 (2011): 4249–61.

201 eggs fell nearly 80 percent: Bruce L. Gardner, *American Agriculture in the Twentieth Century: How It Flourished and What It Cost* (Cambridge, MA: Harvard University Press, 2002).

202 two-thirds smaller than it was: Frank Mitloehner, "Testimony Before the Committee on Agriculture, Nutrition and Forestry," U.S. Senate, May 21, 2019.

202 takes up to twenty cows: Mitloehner, "Testimony Before the Committee on Agriculture."

202 "starvation and misery is restored": Richard Dawkins, *River Out of Eden: A Darwinian View of Life* (New York: Basic Books, 1995), 131.

203 first week of March: Daniel Schmidt, "Death in the Deer Woods: Starvation Is Never a Pretty Sight," *Whitetail Wisdom,* December 16, 2013.

203 give the attacking chick: "Siblicide in Nature: Study of Galapagos Seabird Finds Death Can Ensure Species Survival," Wake Forest University, news release, EurekAlert!, December 6, 1996.

204 more than tripled since 1970: Danielle Nierenberg and Laura Reynolds, "Farm Animal Populations Continue to Grow," Worldwatch Institute,

May 23, 2012, https://link.springer.com/chapter/10.5822%2F978-1
-61091-457-4_13.

204 recycling nutrients: Joel Salatin, "Joel Salatin Responds to New York
     Times' 'Myth of Sustainable Meat'," *Grist*, April 17, 2012.

204 under wet and rainy conditions: E. N. Sossidou et al., "Pasture-Based
     Systems for Poultry Production: Implications and Perspectives,"
     World's Poultry Science Journal 67, no. 11 (2011): 47–58.

205 mortality rates three times as high: A. Phelps, "Alternative Systems to
     Cages Need Time, Say Researchers," *Feedstuffs*, 1991.

205 on grain in a feedlot: Daimon C. Meeh et al., "Feeding a Population
     with Smaller Scale and Alternate System Production: An Examination
     of Farm Requirements with a Multi-Species Pasture System to Feed 10
     Million People," *Renewable Agriculture and Food Systems* 29, no. 2 (June
     2014): 176–85.

206 "death need not entail suffering": Michael Pollan, *The Omnivore's
     Dilemma: A Natural History of Four Meals* (New York: Penguin, 2006), 327.

207 branded, castrated, then dehorned: D. T. Mills, "Assessment of the
     Current On-Farm Welfare of Kenyan Beef Cattle as Part of an Evalu-
     ation of the Potential of Developing Countries to Access Niche High-
     Welfare Beef Export Markets in the EU," Interim Report, ILRI, 2012,
     Nairobi, Kenya.

207 "do not save an old man": S. S. Ole Sankan, *The Maasai* (Nairobi, Kenya:
     Kenya Literature Bureau, 1971).

208 "very rich people, with many resources": Delia Grace, interview with
     the author, November 21, 2018.

209 fast-growing birds are highly profitable: Jacob Bunge, "Foul Nuggets?
     Blame Bigger Birds," *Wall Street Journal*, March 11, 2019.

210 more than six hundred pounds: Kitty Block, "Hollywood Celebrities
     Ask McDonald's to Curb Chicken Abuse," *A Humane World* (blog),
     Humane Society of the United States, September 12, 2018, https://blog
     .humanesociety.org/2018/09/hollywood-celebrities-ask-mcdonalds-to
     -curb-chicken-abuse.html.

210 high carbohydrate intake: Jacquie Jacob, "Sudden Death Syndrome in
     Poultry," *eXtension*, May 5, 2015.

210 slowing the growth of the birds: Billy M. Hargis, "Ascites Syndrome in
     Poultry," Merk Veterinary Manual, accessed January 17, 2020, https://
     www.merckvetmanual.com/poultry/miscellaneous-conditions-of
     -poultry/ascites-syndrome-in-poultry.

211 more than $5 billion a year: University of Georgia, *2018 Ag Snapshots*,
     Center for Agribusiness and Economic Development, 2018.

212 switching their purchases to smaller birds: Bunge, "Foul Nuggets?"

212 billions of added pounds of manure: Gozia Wozniacka, "The Race to Produce a Slower-Growing Chicken," *Civil Eats*, 2019.

212 toward slower-growing birds: Wozniacka, "Race to Produce."

212 replace electrical stunning: Global Animal Partnership, "5-Step Animal Welfare Rating Standards for Chickens Raised for Meat," April 3, 2018, https://globalanimalpartnership.org/wp-content/uploads/2018/04/GAP-Standard-for-Meat-Chickens-v3.1-20180403.pdf.

212 a quarter of the market: Wozniacka, "Race to Produce."

213 the cruelty had stopped: Zlati Meyer, "Tyson's Chicken Cams Will Be Monitored for Animal Cruelty," *USA Today*, June 21, 2017.

213 support for an eventual reform: Wayne Pacelle, "The Long Road to Animal Welfare: How Activism Works in Practice," *Foreign Affairs* 94, no. 4 (July/August 2015): 65–70,71–77.

213 only two farms using gestation crates: Diana Lynne, "Pigs Win Constitutional Protection," *WND*, November 6, 2002.

214 two-thirds of California voters: Sara Shields et al., "A Decade of Progress Toward Ending the Intensive Confinement of Farm Animals in the United States," *Animals*, May 2017.

214 stomping on a sick hen: Shields et al., "Decade of Progress."

214 nullify Prop 2's extended reach: "California's Proposition 12, Farm Animal Confinement Initiative," Ballotpedia, 2018, https://ballotpedia.org/California_Proposition_12,_Farm_Animal_Confinement_Initiative_(2018).

215 Whole Foods Market and Chipotle: Bob Segall, "Crate Controversy: Pig Farmers Face Growing Pressure," news story, WTHR (Indianapolis), April 14, 2016.

215 California is taking a strong lead: Deena Shanker, "Companies Are Rushing to Meet Cage-Free Egg Deadline," Bloomberg (website), March 8, 2019, https://www.msn.com/en-us/money/companies/companies-are-rushing-to-meet-cage-free-egg-deadline/ar-BBUxCrZ.

215 fully cage-free sourcing: Cathy Siegner, "Oregon Law Requires Cage-Free Eggs by 2024," *Food Dive*, August 19, 2019.

215 federal meddling with their own practices: Shields et al., "Decade of Progress."

218 quickly won two seats: M. M. van Huik and B. B. Bock, "Attitudes of Dutch Pig Farmers Towards Animal Welfare," *British Food Journal* 109, no. 11 (2007): 879–90.

218 "welfare of animals as sentient beings": C. C. Croney and S. T. Millman, "Board Invited Review: The Ethical and Behavioral Bases for

Farm Animal Welfare Legislation," *Journal of Animal Science* 85 (2007): 556–65.

219 In other words, toys: Monique Mul et al., "EU-Welfare Legislation on Pigs," Report 273, Wageningen University & Research, March 2010.

219 58 percent higher: Robert Hoste, "International Comparison of Pig Production Costs 2015," Results of InterPIG, Wageningen University & Research, April 2017.

219 not housing costs: Hoste, "Comparison of Pig Production Costs."

220 filled with different kinds of food: Aart van Bezooijen, " 'Toys for Pigs' by Sharon Geschiere Wins the First Design to Business Award," *Core 77*, July 1, 2008.

224 next generation of farmers: Andy Eubank, "Hoosier to Be Honored as 'Champion of Change' for Agriculture," *Hoosier Ag Today*, July 29, 2014.

225 animals to turn around: "A Comprehensive Review of Housing for Pregnant Sows," Task Force Report, *Journal of the American Veterinary Medicine Association* 227, no. 10 (November 15, 2005): 1580–90.

225 "foraging, movement, and postural changes": "Comprehensive Review of Housing," 1583.

Chapter 8: THE BRAVE NEW FUTURE OF FOOD

230 had fallen essentially to zero: Steven Pinker, *Enlightenment Now: The Case for Reason, Science, and Human Progress* (New York: Viking, 2018), 73.

230 11 percent in 2018: Food and Agriculture Organization of the United Nations, *State of Food and Nutrition Security in the World, 2019*, FAO website, http://www.fao.org/state-of-food-security-nutrition/en/.

231 kept most of the world's food producers: Intergovernmental Panel on Climate Change (IPCC), *Climate Change and Land*, IPCC website, August 2019, https://www.ipcc.ch/srccl/.

231 "very low food security": Alisha Coleman-Jensen et al., "Household Food Security in the United States in 2018," USDA, ERR-270, September 2019, 9, https://www.ers.usda.gov/publications/pub-details /?pubid=94848.

231 four out of ten American adults: Cheryl D. Fryar et al., "Mean Body Weight, Height, Waist Circumference, and Body Mass Index Among Adults: United States, 1999–2000. Through 2015–2016," National Health Statistics Reports, December 20, 2018; "Study: The Average American Has Grown Wider, but Not Taller," *HealthDay News*, December 20, 2018.

231 increased by almost half since 2000: World Health Organization, "Obe-

sity and Overweight," February 16, 2018, https://www.who.int/news-room/fact-sheets/detail/obesity-and-overweight.

231 population of overweight people: "Trends in Adult Body-Mass Index in 200 Countries from 1975 to 2014," *Lancet,* April 2, 2016.

232 18 percent of total food calories: Joseph Poore and T. Nemecek, "Reducing Food's Environmental Impacts Through Producers and Consumers," *Science,* June 1, 2018.

232 good news for habitat protection: Dan Blaustein-Rejto, "Achieving Peak Pasture," Breakthrough Institute, 2019, https://thebreakthrough.org/articles/achieving-peak-pasture.

232 on pastures or in feed lots: David Richards et al., "World Population Day 2017: IFPRI Models Impact of Population Growth on Demand for Food," International Food Policy Research Institute (IFPRI), July 10, 2017, https://www.ifpri.org/blog/world-population-day-2017-ifpri-models-impact-population-growth-demand-food.

232 beans, peas, or lentils: Janet Ranganathan et al., "How to Sustainably Feed 10 Billion People by 2050, in 21 Charts," World Resources Institute, December 5, 2018, https://www.wri.org/blog/2018/12/how-sustainably-feed-10-billion-people-2050-21-charts.

232 total greenhouse gas emissions: Pierre J. Gerber et al., *Tackling Climate Change Through Livestock: A Global Assessment of Emissions and Mitigation Opportunities,* Food and Agricultural Organization of the United Nations, 2013, http://www.fao.org/3/a-i3437e.pdf.

233 house with a pig inside: Weijia Huang and Dekuan Huang, "Why the Character for 'Family' Has a Pig Inside a House," *China Daily USA,* October 7, 2011.

233 "chicken in his pot": Carolyn Harris, "The Queen's Land," *Canada's History* 97, no. 4 (2017): 34–43.

233 valued ritual of manly prowess: Anne DeLessio-Parson, "Doing Vegetarianism to Destabilize the Meat-Masculinity Nexus in La Plata, Argentina," *Gender, Place & Culture* 24, no. 12 (2017): 1729–48.

233 somewhere between 29 and 70 percent: Marco Springmann et al., "Analysis and Valuation of the Health and Climate Change Cobenefits of Dietary Change," *PNAS,* April 12, 2016.

234 cutting their consumption the most: Springmann et al., "Analysis and Valuation."

234 reduced consumption of animal-based foods: Janet Ranganathan et al., "Shifting Diets for a Sustainable Food Future," World Resources Institute, April 2016, https://www.wri.org/publication/shifting-diets.

234　to feed the added two billion people: Ranganathan et al., "Shifting Diets."

234　"reduce your impact on planet Earth": Michael Pellman Rowland, "The Most Effective Way to Save the Planet," *Forbes* website, June 12, 2018, https://www.forbes.com/sites/michaelpellmanrowland/2018/06/12 /save-the-planet/#510bfc1a3c81.

235　reduced by more than half: *Food, Planet, Health: Healthy Diets from Sustainable Food Systems,*" adapted summary of *Food in the Anthropocene: The EAT-Lancet Commission on Healthy Diets from Sustainable Food Systems,* 2019. https://eatforum.org/content/uploads/2019/01/EAT -Lancet_Commission_Summary_Report.pdf.

235　world's leading nutrition scientists: Liz Crampton, "Lancet Report Opens Fresh Debate About Meat," Morning Ag, Politico, January 18, 2019.

235　scarcity, not excess, remains a leading problem for many: Kalle Hirvonen et al., "Affordability of the EAT-*Lancet* Reference Diet: A Global Analysis," *Lancet Global Health* 8, no. 1 (January 1, 2020): E59—E66.

235　3 percent are completely vegan: Maura Judkis, "You Might Think There Are More Vegetarians Than Ever. You'd Be Wrong." *Washington Post,* August 3, 2018.

236　"consumption of red or processed meats": Alison Auld And Ryan Mcnutt, "Behind the Beef: Dal-Led Research on Red and Processed Meats Challenges Orthodoxy, Stirs Controversy," *Dal News,* October 1, 2019.

236　consumption that much more difficult: Tara Parker-Pope and Anahad O'Connor, "Scientist Who Discredited Meat Guidelines Didn't Report Past Food Industry Ties," *New York Times,* October 4, 2019.

236　"animals will need to be killed": Richard Branson, "Clean Meat Is the Future of Meat," Virgin website, February 13, 2018, https://www .virgin.com/richard-branson/clean-meat-future-meat.

236　demand for cow-based products: Catherine Tubb and Tony Seba, "Rethinking Food and Agriculture 2020–2030," RethinkX, September 2019, https://www.rethinkx.com/food-and-agriculture.

237　from $4.6 billion to $85 billion: Cathy Siegner, "Plant-Based Meat Market Forecast to Reach $85 Billion by 2030, Report Says," *Food Dive,* July 22, 2019.

237　sales of authentic dairy milk: Cathy Siegner, "Why Lab-Created Milk Is a Threat to Dairy Farmers," *Food Dive,* February 26, 2019.

238　cheese, yogurt, and ice cream: Chase Purdy, "A Tech Startup Is Making

Convincing Cow-Free Milk by Genetically Engineering Yeast," *Quartz,* December 20, 2017.

238 equivalent of one million real eggs: Megan Poinski, "JUST Egg Cracks the Substitute Category Wide Open," *Food Dive,* February 21, 2019.

238 three-quarters of the global sweetener market: Cathy Siegner, "Ain't Nothin' Like the Real Thing? Analysts Look at the Long Game for Meat Alternatives," *Food Dive,* August 2, 2019.

238 in just the last two years: Cathy Siegner, "$16B Invested in Plant-Based and Cell-Cultured Meat Since 2009," *Food Dive,* May 7, 2019.

238 valued at $2 billion: Christopher Doering, "Impossible Foods Raises $300 Million as Exec Touts Long Runway for Growth," *Food Dive,* May 13, 2019.

239 valuable client relationships: Cathy Siegner, "Lightlife Foods Launches a Plant-Based Burger," *Food Dive,* January 24, 2019.

239 "want to convert the world": Emma Liem, "Plant-Based Meat Sizzles at NRA Show as Brands Eye Retail," *Restaurant Dive,* March 21, 2019.

239 says it wants to replace animals: Cathy Siegner, "Impossible Burger Will Be Sold in Grocery Stores Next Year," *Grocery Dive,* November 9, 2018.

239 "move quickly into the marketplace": Christopher Doering, "Impossible Foods Raises $300M as Exec Touts Long Runway for Growth," *Food Dive,* May 13, 2019.

240 three hundred million egg whites a year: Lilianna Byington, "Why Kellogg's MorningStar Farms Is Going 100% Plant Based," *Food Dive,* March 13, 2019.

240 "separately under a suitable medium": Kat Eschner, "Winston Churchill Imagined the Lab-Grown Hamburger," Smithsonian.com, December 1, 2017, https://www.smithsonianmag.com/smart-news/winston-churchill-imagined-lab-grown-hamburger-180967349/.

240 first cultured pork sausage: Deena Shanker and Lydia Mulvany, "We'll Always Eat Meat. But More of It Will Be 'Meat,'" Bloomberg Businessweek, January 25, 2019, https://www.bloomberg.com/news/articles/2019-01-25/we-ll-always-eat-meat-why-more-of-it-won-t-be-meat-quicktake.

240 duck tasted as advertised: Amanda Little, *The Fate of Food: What We'll Eat in a Bigger, Hotter, Smarter World* (New York: Harmony, 2019), 177.

241 and Meat the Future: Shenggen Fan, "Alternative Meat Can Sustain Food Systems," IFPRI blog, November 26, 2019, https://www.ifpri.org/blog/alternative-meat-can-sustain-food-systems.

241 "meat, fish and dairy foods": Pat O. Brown, Impossible Foods, "An Open Letter from Our CEO," August 10, 2017, https://www.facebook.com/ImpossibleFoods/posts/an-open-letter-from-our-ceoto-our-communitythe-new-york-times-published-an-aug-8/1524134577643350/.

241 96 percent less dependent: Cathy Siegner, "Impossible Burger Boasts Much Smaller Carbon Footprint Than Beef," Food Dive, March 22, 2019.

242 product lived up to its name: Pat Sharpe, "Plant-Based Burgers That Taste Like Meat? That's Impossible," Texas Monthly, June 22, 2017.

242 the form of fresh ground beef: M. Shahbandeh, "Category Share of Beef Sales in the United States in 2019, by Cut Type," Statista, October 22, 2019, https://www.statista.com/statistics/191269/fresh-beef-category-share-in-2011/.

242 "This is a f——ing cow!": Alexandra Deabler, "Burger King Pranks Customers with Vegetarian 'Impossible Whopper,'" Fox News, April 1, 2019.

242 beans, lentils, or sunflower seeds: Frank B. Hu, Brett O. Otis, and Gina McCarthy, "Can Plant-Based Meat Alternatives Be Part of a Healthy and Sustainable Diet?," JAMA 322, no. 16 (October 2019): 1547–48.

243 "not just a niche product": Nathaniel Popper, "Behold the Beefless 'Impossible Whopper,'" New York Times, April 1, 2019.

243 its Oakland, California, plant: Doering, "Impossible Foods Raises $300m."

243 "make vegetables out of meat?": Corinne Reichert, "Arby's Is Making Vegetables Out of Meat," CNET, June 28, 2019, https://www.cnet.com/news/arbys-is-making-vegetables-out-of-meat/.

243 reached a competitive price point: Haley Swartz, "The Role of Plant-Based, Meatless Meats in Sustainable Diets," Food Climate Research Network, July 27, 2017, https://www.fcrn.org.uk/fcrn-blogs/role-plant-based-meatless-meats-sustainable-diets.

243 more than two hundred dollars: Marta Zaraska, "Meeting Meat-Eaters Halfway," Breakthrough Journal, March 2019.

244 "cell-based foods as well": Nathaniel Popper, "You Call That Meat? Ranchers Beg to Differ," New York Times, February 9, 2019.

244 "eating meat doesn't have to be a problem": Cathy Siegner, "Applegate Farms Launches Sausage Line Sourced from Regenerative Agriculture," Food Dive, February 19, 2019.

245 even to Beyond and Impossible burgers: Mariko Thorbecke and Jon Dettling, "Carbon Footprint Evaluation of Regenerative Grazing at White Oak Pastures, Results Presentation," Quantis, February 2019.

245 the emissions became negative: Paige L. Stanley et al., "Impacts of Soil Carbon Sequestration on Life Cycle Greenhouse Gas Emissions in Midwestern USA Beef Finishing Systems," *Agricultural Systems,* May 2018.

245 "which is the ultimate goal": Alice Robb, "Bloody, Meaty Veggie Burgers? Vegetarians Don't Want That," *New Republic,* October 13, 2014.

245 "because of the processing": Alex Trembath, "The Fake Backlash to Fake Meat," *OneZero,* August 12, 2019.

246 "highly processed foods": Jade Scipioni, "Whole Foods CEO on Plant-Based Meat Boom: Good for the Environment But Not for Your Health," CNBC, August 21, 2019,

246 "disodium inosinate": Advertisement, "What's Hiding in Your Plant-Based Meat?" *New York Times,* October 28, 2019.

246 "we need to be careful": Quoted in Queena Kim, "Plant-Based Hamburger Leaves 'Blood' on the Plate," *Marketplace,* October 15, 2014.

246 "Doesn't mean I'm against it": Kate Smith, "Fake Vegan Meatballs Might Save the World Says Author, Michael Pollan," *Live Kindly,* December 4, 2018.

246 "capitalize on animal welfare concerns": "'Bleeding' Veggie Burger Has 'No Basis for Safety,' According to FDA," ETC Group website, August 8, 2017.

247 fed with a nutrient mix: Cathy Siegner, "Plant-Based Tuna Launches at Whole Foods and Thrive Market," *Grocery Dive,* February 21, 2019.

247 faux fish will also be a part: Clare Leschin-Hoar, "Seafood Without the Sea: Will Lab-Grown Fish Hook Consumers?," *The Salt,* National Public Radio, May 5, 2019.

248 Probiotics and CLA: Hank Cardello, *Stuffed: An Insider's Look at Who's (Really) Making America Fat and How the Food Industry Can Fix It* (New York: Harper Collins, 2009).

248 nut butters, soups, and nutrition bars: Monica Watrous, "Whole Foods Names Top 10 Trends for 2019," *Food Business News,* November 15, 2018.

248 from a health-care background: Jessi Devenyns, "Big Food Filling C-Suite Ranks with a New Kind of CEO," *Food Dive,* August 10, 2018.

248 bottled water drink named LifeWTR: Christopher Doering, "PepsiCo Pivots Away from Sugary Drinks with $3.2 Billion Sodastream Buy," *Food Dive,* August 20, 2018.

249 about half of its total revenue: "GMA Reboot: 'We Are Not the Food Industry,'" Morning Ag, Politico, March 27, 2019.

249 committed to consumer transparency: Cathy Siegner, "Danone, Mars,

Nestle, and Unilever Launch Sustainable Food Policy Alliance," *Food Dive*, July 13, 2018.

249 other healthy options: Margarita Raycheva, "Food Retail Industry Feels Pressure to Offer Healthier Checkouts," *IEG Policy*, October 12, 2018.

249 nutrition balance, dietary health, or obesity: Jaewon Kang, "A Taste of AI," *Wall Street Journal*, October 10, 2019.

250 "we've really got nothing": Greg Drescher, Speech delivered at Culinary Institute of America, May 21, 2019.

250 sauces they desire: Bee Wilson, "For Your Mouth Only: Welcome to the Era of Personalized Food," *Economist*, February/March 2019.

250 headquartered in Columbus, Ohio: "Print Pizza Any Shape You Want," *Fine Dining Lovers*, March 3, 2017.

251 size of the nugget coming out: Annie Gasparro and Jesse Newman, "The Future of Food," *Wall Street Journal*, October 3, 2018.

251 today's consumption of digital music: Amit Zoran and Marcelo Coelho, "Cornucopia: The Concept of Digital Gastronomy," *Leonardo* 44, no. 5 (2011): 425–31.

251 will have the edge: Gareth Hockley and Mathew Lincez, "What Connected Culinary Could Mean for Big Food," *Idea Couture*, July 19, 2017.

251 farther down an ecomodernist path: Rob Mitchum, "The Big Data Harvest," Envision, Purdue College of Agriculture, Fall 2017.

252 vegetable fields dry and unplanted: Eris Holthaus, "The Thirsty West: 10 Percent of California's Water Goes to Almond Farming," *Slate*, May 14, 2014.

252 only as much as needed: Matthew J. Grassi, "Inside California Irrigation: Winters Farming," *Precision Ag*, January 9, 2018.

253 see more than the human eye: Markus Weber, "Agricultural Drones: From Detection to Diagnosis," *PrecisionAg*, January 2, 2018.

254 used on herbicide-tolerant crops: Matthew J. Grassi, "How Blue River's See & Spray Technology Could Change Agriculture Forever," *PrecisionAg*, August 5, 2017.

254 "the cows did that": Yifang Wang, "Facial Recognition Software Meets Its Match: Farm Animals," *Wall Street Journal*, May 1, 2019.

254 possibly even farmed fish: Gasparro and Newman, "Future of Food."

254 may not pay off: Grassi, "Inside California Irrigation."

255 acres of U.S. cropland: Karl Plume, "Monsanto's Climate Corp to Expand Digital Farming Platform," Reuters, August 17, 2016.

255 supplying advanced aerial imagery: Matt Hopkins, "The Climate Corp., Deveron Form Drone Analytics Partnership," *PrecisionAg*, November 18, 2017.

255 "blinds its practitioners": Quoted in Jayson Lusk, *Unnaturally Delicious: How Science and Technology Are Serving Up Super Foods to Save the World* (New York: St. Martin's Press, 2016), 106.

255 with sub-inch accuracy: Doug Weist, "Sub-Inch GPS," FarmTech website, 2015, accessed January 22, 2020, https://farmtech.us/sub-inch-gps/.

255 insects resistant to the chemicals: Harold van Es et al., "Digital Agriculture in New York State: Report and Recommendations," Cornell University, College of Agriculture and Life Sciences, Cornell University, November 2016.

255 without any reduction in yield: Lusk, *Unnaturally Delicious*.

256 GPS auto-steering: David Schimmelpfennig, "Farm Profits and Adoption of Precision Agriculture," USDA, ERS Report 217, October 2016.

256 with no loss of yield: Manik Kundu and Biswapati Mandal, "Mani-Agricultural Activities Influence Nitrate and Fluoride Contamination in Drinking Groundwater of an Intensively Cultivated District in India," *Water, Air, and Soil Pollution* 198 (March 2009): 243–52.

257 gain an added $144 per hectare annually: Dharini Parthasrathy, "Laser Technology to Level Farm Land Saves Water and Energy," CGIAR Research Program on Climate Change, Agriculture and Food Security, May 25, 2015.

257 different depth levels in the soil: Richard Stirzaker, "Turning Water into Food: A Soil Water Sensor for Resource Poor Farmers," Australian International Food Security Centre (AIFSRC), 2012.

258 done by Nicaraguans: John Seabrook, "The Age of Robot Farmers," *New Yorker*, April 8, 2019.

258 two-thirds of all hired workers: Economic Research Service (USDA), "Farm Labor," October 23, 2019, https://www.ers.usda.gov/topics/farm-economy/farm-labor/.

258 discovered the work was too hard: Seabrook, "Age of Robot Farmers."

258 also on the verge: Philip Martin, *Importing Poverty? Immigration and the Changing Face of Rural America* (New Haven, CT: Yale University Press, 2009).

259 more space to grow: Gosia Wozniacka, "AND NOW: Robots Are About to Take All the Farm Jobs," *Business Insider*, July 15, 2013.

259 easier for the robots: Matt Simon, "Why Robots Should Shake the Bejeezus Out of Cherry Trees," *Science*, January 24, 2018.

259 identify which tomatoes are ripe: Hiawatha Bray, "Farm Robots: The Next Growth Industry?," *Boston Globe*, March 29, 2019.

261 the shortages persist: Michael Larkin, "Labor Terminators: Farming

Robots Are About to Take Over Our Farms," *Investor's Business Daily,* August 10, 2018.

261 had increased wages: California Farm Bureau Federation, "Survey: California Farms Face Continuing Employee Shortages," April 30, 2019.

262 covers eight acres in a day: Harvestcroo.com, "About Harvest Croo," Harvest Croo Robotics, accessed January 2020, https://harvestcroo.com/about/.

263 "unless you have to": Andy Fell, "Smart Farm," Food and Agriculture News, University of California (Davis), January 24, 2018.

264 multiple layers of clothing and earmuffs: Marnette Federis, "How Immigrant Workers Are Preparing for Automation in Agriculture," *PRI's the World,* October 17, 2019, https://www.pri.org/stories/2019-10-17/how-immigrant-workers-are-preparing-automation-agriculture.

Epilogue: STRAIGHT TALK TO COMMERCIAL FARMERS

268 "needs of farmers in the Midwest": Bernard Weinraub, "Campaign Trail; For Quayle, a Search for Belgian Endive," *New York Times,* September 20, 1988.

268 "people telling them to go organic": Jeffrey Goldberg, "Central Casting," *New Yorker,* May 21, 2006.

269 "any developed nation in the world": Quoted in Carol Spaeth-Bower, "Chairman Conaway Introduces Agriculture and Nutrition Act," *Wisconsin State Farmer,* April 12, 2018.

269 "we all want the same thing": Andrew Lawler, "Has the Food Movement's Moment Finally Arrived?" *Slate,* November 17, 2014.

270 "consumers in the cities": American Farm Bureau Federation, 2018 Annual Convention, Farm2Table Food Forum, January 7, 2018.

271 transparently self-serving reasons: Quoted in "Farm Bureau Takes Exception to Lunch Regulations," *Sidney Herald,* September 29, 2012.

271 "OK with your kids eating crap": Peter Robison and Linda Mulvany, "Big Dairy Is About to Flood America's School Lunches with Milk," *Bloomberg Businessweek,* January 9, 2019.

272 "audience of commodity farmers": Eric Mortenson, "American Farm Bureau Federation Holds Steady," *Capital Press,* January 14, 2015.

273 political contributions to Republicans: Center for Responsive Politics, "Food & Beverage: Long-Term Contribution Trends," Open Secrets.org, accessed January 22, 2020, https://www.opensecrets.org/industrie/totals.php?cycle=2018&ind=N01.

273 90 percent of the vote: Mitch Smith, "Frustration Mounts Among

Farmers as China Trade Talks Break Down," *New York Times,* May 10, 2019.

274   the "healthier choice" foods: Bridget Kelly and Jo Jewell, *What Is the Evidence on the Policy Specifications, Development Processes and Effectiveness of Existing Front-of-Pack Food Labelling Policies in the WHO European Region?,* World Health Organization, 2018, http://www.euro.who.int/en/publications/abstracts/what-is-the-evidence-on-the-policy-specifications,-development-processes-and-effectiveness-of-existing-front-of-pack-food-labelling-policies-in-the-who-european-region-2018.

275   so long as it was not deceptive: Mary L. Azcuenaga, "The Role of Advertising and Advertising Regulation in the Free Market," Federal Trade Commission, April 8, 1997.

275   prohibiting any FTC action: Mary Story and Simone French, "Food Advertising and Marketing Directed at Children and Adolescents in the US," *International Journal of Behavioral Nutrition and Physical Activity* 1, no. 3 (2004): 1–17.

275   killing the effort once again: Robert Paarlberg, *The United States of Excess* (New York: Oxford University Press, 2015).

276   exceed guideline limits: World Cancer Research Fund International, "Restrict Food Advertising and Other Forms of Commercial Promotion," NOURISHING Framework, October 2018, https://www.wcrf.org/sites/default/files/Restrict-advertising.pdf.

276   "We are not Denmark!": Catherine Boyle, "Clinton and Sanders: Why the Big Deal About Denmark?," CNBC, October 14, 2015.

Index

Page numbers of illustrations appear in italics.

Adamchak, Raoul, 183
AeroFarms, Newark, N.J., 110, *110*
Africa, 7, 139–40, 145, 164–66, 231
  gene editing, 189, 192–93
  GMOs, 171, 178–81, 193
  livestock, 15, 205–8, 232, 234, 244
  new tools for small farms, 256–57
  rural hunger, poverty, 3–4, *4*, 139,
    158, 164–65, 181, 194, *230*
  Yudelman and, 170
  See also green revolution; *specific*
    countries
Agnew, Eleanor, 129
Agricultural Course (Steiner), 119
Agricultural Testament (Howard),
  119–20
Agriflora company, 179
agroecology, 14, 140–42, 150, 151,
  152–59, 160, 161, 166, 170, 267
Ahold Delhaize, 46, 60, 63, 249
Alcott, Bronson, 11–12, *12*, 82
Alcott, Louisa May, 11–12
Aldi, 249
Aleph Farms, Israel, 240
Alliance for a Green Revolution in
  Africa, 145

Altieri, Miguel A., 153, 155, 156
Amazon, 251
Animal Liberation (Singer), 206
Applebee's, 13, 66–69, *68*
Applegate Farms, 244
Aramark, 212, 213
Arby's, 243
Argentina, 176
Asia, 231
  "East Asian Miracle," 229
  GMOs, 171, 178–79, 181–82
  green revolution, 141–42, 144, 150,
    155, 228
  new tools for small farms, 256–57
  rural hunger, poverty, in, 165, *230*
  See also specific countries
Ausubel, Jesse, 36
Avocado, Nikocado, 66

Back from the Land (Agnew), 129
back-to-the-land movement, 128–30
Baker, Rodney, 99
Balfour, Lady Eve, 121–22
Baltimore, Md., urban farming, 108
"Baltimore Food Hub," 107
Barber, Dan, 20

Bassey, Nnimmo, 193
Beeson, Kenneth, 130
Belasco, Warren, 128, 129
Benedict, Neb., 39
Berry, Wendell, 26, 81–82, 101, 255
Beyond Burgers and Beyond Meat,
   69–70, 237, 238, 240, 242, 245
Bible, Geoffrey, 54
Bill and Melinda Gates Foundation,
   145, 192
Biodynamic Association (BDA), 118
biotech food, 168–94
   companies developing, 171–72
   CRISPR, 170, 185–88, 187
   Europe and, 168, 171, 173, 185,
      188–90
   gene editing, 15, 172, 184–94
   GMOs, 168–83
   opponents, 172, 173, 178–82
   Paarlberg's interest in, 170–71
   Ronald and, 182–83
   Trump deregulation and, 187
Bittman, Mark, 5, 7, 245, 269
BlueNalu, 247
Blue River Company, 260
   LettuceBot, 258–59, 260
   See & Spray, 253, 258, 260
Bon Appétit, 212
Borlaug, Norman, 143, 145–47, 146,
   151, 158
Bosch, Carl, 116–17, 120
Branson, Richard, 236, 238, 239
Brazil, 85, 95, 150, 170, 171, 176,
   219
Brin, Sergey, 238
Brooklyn Grange, N.Y.C., 109
Brown, Cheryl, 87
Brown, Patrick, 241
Bumble Bee, 247
Burger King, 72, 213, 214, 242, 243
Burt, Austin, 192
Butz, Earl, 24

Cadbury, 51
Cahillane, Steve, 248
Cainthus company, 254
California, Propositions 2 and 12,
   195, 214, 215–17
Camden, N.J., urban gardens, 107
Canada, 103, 128, 160–61, 172, 186,
   219, 224, 239, 242
Cardello, Hank, 53–54
Cargill, 239, 240, 254
Carl's Jr. restaurants, 242
Carson, Rachel, 113, 124–26, 125,
   137
cell-grown meat and seafood, 237,
   238, 240–41, 243–44, 247
Center for Food Integrity, 190
Central Valley, Calif., 91, 263
Charles, Prince of Wales, 122, 152
Chavez, Cesar, 263
Chavez, Hugo, 166
Cheesecake Factory, 73
Chef 3D printer by BeeHex, 250
Chesapeake Bay, 37–38
Chile, 91, 150, 153, 153, 275
China, 91, 120, 137, 161–62, 170, 192,
   224, 233, 273
   GMO rice and maize seeds, 171
   green revolution and, 144
   hunger, poverty, in, 121, 228, 231
   meat alternatives in, 241
   organic food exports, 134, 137
   obesity in, 231
Chipotle, 71–72, 98, 212, 215, 245
Choice Market, 60
Churchill, Winston, 240
Clark Farm, Carlisle, Mass., 82–86,
   87–89, 89, 138
climate change, 201–2, 230–32, 237,
   244–45, 265
Climate FieldView, 255
Clinton, Bill, 24
Clinton, Hillary, 276

Coca-Cola, 48, 53, 56
Cochrane Collaboration, 74
Cockburn, Alexander, 146
College of Tropical Agriculture
    (CSAT), Mexico, 151
community supported agriculture
    (CSA), 5, 12, 13, 14, 81–89, 101–2,
    109, 135
Compassion by the Pound (Norwood),
    195
ConAgra, 56, 135, 239, 240, 249
Conaway, Mike, 269
Conway, Sir Gordon, 149, 169–70
Coody, Lynn, 133
corn and soybean production, 9,
    22–25, 35, 124
  gene-edited crops and, 191
  Nidlinger Farms, Ind., 30–34
  organic farming and, 130
  smart seeds and, 32–33
Costa Rica, 258
Costco, 135, 215
CRISPR, 170, 185–88, 187, 190, 193
  Anopheles mosquitoes, 192–93
  -Cas9, 186, 192
  medical applications, 186
  precision guided sterile insect
    technique (pgSIT), 193
  regulatory status, 186–90
  used on human embryos, 192
Cuba, 156–57, 159
Culinary Breeding Network, 20
CVS Pharmacy, 49
Cywinski, John, 67

Danone North America, 249
Dawkins, Richard, 202
DeGregori, Thomas R., 149
de Schutter, Olivier, 141, 159
Desrochers, Pierre, 100
Detroit, Mich., 107
  RecoveryPark Farms, 107–8

DiCaprio, Leonardo, 238
Diet for a Small Planet (Lappé),
    182–83
Dimitri, Carolyn, 106
Donatos pizza chain, 250
Dorito Effect, The (Schatzker), 19
Drescher, Greg, 249–50
Dr Pepper Snapple, 56
Dukakis, Michael, 267–68
Dunkin' Donuts, 72, 73, 242
Dupont company, 171–72

Earthbound Farm, Calif., 134
Earth First, 183
EAT-Lancet Commission, 234–36
ecomodernism, 10, 38, 251–56
Editas biotech company, 186
Ehrlich, Paul, 142
El Pilar Forest Garden Network,
    Belize, 154
environmental concerns
  agricultural land and, 232, 234
  animal products and, 37, 232, 234
  aquifer depletion, 36
  biodiversity and, 149
  black plastic "mulch" and, 138
  CSA and, 88–89, 100–101
  Dust Bowl of the 1930s and, 29
  excessive eating and, 231–32
  factory farms and, 201–2
  farm animals and, 201–2, 225–26,
    232, 237, 244
  faux meats and, 237–38, 241
  fertilizer runoff, damage from, 37
  gene editing and, 193
  GMO seeds and, 32–33
  green revolution and, 145, 147, 149,
    159–60
  high-yield farming and, 141
  "holistic" grazing and, 244
  insecticides and herbicides, 124,
    125, 127–28

environmental concerns *(continued)*
 locally sourced food, 100–101
 milpa farming, 153–54
 modern farming and, 9, 28–38, 44,
  174
 organic farming and, 5, 113, 126,
  131, 138
 PA and, *31, 32–35, 34,* 44, 255
 preindustrial farming and, 29
 soil erosion, 35, 152
 sustainability and, 130, 241
 water use and, 35, 36, 157, 160, 252,
  254, 257
 wheat production and, 36
Environmental Protection Agency
 (EPA), 36, 126, 127, 128, 131, 132,
 187
Ethiopia, 165–66, 178
Europe
 biotech food, 168, 171, 173, 185,
  188–90
 Blair House Agreement, 162
 farm animal welfare, 6, 18, 212,
  217–23
 food ads and children, 275–76
 France, Label Rouge, 212
 front-of-package nutrition guidance
  system, 273–74
 gene-editing/CRISPR crops,
  172–73, 185, 188–89
 globalization and, 162
 GMOs, 168, 171, 174–76, 179, 181,
  185, 188
 meat consumption and, 233
 meat contamination and, 174
 obesity rates vs. U.S., 18, 274
 organic farming and, 189
 Treaty of Amsterdam, 218
European Peasants' Coordination
 (CPE), 162
Evenson, Robert, 145

factory farms (livestock industry), 6,
 196, 197
 animal welfare, 98, 202–5, 210–27
 beef cattle production, 200–201
 breeding practices, 211–12, *211*
 certification systems, 212
 chickens, 199, 209–13, *209, 211*
 concentrated animal feeding
  operations (CAFOs), 15, 98
 confinement systems, 6, 98–99, 198,
  199, 200, 202–4, 209
 crate-free pork, 214–15
 egg producers, 198–99, 204–5, 214,
  215
 environmental impact, 37, 201–2
 food safety and, 98–99
 labor and, 42, 198, 201, 205
 lower consumer costs and, 205
 market competition and, 198
 meat exporting, 224
 milk production, 198, 200, 202
 organic dairy farms, *137,* 138
 organic egg production, 135–36
 overbreeding and, 203
 pig industry, 199–200, 213–15
 progressive pig farms, 23, 217–27
 reduced costs of, 201
 slaughtering, 199, 203, 211, 212
 social benefits of, 201
 waste disposal, *225–26*
 See also farm animals
family farms, 4, 6, 39, 40–43, 44
 average price per acre, 44
 commercial farms as, 269
 farming communities, 40–41
 income/net worth and, 28, 43
 lifestyle farms, 38–44, 97, 207, 265
 local food and, 76, 77–111
 loss of, 39–40, 42, 200
 percentage of farms, 43
 progressive pig farm, 15, 223–27

service providers for, 254–55
See also specific farms
Famine in England (Wallop), 121
Famine 1975! (Paddock and Paddock), 142
Fanjul brothers, 24
Farmageddon (Lymbery), 5
farm animals, 15, 20, 195–227
  agricultural land and, 232, 234
  animal welfare groups, 213–17, *217*
  antibiotic free (ABF) meats, 72
  beef cattle, 200–201, 205
  CAFOs and, 15, 98–99
  chickens, 15, 199, 209–13, *209, 211*
  CSA farming model and, 84, 85
  dairy cows, 198, 200
  Depression-era rhyme, 42
  egg-laying hens, 195, 198–99, 204–5, 214, 215
  facial recognition and, 254
  family farms and, 41–42
  FDA and, 191
  faux products and, 6, 10, 15, 69–70, 232–47
  4-H club and, 196–97
  gene editing and, 186–87, 191–92
  GMO animals, 191
  grazing systems, 244–45
  greenhouse gas emissions and, 201–2, 232, 244
  market competition and, 198
  measuring happiness in, 208
  meat animals not named, 207
  mistreatment, 13, 195, 197, 203–4
  number of, 204
  organic farms, 113, 135–38, *137*
  outdoors or indoors, 198, 208–9
  parasites, pathogens, and, 99
  pastoralist communities, 205–7
  pasture, barnyard systems, 204–5

  pigs, 15, 199–200, 204, 206, 209, 214–15, 217–27, 244, 269
  replaced by machines, 197–98
  slaughtering, 206, 207, 208
  stressed animals, 208, 224–25
  traditional animal husbandry, 196–98, *196*, 204
  veal calves, 214
  welfare regulations, 6, 12, 13, 195, 214, 215, 217–23, 265
  Whole Foods rating system, 85
  wild animals vs., 202–3
  See also factory farms
Farm Bill of 2018, 269, 272
Farm Bureau, 270
FarmedHere, Chicago, Ill., *110*, 111
farmers markets, 5, 6, 9, 12, 14, 76, 97, 81, 88, 101–5, *104*, 135
Farmer-to-Consumer Direct Marketing Act of 1976, 104–5
Farm Foundation, 271
farming, 4, 6–7, 12, 20, 29, 31, *35*, 38, 41
  African American past and, 81
  agroecology, 14, 139–42, 150, 151, 154–59, 161, 166, 170
  ancient systems, 151–53
  biotech methods, 168–94
  CSA, 5, 13, 12, 14, 78, 81–89, 101–2, 109, 135
  ecomodernism, 10, 38, 251–56
  falling farm population, 38, 124
  farm animals, 195–227
  farm laborers, 258, 261, 263–64
  farm wages, 91, 261
  food's nutrient content and, 19–20
  government subsidies, 9, 19, 22, 28
  hard physical labor of, 7, 40, 85, 140, 198, 258, 263–64
  high-yield seeds, 142–49

farming *(continued)*
  industrial or commercial
    agriculture, 17–44, 251–56
  locally sourced food, 12–13, 18,
    77–111
  machines, 257–64, *260*, *262*
  organic farming, 5, 6, 112–38
  productivity, 29–30, *30*, 34–35
  rural hunger, poverty, and, 6, 7,
    139–67
  science-based methods, 29, 31–35,
    31, *34*, 140, 159 (*see also* precision
    agriculture)
  social values and, 39
  USDA definition of a farm, 38
  See also agroecology; factory
    farms; farm animals; industrial or
    commercial agriculture; organic
    farming
farm-to-table restaurants, 10, 87
fast-food chain restaurants, 10, 50
  animal welfare and, 213, 214–15
  antibiotic free chicken and, 71–72
  calories on menus, 72–74, *73*
  chains designated healthy, 70–71
  dimethylpolysiloxane used, 65
  excessive calories and, 65–66, 71
  excessive salt and, 71
  food cooked elsewhere and, 65
  healthier foods and, 71–72
  meat substitutes used at, 242
  portion sizes, 20, *21*, 71
  progressive change and, 70–71
  study of items (2019), 71
  types of restaurant goers and, 70
  See also restaurant chains
Fast Food Nation (Schlosser), 18–19
faux meat, milk, fish, and eggs,
    6, 10, 15, 69–70, 216, 232–47,
    265
Fearing, Jennifer, and Fearless
    Advocacy, 216–17, *217*

fertilizers, 9, 14, 116, 121, 150
  Cuba and, 157
  green revolution and, 150, 155
  new tools for small farms, 256–57
  nitrogen, 6, 35, 36, 37, 116–17, 121,
    123, 124, 137, 155
  organic, 14, 113, 114
  PA and, 9, 13, 33, 34, 255–57
Field to Market study (2016), 36
Finless Foods, 247
Food, Inc. (film), 8, 22
food companies, 18–19, 45–65
  added sugars, 51, 52, 54–55
  advertising and marketing, 13,
    47–49, *47*, 52, 56, 60
  Big Ag and, 15, 270–73
  checkout-free technology, 60
  children, teens targeted, 13, 53,
    275–76
  consumer preferences and, 55
  diet quality gap and, 75
  excessive eating and, 45–46, *46*, 48,
    51–54
  faux-meat sector investments,
    239
  food labels and, 60–65, 273–74
  health claims and, 248
  healthy products, 55, 56, 58–59,
    247–50, 270
  lobbyists and, 24, 57, 58, 275
  obesity and, 45, 52, 55
  organic products, 11, 134, 244
  political affiliation of, 273
  poultry companies, 210
  processed foods, 13, 26–27, *27*
  product development, 51–52
  reduced sugar or sugar-free
    products, 55
  snacks, 45, 51
  sugary beverages, 56–58, 75
  ten largest, 56
  ultraprocessed foods, 95

unhealthy products, 13, 51–52, 56
See also specific companies
food costs, 10
    federal policies and, 9, 23–25
    junk vs. healthy foods, 27–28
    organic foods, 112, 115–16, 133, 136
    processed foods and, 26–27, 27
    restaurant eating and, 136
food delivery apps (Uber Eats,
    Grubhub, DoorDash), 55–56, 72
food deserts, 50–51
food imports, 23, 24, 78, 79, 91, 131,
    137, 141, 156, 157, 165
Foodini, 250–51
food labels, labeling laws, 60–65, 96,
    184, 244, 273–74
    Facts Up Front, 61–62, 65
    Guiding Stars, 63–65, 64, 274
Food Lion markets, 63
Food Marketing Institute, 53, 65, 193
food movement, 7–10, 12–13, 102,
    105–6, 245–46, 265
"Food Movement, Rising, The"
    (Pollan), 7
Food Network, 70–71
Food Policy Councils (FPCs), 103
Food Politics (Nestle), 19
Food Quality Protection Act, 127
food safety, 4, 96–100
    adoption of HACCP systems, 97
    Alar on apples, 131, 133, 173
    consumers ignoring science, 173
    factory farms and, 98–99
    gene-edited crops and, 173
    GMOs and, 176–77, 181, 184
    home raised poultry, 99–100
    incidences of illness, 96
    locally sourced food and, 96–98
    meat and, 99
    pigs, diseases of, and, 99
    radiation technique and, 169
    what causes problems, 96

Food Safety Modernization Law,
    97–98
food sovereignty, 14, 160–61,
    166–67
food swamp, 45–76
    food companies and, 45–59
    as predictor of obesity, 50
    promising trends, 74–76
    restaurant chains and, 65–74
    supermarket products, 59–65
food transport, 5, 78, 90–91, 100
Fooducate, 48, 93
4-H club, 196–97, 196, 204
Fresco, Louise O., 113
Friends of the Earth, 158, 163, 171,
    173, 180, 188, 246
Frito-Lay, 51, 52, 55, 272
Frosted Flakes, 93
Fruitlands, 11–12, 12
fruits and vegetables, 17
    American diet and, 22, 28, 74
    availability per capita, 92
    delocalization and, 89–90, 91
    "Dirty Dozen" report, 132–33
    farm land use and, 22, 25–26
    federal policies and, 9, 23, 25–26
    food safety, 96–100, 115, 131–33
    gene-edited varieties, 191
    immigrant farm labor and, 81, 258,
        261, 263–64
    imports, 23, 91–92
    locally sourced, 6, 84, 89
    organic produce, 115
    packinghouses, 264
    prices and, 23, 25–26, 27
    processed, 90, 92, 94
    recommended daily amount, 47
    robotic harvesting, 15, 258–65, 260,
        262
    shelf tag systems and, 64
    spoilage problem, 88, 94
    USDA Thrifty Food Plan and, 28

Funes-Monzote, Fernando, 156
future of food, 228–66
  AI-enabled products, 249
  America's dietary health, 247–51
  animal products and, 232–34
  excessive eating and, 231–32, 233
  faux animal products, 232–47
  healthier food choices, 247–50
  historical predictions, 228, 237
  PA and new technology, 251–56
  personalized foods, 250–51
  planetary health diet, 234–36
  population increase, 228–29, 229
  retreat of hunger and, 228–30
  robotic harvesting, 15, 257–65, 260,
    262
  3D food printing, 250–51
  undernourishment, 230–31, 231

Gasteratos, Kristopher, 244
Gates, Bill, 183, 238
gene editing, 15, 172, 184–94
  Africa and, 189
  of animals, 186–87, 191–92
  critics of, 189
  FDA and, 191
  first gene-edited meal, 187
  first U.S. product marketed, 187
  of humans, 192
  of insects, 192–93
  of plants, 186–88, 190–91
  potential dangers of, 193, 194
  regulations and, 188–90
  transgenic GMO methods vs., 190
  USDA and, 186, 187
General Mills, 54–55, 56, 272
Genoways, Ted, 39
Gen Z, 102
Georgia, 210–11, 258
Ghana, 178
Ghingo, John, 244
Glickman, Dan, 272

Gliessman, Stephen R., 151
Global Animal Partnership and
  GAP-certified farms, 212
globalization, 6, 161–62, 164–66
glyphosate (Roundup), 128
GMOs (genetically engineered
  crops), 14–15, 168–83, 190
  Asia, Africa, and, 178–82, 193
  benefits, 176, 177, 183
  biotech companies and, 171–72
  bogus allegations and, 176
  Bt crops, 174, 183
  European regulation of, 168,
    174–75, 179, 181, 185
  farming chemical use and, 35
  food safety and, 176–77, 181, 184
  as Frankenfoods, 171
  livestock and, 191
  mandatory labeling and, 184
  opponents, 14, 168–70, 173, 176,
    179, 181, 184
  Paarlberg and, 170–71, 178–79
  Ronald and, 182–84
  Roundup Ready crops, 174
  salmon variety, 191
  U.S. regulation of, 168, 176–77
Good Catch Foods, 247
Grace, Delia, 206–7, 208
Greene, Julie, 46, 48, 51
Green Meadows Farm, Mass., 83
Greenpeace, 141, 158, 171, 180,
  189
green revolution, 141–51, 228–29
  agroecology vs., 141, 155
  benefits, 141–45
  critics of, 145–46, 147, 151, 158
  crop diversity and, 149
  crop yields, increasing, 150
  environmental impact, 145, 147,
    149, 159–60
  high-yield seeds and, 142–49
  interests of poor peasants and, 166

Grocery Manufacturers Association
(GMA), 248–49, 270, 275
  SmartLabel system and, 65
Guatemala, agroecology and, 155
Guiding Stars, 43, 63–65, 64, 274

Haber, Fritz, 116–17, 120
Hale, Bill, and Hale Group, 68
Hamburg, Margaret, 61
Hamburgers in Paradise (Fresco),
113
Hannaford supermarkets, 63, 64
Harper, Caleb, 111
Harris, Will, 245
Harvard University, 3, 4, 5, 8
  Chan School of Public Health,
  74–75, 132, 235
Harvest CROO Robotics, 262–63,
262
Hazard Analysis and Critical Control
Point (HACCP), 97
Healthy, Hunger-Free Kids Act, 271
He Jiankui, 192
Herbruck's farm, Mich., 135–36
Hershey, Lewis B., 18
Hershey company, 60
Hess, Rudolf, 118
Hilltop Farm, Pittsburgh, Pa., 107
Hippie Food (Kauffman), 129
H. J. Heinz, 135
home gardening, 123
  at the White House, 8–9, 103–4,
  105, 271
  World War I and II and, 103–4
Homegrown Paleo Cookbook, The
(Rodgers), 84
Honduras, agroecology and, 155
honeybees, 127–28
Horticulturae, 159
Howard, Albert, 119–21, 122
  "Nature's farming," 120, 140
Howdy Doody (TV show), 93

Humane Society of the United States
(HSUS), 213–17, 226–27
  cooperation with United Egg
  Producers, 215–16
  reforms initiated by, 195, 213–17

Illinois Farm Bureau, "Adopt-
a-Legislator" program, 269
Impossible Burgers, Impossible
  Foods, 237, 239–43, 245, 246
  Impossible Whoppers, 242, 243
  The Return (film), 246
India, 121, 142–46, 149
  crop diversity in, 149
  environmental concerns, 147
  globalization and, 162
  GMO crops and, 181–82
  green revolution and, 142–50,
  228–29
  high-yield wheat and rice, 142–45,
  147–48
  soil depletion and, 121
  water management, 257
Indonesia, 147, 258
industrial or commercial agriculture
  (Big Ag), 5, 7, 11, 13–14, 16, 17–44
  benefits to farmers, 41–43
  corn and soybeans, 13, 22–25, 30–34
  criticism, straight talk, 15, 267–76
  critics, 5, 7–8, 22, 23, 28, 35, 269
  dietary health and, 18–19, 267,
  270–73, 276
  ecomodernism and, 251–56
  environmental impact, 9, 28–30, 30,
  32–33, 34, 35, 36, 44
  as family farms, 269
  farm size increase and, 41
  federal policies, 23–25, 268–69
  future of, 251–56
  grain exports, 24–25
  impact on communities, 38–44
  irrigation systems, 35, 36, 251–53

industrial or commercial agriculture (Big Ag) *(continued)*
  monocultures and, 14, 130
  Nidlinger Farms, Ind., 30–34
  organic growers, 134, 138
  PA and science-based methods, 9–10, 13, 30–35, 44, 124, 127, 251–56, 276
  percentage of farms, 39, 43
  percentage of sales, 13, 39, 43, 256
  politics and, 267–69, 272–73
  processed foods, 26–27, 27
  produce farms and spoilage, 88
  productivity, 29–30, 30, 35
  quantity of food produced, 28–29
  relationship to Big Food, 270–73
  robotics and, 15, 257–64, 265
  wheat production, 24–25, 36
insecticides and herbicides
  agricultural tech and, 253–54
  biocides, 137
  cancer scares and, 131, 133, 173
  Carson and, 124, 125, 126, 137
  DDT, 113, 125, 126
  declining use of, 9, 35, 36
  federal regulations, 126–27, 132
  glyphosate (Roundup), 128, 174
  honeybees and, 127–28
  Indonesia, problems with, 147
  integrated pest management, 127
  organic farming and, 116, 137
  residue in foods, 127, 131–33
Institute for Gene Ecology, Norway, 179, 180
Intergovernmental Panel on Climate Change (IPCC), 231
International Livestock Research Institute (ILRI), Nairobi, Kenya, 206
International Monetary Fund (IMF), 161, 162

International Wheat and Maize Improvement Center, Mexico, 149
In't Hout, Corstiaan and Pietertje, 80
Intrexon company, 188
irrigation systems, 35, 36, 157, 251–53, 257
Itzkan, Seth, 246

Jack in the Box, 72
Jackson, Wes, 130
James, Walter, 122
Jansson, Stefan, 186, 187, 189
Jaramillo, Mauricio, 144
John Deere Company, 34, 260
Just Egg, 238
Just Inc., 240, 243

Ka-shing, Li, 238
Katcher, Joshua, 242
Katz, David, 62–63
Kauffman, Jonathan, 129
Kellogg's, 47, 48, 56, 135, 240, 248, 272
Kenya, 171, 178, 181, 206–7
Kerry, John, 267, 268
Kerry, Teresa Heinz, 268
Kessler, David, 52
KFC, 72, 98, 211
Kiess, Duane, 33, 34
King Corn (film), 22
Kingsolver, Barbara, 7, 8
Koch Foods, 210
Kraft Heinz, 54, 55, 56, 272
Kroger, 135, 191, 215, 238
Kumanyika, Shiriki, 56

Lake Erie Bill of Rights, 37
Lappé, Frances Moore, 182–83
Latin and Central America
  addressing poverty in, 150, 155
  agroecology and, 151, 154–55
  ancient farming in, 151–54, 153

fertilizer use, trends, 155
food labels, 274
GMOs and, 171
green revolution and, 150, 155
landowning inequities, 150–51, 155, 163, 164
loss of forested areas, 151
manual labor in farming and, 258
meat consumption and, 233
See also specific countries
La Via Campesina (LVC), 156, 161–67
Declaration of Nyeleni, 163–64
European NGOs funding, 162–63
food sovereignty and, 163–64
Venezuela, H. Chavez and, 166–67
Legan, Mark, 223–27, 246–47
Legan, Phyllis, 223, 224
Legan farm, Ind., 223–27
Leno, Jay, 272
Lightlife Foods, 238–39
Limits to Growth (Meadows), 130
Little, Amanda, 243
Little Beet, 71
Living Soil, The (Balfour), 122
Loblaw (Canadian grocer), 63
Local Farms, Food, and Jobs Act, 129
locally sourced food, 3, 8, 14, 76, 77–111, 170
advocates, 79–82, 101, 103, 105
benefits, 82
Clark Farm and, 82–86
defining, 78
environmental impact, 100–101
Farm to School Grant, 105
history of, 79, 80, 89–91, 161
home raised poultry, 99–100
Maine clambake, 77–78
nostalgia and tourism, 81
on-farm sales, 78
percentage of sales, 13, 78–79
pick your own, 78, 81
political support for, 105–6

portion of national diet, 78
prices and, 83–84
problems with, 6, 85–86, 88, 89, 92, 100–101
restaurant sales, 87, 98, 107–8
Rhode Island and, 103
roadside stands, 78
safety of, 96–100
small-scale specialization, 87–88
social benefits, 101–2
urban agriculture, 14, 106–11
USDA programs and, 105
"locavore," 8, 78, 79
Look to the Land (James), 122
Lovelock, James, 141, 145
Lusk, Jayson, 255
Lymbery, Philip, 5
Lynas, Mark, 168, 169–70, *169*, 173–74, 183, 184

Machado, Fernando, 242–43
Mackey, John, 245–46
Maduro, Nicolás, 166
maize, 3, 4, 144
gene-edited, 186, 189, 190
GMO, 171, 177, 178, 180, 181
green revolution, 144, 148, 149
Malaysia, 56, 258, 275
Malthus, Thomas Robert, 228, *229*, 232
Mann, Charles, 145–46
Mars, Inc., 56, 249
Maumee River watershed, 37
Mayer, Jean, 130
Mazourek, Michael, 20
McBride, Jim, 63, 64
McBride, Tim, 149
McDonald's, 72, 98, 199, 214, 215
P.L.T. Burger, 242
Melton, J. Michael, 239
Memphis Meats, 238, 240–41, 243
Mercy for Animals, 212

Merrigan, Kathleen, 105

Mexico, 143, *146*, 150–52, 202
  chinampas, 151–52, *152*
  ejido system, 164
  green revolution and, 151
  millennials, 101–2

Miller, Stacy, 87

Minute Maid, 248

Mississippi River dead zone, 37

Missouri, Urban Agricultural Zones
  (UAZs), 108

Mitloehner, Frank, 201

Mondelez, 215

Monsanto Company, 171–72, *172*,
  174, 182, 184, 190, 255

Moore, Patrick, 141, 145

MorningStar Farms, 240
  "Cheezeburger," 240

Mosa Meats, 240

Moskowitz, Howard, 52

Moss, Michael, 51, 55

Mother Earth News, 129

Mudd, Michael, 54

Musk, Kimbal, 111

Nabisco, Oreo cookies, *46*, 52

National Chicken Council, 212

National Organic Program, 136, 138

National Organic Standards Board,
  190

National Restaurant Association
  (NRA), 68
  menu labeling law and, 72–74, *73*
  total sales (2017), 65

Natsios, Andrew, 181

Natural Resources Defense Council
  (NRDC), 131

Nature Conservancy, 154

Nature's Bounty, 248

Nestlé, 56, 215, 239, 240, 247, 248,
  249

Nestle, Marion, 19, 20

Netherlands
  animal welfare and environmental
    regulations, 218, 219, 220, 222, *221*
  food labels, 274
  NGOs funding LVC, 162–63
  Noordman farm, 217–18, 220–23
  Wageningen University & Research,
    113, 220, *221*

New Age Meats, 240, 243

New York City
  Bareburger restaurant, 136
  urban agriculture, 109, *109*, 111
  GreenThumb program, 108

New York Times, 8, 22, 184
  Food for Tomorrow conference,
    269

Niccol, Brian, 245

Nidlinger, J.D., 33

Nidlinger, John, 30–34, *31*, 124, 168

Nidlinger, Nan, 30

Nidlinger Farms, Ind., 30–34, *34*, 37,
  44, 124, 168

Nigeria, 139–40, 178, 193

Noordman, Herbert and Annemarie,
  218, 220–23

Noordman farm, Netherlands,
  217–18, 220–23

Nooyi, Indra, 56, 248

North American Meat Institute, 235

Norwood, Bailey, 195, 210

NOVA Food Classification
  System, 95

nutrition, 9, 15, 16, 17–20, 74–76,
  93–94
  animal products and, 15, 18, 201,
    232–34
  Big Ag and, 15, 267, 270
  Big Food and, 13, 26–27, *27*, 45–59
  calorie restriction and, 21
  cell-grown meat products, 237, 238
  chain restaurants and fast food,
    65–74

consumers and healthier choices, 4, 55, 56, 58–59, 247–50, 270
countercultural impact on, 129
dieting and, 53
diseases of deficiencies, 17–18, 93–94
diseases of overeating, 228, 231, 266
excessive grains, protein, sugar, salt, saturated fat, 22, 74, 75, 274–75
fats and, 21, 66–67, 68, 74, 75
faux foods, 6, 10, 15, 69–70, 236–40
food deserts and, 50–51
food imports and, 91–92
food labels, 60–65, 64, 96, 184, 244, 273–74
food programs, 18, 26, 105, 231, 271, 272
fortified foods, 93–94
future of America's dietary health, 247–51, 265
global eating patterns and, 233–34
green revolution and, 145
"intuitive eating," 74
junk food, 27–28, 272
national menu labeling, 72–74, 73
nineteenth-century foods, 80
obesity and, 9, 18, 19, 20, 45–46, 50, 52, 55, 271, 273
organic foods, 113, 133, 136
promising dietary trends, 74–75
snacks, increase in, 45
socioeconomics and diet, 75–76
supermarkets and, 59–65
unbalanced diet and, 21–22
unhealthy choices, 13, 51–52, 56, 265–66
unsound medical advice and, 21
USDA "Thrifty Food Plan," 28
U.S. low rankings in, 18
NuVal, 62–63

Obama, Barack, 9, 57, 103, 195, 224, 275
Obama, Michelle, 8–9, 50, 104, 105, 271
Omnivore's Dilemma, The (Pollan), 8, 204
online food purchases, 59–60, 71, 72, 102
Organic Consumers Association, 136, 184
organic farming, 6, 14, 112–38, 268
    absolutism of, 114–15, 124, 127
    anti-gene-edited crops, 190
    back-to-the-land and, 128–30
    BDA and, 118
    certification, 85, 105, 112, 130, 134
    Clark Farm, Mass., 82–86, 138
    cost, 130
    critics, 130–31
    dairy farms, 138
    Earthbound Farm, Calif., 134
    egg production, 135–36
    environmental impact of, 5, 113, 126, 131, 138
    EU movement, 189
    farm animals and, 113, 115
    farm land, 6, 10–11, 14, 112, 115
    fertilizers and compost, 6, 112, 114, 116–20, 124, 161
    German biodynamic farms, 118
    history of, 116–26, 123
    hydroponics and, 138
    industrial scale vs. smaller, diverse farms, 113, 134, 138
    labor and, 14, 85, 112, 124
    lack of science and, 14, 113–14
    National Organic Program, 134
    natural vs. synthetic rule, 114, 124, 127, 134, 137
    NGOs endorsing, 158
    preindustrial methods and, 116
    reform recommended, 137

organic farming (continued)
  restaurant eating and, 136
  USDA study (1980), 130
  yields, 126, 131
Organic Farming and Gardening
  magazine, 122, 123, 129
organic foods, 3, 112, 170
  cancer scares and, 131, 133
  dairy products, 115–16
  food companies and, 135
  imports, 134, 136–37
  Million Women Study and, 132
  most popular produce, 115
  nonlocal sources, 134
  nutrition and, 113, 133, 136
  popular beliefs and, 113–14
  price, 112, 115–16, 133
  as processed food, 135, 135
  retailers, 134, 135
  retail sales, 11, 14, 112, 115, 136
Organic Foods Production Act of
  1990, 133–34, 136
Organic Front, The (Rodale), 122
Oscar Mayer, 214–15

Pacelle, Wayne, 213
Packaged Facts, 78–79
Paddock, William and Paul, 142
Panera Bread, 71–72, 212
Participatory Ecological Land Use
  Management (PELUM), 180–81
Paul, Katherine, 136
Pay Dirt (Rodale), 122
Pelto, Gretel and Pertti, 90
People for the Ethical Treatment of
  Animals (PETA), 195, 211
PepsiCo, 48, 55–56, 215, 248
Perdue, Sonny, 271
Perdue Farms, 210, 212
Perfect Day, 238
Peru, 152–53, 153, 155
Pete and Gerry's egg farm, 135

Peterson, John, 87
Pilgrim's Corporation, 210
Pillsbury Company, 54–55, 97
Pingree, Chellie, 105, 129
Pinker, Steven, 229
Pinstrup-Andersen, Per, 143–44
Pioneer Valley, Mass., 91
Pizza Hut, 70
Pollan, Michael, 7, 8, 22, 24–25,
  79–80, 101, 204, 246, 269
Polyface Farm, Va., 204
Poore, Joseph, 234
Popeye's, 213
Population Bomb (Ehrlich), 142
potatoes, 17, 100–101, 186
Pratt, Katie, 197
precision agriculture (PA), 9–10,
  31–35, 34, 44, 251–64, 253, 260, 262,
  276
  environmental benefits, 31, 32–35,
  127, 160, 255, 265
  future of food and, 251–56, 265
  GMO seeds and, 32–33, 127
  Nidlinger Farms, Ind., 31–34
  service providers for smaller farms,
  254–55
preindustrial farming methods, 7, 10,
  13, 29, 36, 80, 81
  environmental damage and, 9, 29
  Fruitlands, 11–12, 12
  Yale's Sustainable Food Program
  and, 80
Prentice, Jessica, 78, 79
Pretty, Jules, 160
Prevention magazine, 123
processed foods, 17, 92–96, 93
  farm production and, 26–27, 27
  faux animal products as, 245–46
  food safety and, 96
  fortification of, 93–94
  GMOs in, 177
  labeling of, 96

meats, 18
  organic, 135, *135*
  ultraprocessed problems, 95

Quelch, John, 98

Raley's, 249
Reagan, Ronald, 161
Reiley, Laura, 102–3
restaurant chains, 13, 65–74
  animal welfare and, 212–13
  big chicken buyers, 212, 213
  calories on menus, 13, 72–74, *73*
  dietary health and, 13, 19, 65,
    66–67, *68*, 70, 75
  food safety and, 98
  "ghost kitchens," 72
  locally sourced food, 98
  national sourcing, 98
  plant-forward menus, 69, 250
  portion sizes, 20
  potatoes and profits, 69
  prepared foods at, 69
  types of restaurant goers and, 70
RethinkX, 236
rice, gene-edited and high-yield, 143,
  144, 186, 190–91
Rice Research Institute, Philippines,
  144
Rockefeller Foundation, 178–79,
  182
Rodale, Jerome I., 122–24, *123*, 125,
  126
Rodgers, Andrew, 82–86, 87–89, *89*,
  138, 235
Rodgers, Diana, 83, 84, 235
Rodriguez, Ray, 263–64
Ronald, Pamela, 182–84
Roosevelt, Eleanor, 103–4
Root AI, Virgo robot, 259
Rosset, Peter, 156
Row 7 Seed Company, 20

rural hunger and poverty, 6, 139–67
  Africa, 139–40, 165–66
  agroecology and, 14, 140–42,
    156–59, 166
  Central and South America, 150–55
  China, 121, 144
  climate change and, 230–31
  EAT-*Lancet* benchmark diet, 235
  falling rates of, 229–30
  food sovereignty, 160–61, 166
  government investments and, 145
  green revolution and, 141–45,
    147–49, 159–60, 166
  high-yield seeds and, 142–44, *146*
  India, 121, 141–45, 147–48
  meat consumption and, 233
  Mexico, 143
  outsider's visions of, 161
  science-based farming methods
    and, 7, 141, 145, *146*, 159–60
  small farms and, 144–45
  Sustainable Agricultural
    Intensification (SAI) and, 160
  undernourishment, 230–31, *231*
Ruskin, Gary, 184

Safeway, 191
Salatin, Joel, 204, 205
Sanders, Bernie, 276
Sanford, Albert, 40
San Francisco, Urban Agriculture
  Incentive Zones Act, 108
Sanger, Stephen, 54
Savage, Steven, 126
Savory, Allan, 244
Schatzker, Mark, 19
Schlosser, Eric, 18–19
Schneider, Mark, 248
Seifer, Darren, 250
Shewfelt, Robert, 96
Shimizu, Hiroko, 100
Shiok company, Singapore, 247

Shiva, Vandana, 146, 147–48, 150, 246
Sikazwe, Emily, 179
Silent Spring (Carson), 113, 125, 126, 137
Singer, Peter, 206
Singh, Manmohan, 181–82
Site Specific Technology Software (SST), 254
60 Minutes (TV show), 131
slow food, 3–4, *4*, *5*
Slow Food USA, 3
Smale, Melinda, 149
Smil, Vaclav, 116
Smithfield company, 224
Smuckers, 55
Sodexo, 213, 215
Specter, Michael, 115
Starbucks, 71, 72, 212
Starr, Amory, 101–2
Steiner, Rudolf, 117–18, 119, 122, 123, 126
Stone Barns Center for Food and Agriculture, restaurant, 10
Story of Agriculture in the United States, The (Sanford), 40
Subway, 212, 213
sugar, 9, 24, 75
  labeling of added sugars, 249
  Milkybar Wowsomes, 248
  substitutions for, 238, 248
  sugary beverages, 13, *21*, 56–58, 70, 74, 75, 272, 274–75
supermarkets, 5, 59–65
  advertising and marketing in, 46–48, *46*, 60
  animal welfare and, 214–15
  anti-GMO policies, 191
  food imports and, 91–92
  food safety and, 97
  as grocerants (in-store eating), 49
  healthy eating and access, 50–51

  leverage over food companies, 60
  locally sourced food, 78
  nutritional information and, 13, 46, 62–65, *64*
  online shopping, 59, 102
  origins and growth, 90
  "rescue" projects, 94
  socioeconomics and, 75
  unhealthy products in, 51
  wellness initiatives, 249
Super-Size Me (film), 20
Sustainable Agricultural Intensification (SAI), 160
Sustainable Food Policy Alliance, 249
sustainable food production, 3, 130, 160, 234–35
Sweden, gene editing and, 186, *187*
Sweetgreen, 71
Syngenta AG, 171–72

Taco Bell, 70, *73*
Tanzania, 178
Target, 191
Tata Group, 192
Taylor, Jim, 243
Thatcher, Margaret, 161
This Blessed Earth (Genoways), 39
Tim Hortons, 238
Tomorrow's Table (Ronald and Adamchak), 183
Trader Joe's, 191, 240
Trillin, Calvin, 115
Trimble, Stanley, 29
Tropicana, 248
Trump, Donald, 187, 261, 273, 275
Tsongas, Paul, 268
Tyson Foods, 69–70, 98, 210, 212–13, 239

Uganda, 3–4, *4*
ultraprocessed foods, 95–96

Unilever, 56, 249
United Kingdom
  food advertising to children and,
    275–76
  food labels, 61, 274
  front-of-package nutrition guidance
    system, 273–74
  Million Women Study, 132
  Soil Association, 180
United Nations (UN), 158, 230
  agroecology promoted by, 14, 141,
    156, 157–58, 159
United Nations Food and
    Agricultural Organization (FAO),
    148–49, 150, 153, 156–57, 173,
    232
  Paarlberg at Rome event, 157–58
United States
  American diet, 21–23, 74, 90
  American taste preferences, 28, 236,
    249
  animal product consumption, 234,
    235
  average per capita calorie
    consumption, 20
  beef sales as ground beef, 242
  biotechnology companies, 171
  excess consumption of sugary
    beverages, 274–75
  falling farm population, 38
  farm subsidy policies, 9, 22, 23
  farm wages, 91, 261
  food programs (Food Stamps,
    SNAP), 18, 26, 231, 272
  food advertising to children and,
    275–76
  food costs and, 9, 23–25
  front-of-package nutrition guidance
    system, 273–74
  GMOs and, 168, 176–77
  Great Migration, 263
  immigrant farm labor, 81, 258, 261,
    263–64
  influence of Fanjul brothers, 24
  livestock industry, reaction to
    EAT-Lancet study, 235
  nutritional challenges ranking, 18
  obesity in, 9, 18–21, 19, 231, 274
  politicians and agriculture,
    267–68
  vegetarians/vegans in, 235
  See also specific agencies
University of California, Berkeley,
    Kiwi Campus, 102
University of California, Davis
  agricultural research and, 182
  Fragile Crop Harvest-Aiding
    Mobile Robot (FRAIL-bot),
    259–60, 261
  gene-edited animal research, 191
  Institute for Food and Agricultural
    Literacy, 182
  rice seed varieties, 182
University of California, Santa Cruz,
    263
urban agriculture, 106–11, 109, 110
  foundations supporting, 107
  USDA office for, 109
USAID, 154
U.S. Department of Agriculture
    (USDA)
  Animal and Plant Health Inspection
    Service (APHIS), 186
  Census of Agriculture, no-till or
    reduced till methods, 35
  Conservation Reserve Program
    (CRP) and land idling, 24–25
  decline in food contamination, 99
  definition of a farm, 38
  definition of "family farm," 44
  Dietary Guidelines for
    Americans, 22

U.S. Department of Agriculture (USDA) *(continued)*
  direct farm-to-consumer sales, total retail value (2017), 78
  fake organic products and, 137
  funding of scientists, 182
  gene-edited crops and, 186, 187
  Guiding Stars and, 65
  junk vs. healthy foods prices, 27–28
  "Know Your Farmer, Know Your Food" program, 9, 105
  locally sourced food defined, 78
  Low-Input Sustainable Agriculture (LISA), 130
  Office of Urban Agriculture, 109
  organic certification, 85, 105, 112, 130, 134, 136
  organic farming and, 10–11, 105, 126
  Payment in Kind program, 25
  programs for locally sourced food and farmers markets, 105
  "Report and Recommendations on Organic Farming" (1980), 130
  restricting NuVal system, 63
  spatial yield mapping study, 256
  Specialty Crop programs, 26
  "Thrifty Food Plan," 28
  "victory gardens" and, 103
U.S. Food and Drug Administration (FDA)
  Facts Up Front program, 61–62
  food irradiation and, 169
  gene editing and, 187, 191
  Guiding Stars and, 65
  health claims rules, 248
  labeling of added sugars, 249
  National Consumers League complaint against NuVal, 62
  partially hydrogenated oils banned, 75
  promising dietary trends, 74–75
USRTK (U.S. Right to Know), 184, 190

Van Eenennaam, Alison, 191
vegetarians/vegans, 234–35, 242, 245–46
Veggie Grill, 71
Veneman, Ann, 272
Venezuela, 166–67
Violence of the Green Revolution, The (Shiva), 147–48
Vision Robotics, 259
Vita Mojo, London, 250
Vougioukas, Stavros, 259–60, 261

Wageningen University & Research, Netherlands, 113, 220, *221*
Wallop, Gerard, 121
Wall Street Journal, 273
  "The Future of Food," 249
Walmart, 59, 135, 191
Waters, Alice, 5, 7, 9, 10, 48, 105, 129
Wayne Farms company, 210
Webster, Bruce, 210–12
Wegmans, 49
wheat production, 24–25, 36, 142
  gene-edited crops and, 186, 190
  high-yield varieties, 142–43, *146*
  organic farming and, 115
  PA and reduced fertilizer use, 255
  synthetic nitrogen use and, 124
White, Noel, 239
White Oak Pastures, Ga., 245
Whole Foods, 49, 78, 134, 191, 212, 215, 245, 247, 251
  animal welfare rating system, 85
  top ten food trends for 2019, 248
Wild Oats, 134
Willett, Walter, 235

Wilson, Woodrow, 103
Winson, Anthony, 19, 66
Wonder Bread, 92–93, *93*
World Bank, 158, 161, 162, 164, 165, 170
World Health Organization, 274–75
  on childhood obesity, 231
World Resources Institute (WRI), 188–89, 234
World Trade Organization, 161, 164

Yale-Griffin Prevention Research Center, Katz's shelf tag systems and, 62–63
Yale University, 8, 80
Yang, Yinong, 186
Young, Lisa, 20, *21*
Yudelman, Montague, 170

Zambia, 179–80

Illustration Credits

146 Associated Press

152 Photo by Chris Jackson / Getty Images

153 Rafael Moreno, Blog de Historia General del Peru

169 Photo by Colin McPherson / Corbis via Getty Images

172 Photo by Goran Jakus / Dreamstime.com

187 Photo by Stefan Jansson

196 LivingImages

209 Photo by Chayakorn Lotongkum / Dreamstime.com

211 Image courtesy of Martin Zuidhof, from Zuidhof, et al., "Growth, Efficiency, and Yield of Commercial Broilers from 1957, 1978, and 2005," *Poultry Science,* 93:2970–2982, 2014.

217 Courtesy of Jennifer Fearing; photo by Jay Chamberlin

221 Photo by Robert Paarlberg

229 International Bank for Reconstruction and Development

230 OurWorldinData.org

243 Photo by Robert Paarlberg

253 Photo by Avichai Morag / Getty Images

260 Photo courtesy of Stavros G. Vougioukas

262 Image by Bob Pitzer and Joel Meine